MANUAL OF Oncology therapeutics

MANUAL OF
Oncology therapeutics

KAY SEE-LASLEY, M.S., R.Ph.

Clinical Pharmacist Oncologist,
Lawrence, Kansas

ROBERT J. IGNOFFO, Pharm.D.

Associate Clinical Professor,
Clinical Pharmacist Oncologist,
School of Pharmacy, University of California,
San Francisco, California

The C. V. Mosby Company

ST. LOUIS • TORONTO • LONDON 1981

MOSBY
1906 75 1981
YEARS
A TRADITION OF PUBLISHING EXCELLENCE

Printed in the United States of America

The C. V. Mosby Company
11830 Westline Industrial Drive, St. Louis, Missouri 63141

Library of Congress Cataloging in Publication Data

See-Lasley, Kay, 1948-
Manual on oncology therapeutics.

Bibliography: p.
Includes index.
1. Cancer—Chemotherapy. 2. Antineoplastic agents.
I. Ignoffo, Robert J., 1944- . II. Title. [DNLM:
1. Antineoplastic agents—Therapeutic use. 2. Neoplasms—Drug therapy. QZ 267 S451m]
RC271.C5S43 616.99'4061 81-1998
ISBN 0-8016-4448-8 AACR2

GW/D/D 9 8 7 6 5 4 3 2 01/C/029

CONTRIBUTORS

STEVEN L. BARRIERE, Pharm.D.

Assistant Clinical Professor, School of Pharmacy,
University of California, San Francisco, California

PHILIP D. HANSTEN, Pharm.D.

Associate Professor of Clinical Pharmacy, College of Pharmacy,
Washington State University, Pullman, Washington

SHIRLEY WUNDER, R.N.

Pediatric Hematology/Oncology Research Nurse Coordinator,
Oklahoma Children's Memorial Hospital, Oklahoma City, Oklahoma

NOTE TO THE READER

The information in this book has been carefully reviewed for correctness of dosage and indications. However, the clinician should consult the original literature or package insert for absolute recommendations. Furthermore, some of the medications described do not as yet have final approval by the U.S. Food and Drug Administration or by other foreign countries. Thus the authors and publisher will not be responsible for consequences resulting from the clinical use of this information.

PREFACE

The purpose of the *Manual of Oncology Therapeutics* is to assist health professionals in providing optimal care to patients with neoplastic diseases. We have organized the various sections of this manual so that the user can readily obtain drug information pertaining to the selection, preparation, and monitoring of drugs currently used in cancer chemotherapy. Sections 1 and 2 present a brief discussion of pertinent facts about the cancer problem and the biologic basis of cancer chemotherapy. The core of the manual is presented in Sections 3 through 6, with the emphasis on the proper use of antineoplastic drugs. Over 150 of the most commonly used drug regimens have been outlined for particular adult and pediatric neoplasms. A discussion on hormone therapy follows, explaining the uses of estrogens, antiestrogens, progestins, and corticosteroids in endocrine- and nonendocrine-related malignancies.

The section on drug preparation and administration presents detailed information about the drug acquisition, storage, preparation, stability, incompatabilities, and drug administration of both commonly used and investigational anticancer agents. Section 6, on adverse reactions, lists toxicities both by specific organ and individual agent along with suggested methods for management. Also in this section is a discussion of the application of pertinent pharmacokinetics in the dosage adjustment of anticancer drugs in patients with renal or hepatic failure. The section on ancillary therapy contains current information on the treatment of cancer-related problems such as nausea and vomiting, pain, electrolyte imbalance, malignant effusions, hyperuricemia, drug extravasation, and renal prophylaxis. The section on infections in cancer patients provides information on empiric and specific therapy, along with the clinical use and toxicity of antibiotics used in cancer patients.

The section on drug interactions presents a comprehensive listing of anticancer drug interactions and a discussion of their clinical significance. The final section provides pertinent tables and nomograms for dosage calculation and laboratory monitoring of both pediatric and adult patients.

The information gathered in this manual was taken from the usual reference sources as well as from material supplied by the National Cancer Institute. These are listed at the end of each section. However, in order to keep the bibliography down to a usable level, we have included only those references that we feel will provide the reader with the best discussion of the subject.

We wish to thank the following people for their outstanding input in the development of this manual: Lawrence Trissel, R.Ph., Michael A. Friedman, M.D., Michael DeGregario, Pharm.D., Nancy Ma, Pharm.D., Nancy Nichol, R.Ph., Teresa Flory, R.Ph., and Mara Lewis, R.Ph.

We are grateful for the remarkable effort of Kris Gallagher, Linda Lopez, and Peggy French in the preparation of this manuscript.

We also are indebted to significant others for their encouragement, support, and patience during this endeavor and the Lord Jesus Christ, who brought this manuscript into being and to its completion.

Kay See-Lasley
Robert Ignoffo

CONTENTS

MANUAL OF Oncology therapeutics

Section 1

CANCER STATISTICS

Cancer is a term that encompasses many diseases. These diseases all have one thing in common. They are characterized by abnormal cell growth that results in death of the patient if it continues unchecked.

Cancer is the second leading cause of death in the United States. One in four persons will develop cancer, and two out of three families will experience its presence. It is the leading cause of death in children between the ages of 3 and 14 years.

In 1980 about 785,000 new cases of cancer will be diagnosed in the United States, and about 405,000 patients will die of these diseases. Of the 785,000 newly diagnosed patients, about 262,000 will be alive 5 years or longer because of the treatment they receive. The term "cure" in cancer is generally used when an individual is symptom-free of his disease for 5 years. However, some patients are declared "cured" after 1 year, 3 years, or a period longer than 5 years depending on the type of disease.

Great strides have been made over the years in the treatment of cancer. In the 1900s few patients could expect to live longer than 5 years. In the 1930s the ratio became 1:5, in the 1950s 1:4, and now the ratio is 1:3 persons who will live 5 years or longer. Several cancers are now curable as a result of advances in diagnostic techniques and treatment in recent years. They are acute lymphocytic leukemia, osteogenic sarcoma, Burkitt's lymphoma, Ewing's sarcoma, retinoblastoma, Wilms' tumor, embryonal rhabdomyosarcoma, Hodgkin's lymphoma, histiocytic lymphoma, testicular carcinoma, and choriocarcinoma. New discoveries are made yearly in research, and this list will undoubtedly continue to increase.

Several cancers have increased in incidence since the 1940s, while others have decreased. For example, the overall incidence of cancer of the stomach and uterus has decreased 63% and 37% respectively. In women both bladder and rectal cancer have decreased by about 27%. The most striking increase in incidence has occurred in lung cancer, reaching 133% in men and 108% in women since the mid 1940s. The most common cancer in women is carcinoma of the breast, which has the same incidence as in 1947.

Many factors seem to have influenced the incidence of cancer, especially in Western countries. The major factors appear to be the increased exposure to industrial and environmental chemicals, dietary substances, and smoking. The list of carcinogenic substances is large and will probably grow rapidly in the 1980s because of the enhanced research effort by governmental agencies, such as the Environmental Protection Agency in the United States (Table 1-1).

Lung cancer is the leading cause of death among all cancer patients in the United States. Its primary cause is cigarette smoking. Even though the incidence of lung cancer is increasing, smoking has begun to decrease through public education about its harmful effects. It is expected that the incidence of lung cancer will begin leveling off in future years. There will be 117,000 new cases in 1980 and 101,000 deaths. Lung cancer is a neoplastic disease very resistant to therapy. Some progress has been made in its treatment; however, mortality rates continue to remain high.

Colorectal cancer is the second leading cause of death among cancer patients. In 1980 there will be 114,000 new cases and 53,000 deaths. More than two out of three of these 53,000 deaths could be prevented by an earlier diagnosis. Colorectal cancer is thought to be caused by environmental factors such as the dietary content of an individual.

The third leading cause of death from cancer is breast cancer. However, among women only it is the leading cause of cancer death. In 1980 about 109,000 new cases will appear and 36,000 patients will die. If breast cancer is diagnosed in the early stages when still localized, 85% of patients have a survival rate of 5 years or longer.

The other major types of cancer listed in order of new cases are prostatic

Table 1-1. Common carcinogenic substances in the environment

Polycyclic hydrocarbons	**Antineoplastic drugs**
Benzpyrene	Alkylating agents
Methylcholanthrene	Nitrosoureas
Dibenzanthracene	Antiantibiotics
Aminoazo dyes	Procarbazine
Dimethylamino benzone	**Other**
Aminoazotolerene	Naphthylamine
Hormones	Urethane
Estrone	Aflatoxin B_1
Diethylstilbestrol	Nitrosoamines
Triphenylethylene	Radiation
Oncogenic virus	Parasites
Epstein-Barr	*Schistosoma haematobium*
Herpes hominis type I, II	

carcinoma, cancer of the uterus, urologic carcinomas, oral cancer, pancreatic carcinomas, leukemia, ovarian carcinoma, and skin cancer. All the above statistically have shown a continual increase in survival rates except for pancreatic carcinoma. Its 5-year survival rate is still 1%.

In 1980 about 131,000 patients will die that might have been saved if their disease had been diagnosed at an early stage and they had received treatment during the controllable stages of their disease. Public education, continuing education of health professionals, and the use of screening diagnostic techniques will continue to increase in importance in the attempt to save this group of patients. A greater emphasis on neoplastic diseases, their cause, and treatment will begin to appear in undergraduate and graduate studies in schools of medicine, pharmacy, nursing, and other health-related disciplines in the near future.

Section 2

CELL BIOLOGY AND DETERMINANTS OF RESPONSE

CELL BIOLOGY AND CANCER

Neoplastic cells and normal cells exhibit similar growth patterns. Both types of cells will enter all four stages of development some time during their life cycle. The four stages of cell growth are depicted in Fig. 1. Some normal tissues, such as bone marrow and the gastrointestinal mucosa, have a higher proportion of dividing cells than other tissues. It is the dividing cell, whether normal or neoplastic, that is most sensitive to anticancer drugs. Thus it follows that anticancer drugs should be most effective against tumors with a high proportion of dividing cells.

The proportion of dividing cells in a normal tissue or tumor is termed the growth fraction. Tumor cells in the cell cycle are viable (dividing) when they are present in phases G_0, G_1, S, G_2, and M. High growth fraction tumors are among the most responsive to chemotherapy. Most tumors have growth fractions of between 20% and 70%.[1] Bone marrow and oral mucosa tissue have growth fractions between 20% and 30%.[3] Because platelets and granulocytes arise from bone marrow, bleeding and infection are the primary dose-limiting toxicities from cancer chemotherapy.

The rate of tumor growth is dependent upon the number of dividing cells, not the absolute number of cells; the time it takes for a tumor to double is termed the doubling time. The growth rate for many tumors is described by the Gompertz curve (Fig. 2). This growth pattern indicates that as a mass increases, its growth rate decreases or its doubling time increases. This has been demonstrated in several animal and human tumors.[2] The physiologic explanation for this increase in doubling time and "flattening" of the curve is that the tumor, because of its large size, has outgrown its blood and nutrient supply, which results in slowing of cell growth and reproduction.[2]

In addition to affecting the rate of growth, tumor size will affect the efficacy of chemotherapy. With large tumor masses (greater than 1×10^{10} tumor cells) the ability of anticancer drugs to penetrate into the tumor to pro-

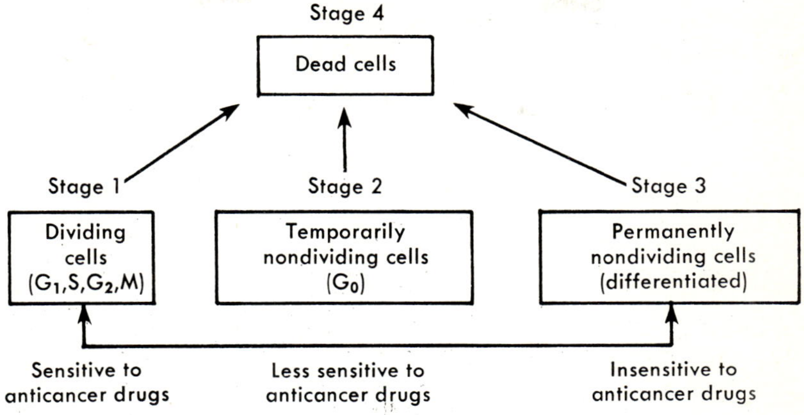

Fig. 1. Stages of cell growth.

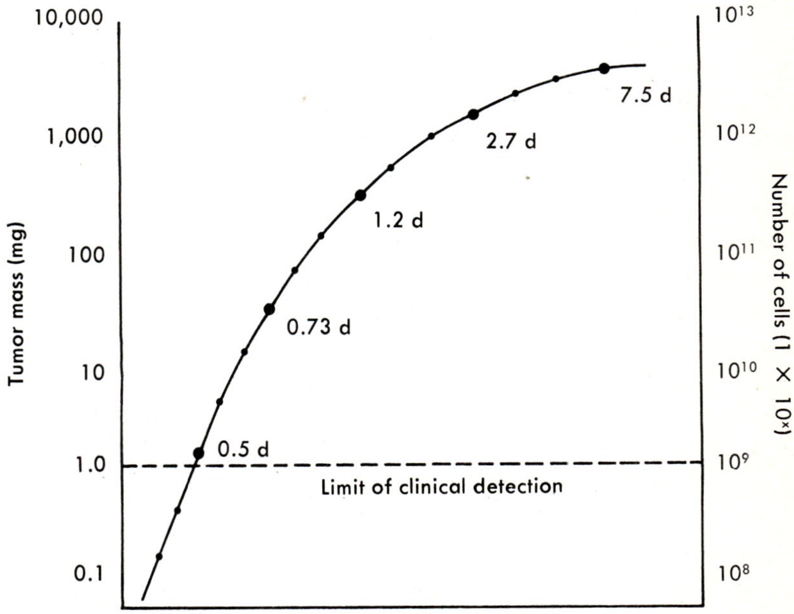

Fig. 2. Gompertzian cell growth. Chart illustrates decreasing growth fraction and increasing doubling time. Doubling times for tumor sizes are indicated next to the curve in days. (Adapted from Schabel, F. M., Jr.: Cancer Res. **29:**2384, 1969.)

duce cell death is diminished. It is also likely that a bulky tumor may have already metastasized to other sites. Thus it follows that the absolute number of tumor cells is an important consideration in determining the length of chemotherapy. Since anticancer drugs kill cells by first-order kinetics (kill a constant fraction rather than a constant amount), the same amount of drug will be required to kill 99% of a small tumor (1×10^9 cells) as to kill 99% of a large tumor (1×10^{12} cells), assuming no change in growth fraction or cell-cycle time. Of course, growth fraction does appear to change with tumor size in most cancers.

These concepts are shown in Table 2-1, in which the doubling time and growth fraction are related to tumor cell number and mass. Even if an effective treatment (99% cell kill) could decrease tumor bulk from 1×10^{12} to 1×10^{10} tumor cells, thereby producing a probable clinical remission, residual disease is present. In this case, therapy must be continued in order to eradicate residual disease.[4] Ideally treatment should be continued until the last tumor cell is eradicated. However, in doing so, therapy suppresses the patient's own immune defenses against the tumor. Thus it is difficult to kill the very last tumor cell.

In order to understand why some drugs are effective in certain tumors, their actions in the cell cycle must be considered. The sites of cell-cycle specificity and nonspecificity are shown in Fig. 3. As implied from the previous discussion, it is those cells that are *not* in the cell cycle that are more likely to survive chemotherapy. These can be either normal cells, such as bone marrow, or tumor cells, the latter of which will regrow after treatment. Thus a primary goal of chemotherapy is to attain selective toxicity to the resting cancer cell while allowing the normal cell to survive. There is evidence that such selectivity exists for most anticancer drugs. For example, the in vitro colony-forming system demonstrates that several anticancer drugs exhibit greater toxicity to lymphoma cells than to bone marrow cells.[5] Fig. 4 shows

Table 2-1. The relationship between tumor size, growth fraction, and doubling time in mouse adenocarcinoma 755 (data from Schabel)

Tumor size	Doubling time	Growth fraction	Cell-cycle time
2 mg	12 hours	100%	—
25 mg	0.7 days	61%	0.48
250 mg	1.2 days	40%	0.57
700 mg	1.8 days	25%	0.61
1.3 g	2.7 days	19%	0.64
5.0 g	7.5 days	7%	0.69

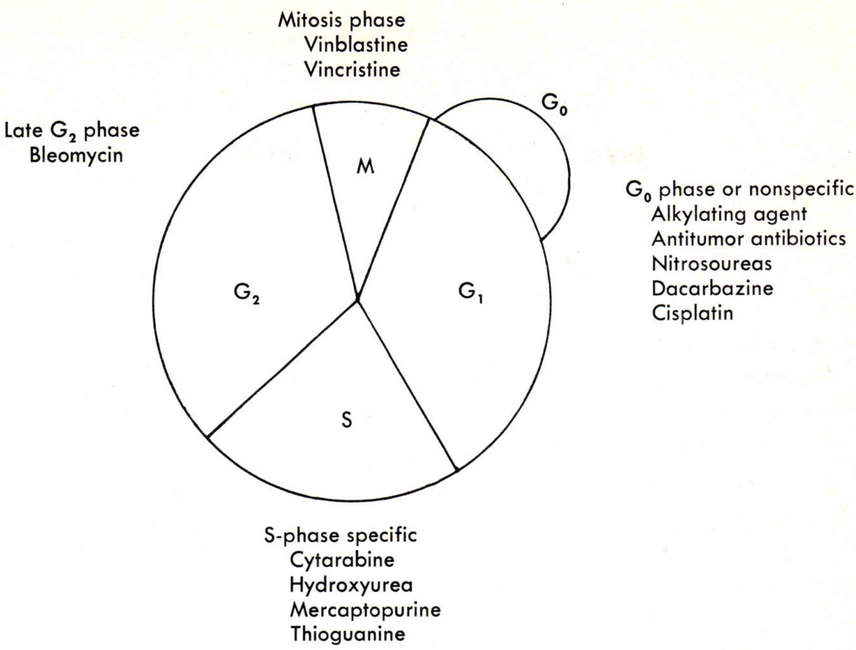

Fig. 3. Cell-cycle specific and nonspecific drug action in the cell cycle. G_0, resting cells; G_1, presynthetic phase; G_2, post-DNA synthetic phase; *M*, mitosis or cell division; and *S*, DNA synthesis. (Modified from Pratt, W. B., and Ruddon, R. W.: The anticancer drugs, New York, 1979, Oxford University Press, pp. 20-42.)

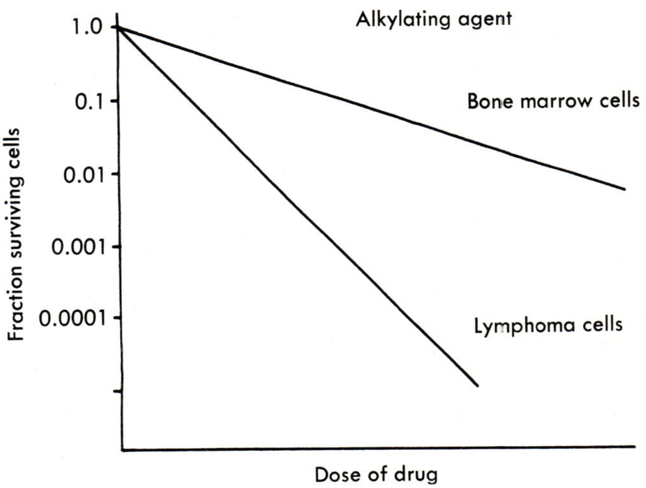

Fig. 4. Drug selectivity. For any dose of drug given, toxicity to lymphoma cells is greater than for normal bone marrow cells. (Adapted from Bruce, W. R., Meeker, B. E., and Valeriote, F. A.: J. Natl. Cancer Inst. **37**:233-245, 1966.)

this differential toxicity in the spleen-colony system for an alkylating agent. This differential toxicity is probably due to the higher growth fraction of lymphoma cells compared to bone marrow cells. Thus a higher percentage of bone marrow cells survive a short exposure to the cytotoxic drug. These results may explain some of the partial selective toxicity observed with the clinical use of cytotoxic drugs. However, the data on cell survival was obtained after single doses of the alkylating agent only and not after multiple doses. The data would undoubtedly be different after subsequent exposure to drugs, because nonproliferating bone marrow cells in G_0 phase might be stimulated to proliferate and thus become more sensitive to therapy. Thus scheduling of drug therapy is an important determinant for successful clinical use of cytotoxic drugs, because sufficient time must be allowed for the recovery of the normal bone marrow cell population.

It would be ideal to administer anticancer drugs on a daily basis, especially if the cell kill by drugs is 75% or more after each dose. If toxicity to normal cells was minimal at this level of cell kill, cure could be achieved in a large percentage of tumors. Unfortunately, clinical use of these drugs requires time for recovery of the host's bone marrow and immune defense mechanisms before further therapy can be given. Intermittent rather than daily chemotherapy is often more effective because it allows time for critical normal cell function to recover before the tumor regrows to its original mass.[4]

Drugs that are more effective in a particular phase of the cell cycle are termed cell-cycle specific agents and are generally effective only against high growth fraction tumors. Even those agents that are cell-cycle nonspecific are more effective against proliferating cells than against nonproliferating cells.

In order to design regimens that will be maximally effective, both the cell-cycle specificity and pharmacokinetics of the drug(s) should be taken into consideration.[6] Therapeutic drug concentrations must be maintained for the length of time required to kill the maximum number of cells in the sensitive phase of the cell cycle. Thus knowledge of the pharmacology of anticancer drugs may assist the clinician in the design of appropriate dosage regimens. An example of this pharmacologic principle can be demonstrated for cytarabine (Ara-C). Since the plasma half-lives for Ara-C are 10 and 120 minutes respectively, the drug should be administered as a continuous infusion to effect adequate exposure to therapeutic concentrations. Adequate exposure in the case of acute myelogenous leukemia (cell-cycle time of 2 to 4 days) would be at least 4 days. The theory in this case is borne out by the improved response rate (38%) in patients receiving 5-day courses of Ara-C as a continuous infusion as compared to the rate of patients receiving five daily injections (20%) and by the longer remission duration (12 months versus 7 months).[6]

RESPONSE TO CHEMOTHERAPY

In order to maximize the patient's chances to respond to chemotherapy, several other clinical factors such as stage of disease, performance status, and prior treatment must be taken into consideration (Table 2-2).

The greatest deterrent to successful anticancer therapy is the development of resistance.[7] Mechanisms of resistance have been well described and are listed in Table 2-3.[3] The use of drugs in combination that have different mechanisms of action has led to improved response rate by delaying the onset of tumor resistance.

However, in using combination drugs, overlapping toxicity, especially

Table 2-2. Clinical factors affecting response to chemotherapy

Stage of disease
Site of disease
Sensitivity to anticancer drugs
Prior therapy
Performance status
Concurrent organ system dysfunction

Table 2-3. Mechanism of resistance to anticancer drugs

Drug	Mechanism
Alkylating agents	Increased DNA repair Decreased drug uptake
Antimetabolites	
Fluorouracil	Decreased uridine kinase Low affinity of thymidylate Synthetase for 5FUdR-MP
Methotrexate	Increased DHFR Low affinity of DHFR for MTX Decreased drug uptake
Mercaptopurine Thioguanine	Decreased hypoxanthine-guanine Phosphoribosyl transferase Increased alkaline phosphohydrolase Altered PRPP aminotransferase
Cytarabine	Increased deoxycytidine deaminase Decreased deoxytidine kinase
Vinca alkaloids	Decreased uptake
Antitumor antibiotics	Decreased uptake
L-Asparaginase	Increased asparagine synthetic capacity Development of antibodies and enzyme

Table 2-4. Karnofsky's performance scale (KPS)

Rating	Status
100	Normal activity
90	Minor symptoms with normal activity
80	Activity with some effort
70	Unable to do heavy work; cares for self
60	Requires assistance; can perform most self-care needs
50	Needs a great amount of assistance
40	Disabled; home care
30	Severely disabled; hospital care
20	Very ill
10	Moribund
0	Dead

myelosuppression, frequently limits the dose from 50% to 75% of their maximum tolerated dose when used as single agents.

Another factor to be considered is the use of drugs that have demonstrated clinical activity against the particular tumor. There are few instances where a nonactive drug will be synergic to the effect of another active agent.

The general status of the patient is important in his response to chemotherapy because of its effect on the dose of the drug and its relation to the stage of disease (performance status). The lower the performance status, the more disabled the patient and the less likely an improvement in the patient's condition. One measure of the performance status (KPS) is derived from Karnofsky's scale (Table 2-4).[8] A KPS of 50% or lower is usually associated with intolerance to chemotherapy, and doses usually must be limited, which lessens the chance of response.

Thus the clinician is faced with the problem of evaluating all the clinical factors in order to develop an effective strategy for the patient.

STRATEGY IN THE CLINICAL USE OF ANTICANCER DRUGS

The choice of an anticancer drug for a particular disease is usually made from the results of clinical trials. Some tumors respond effectively to one drug, while others respond better when treated with combinations of drugs. In most tumors, however, combinations of drugs have not only improved the response rate but also the disease-free interval and survival rates. In a small number of tumors, combination therapy has resulted in decreased response rates.

Section 3 diagrams both the standard and best available regimens for several cancers. Most of these regimens incorporate the following principles of combination chemotherapy: (1) the drugs have demonstrated activity

Table 2-5. Cancers for which adjuvant chemotherapy has been used

Adult tumors	Pediatric tumors
Breast cancer	Embryonal rhabdomyosarcoma
Burkitt's lymphoma	Ewing's sarcoma
Histiocytic lymphoma	Wilms' tumor
Head and neck cancer	
Non–oat cell lung cancer	
Osteogenic sarcoma	
Ovarian carcinoma	
Small cell lung cancer	
Testicular cancer	

Table 2-6. Determinants of a successful adjuvant therapy program

Active chemotherapy for advanced disease (50% CR+PR)
Tumors that are easily diagnosed in early stages
Tumors with a high incidence of microscopic dissemination at the time of diagnosis
The ability of active chemotherapy to achieve total cell kill after decrease of tumor bulk by surgery or radiation

when used alone, (2) they have different mechanisms of action, and (3) overlapping toxicities are minimal.

Another form of chemotherapy uses drugs as adjuvants to surgery and radiotherapy in early stages of disease. The rationale for adjuvant therapy is based on the suspected presence of microscopic disease that cannot be completely eradicated by surgery or radiation.[9] Relapses following surgery or radiotherapy are primarily due to metastases existing before treatment.[10] Thus adjuvant treatment should increase the disease-free or relapse-free interval. Adjuvant therapy is currently being used in several cancers (Table 2-5). However, it appears that certain determinants must be present for adjuvant therapy to effectively eradicate microscopic disease. These determinants are shown in Table 2-6.

Adjuvant therapy of breast cancer has revealed some interesting findings. Bonadonna initially observed a decrease in the release rate for both premenopausal and postmenopausal patients after using CMF (cyclophosphamide, methotrexate, and fluorouracil).[11] Unfortunately the data was reported after only 18 months of follow-up, and at 36 months the relapse curve reached the point of nonsignificance for the treated and placebo postmenopausal patients.[12] The only group where benefit is demonstrated is the premenopausal patient.[13,14]

It appears that prolonged follow-up must be used in the analysis of adjuvant programs, at least for breast cancer. A better predictor for improved response in adjuvant programs may have to be used before preliminary results can be translated into true benefit. No such predictor presently exists.

REFERENCES

1. Steel, G. G.: Cytokinetics of neoplasia. In Holland, J. F., and Frei, E., editors: Cancer medicine, Philadelphia, 1973, Lea & Febiger, pp. 125-140.
2. Schabel, F. M., Jr.: The use of tumor growth kinetics in planning "curative" chemotherapy of advanced solid tumors, Cancer Res. **29:**2384, 1969.
3. Pratt, W. B., and Ruddon, R. W.: The anticancer drugs, New York, 1979, Oxford University Press, pp. 20-42.
4. Skipper, H. E., Schabel, F. M., Jr., and Wilcox, W. S.: Experimental evaluation of potential anticancer agents. XIII. On the criteria and kinetics associated with "curability" of experimental leukemia, Cancer Chemother. Rep. **35:**1-111, 1964.
5. Bruce, W. R., Meeker, B. E., and Valeriote, F. A.: Comparison of the sensitivity of normal hematopoietic and transplanted lymphoma colony-forming cells to chemotherapeutic agents administered *in vivo,* J. Natl. Cancer Inst. **37:**233-245, 1966.
6. Frei, E.: Effect of dose and schedule on response. In Holland, J. F., and Frei, E., editors: Cancer medicine, Philadelphia, 1973, Lea & Febiger, pp. 717-730.
7. Cline, M. J., and Haskell, C. M.: Cancer chemotherapy, ed. 2, New York, 1975, W. B. Saunders Co., pp. 13-27.
8. Muggia, F., et al.: Adjuvant systemic therapy of lung cancer, Cancer Clinical Trials **1:**237, 1978.
9. Carter, S. K., et al.: Integration of chemotherapy into combined modality treatment of solid tumors. I. The overall strategy, Cancer Treat. Rev. **1:**1-13, 1974.
10. Glucksberg, H., et al.: Adjuvant chemotherapy of stage II breast cancer: a comparison of CMFVP versus L-PAM. In Jones, S. E., and Salmon, S. E., editors: Adjuvant therapy of cancer, New York, 1979, Grune & Stratton, pp. 261-268.
11. Bonadonna, G., Brusamolino, E., Valagussa, P., et al.: Combination chemotherapy as an adjuvant treatment in operable breast cancer, N. Engl. J. Med. **297**(8):405-410, 1976.
12. Bonadonna, G., Valagussa, P., Rossi, A., et al.: Are surgical adjuvant trials altering the course of breast cancer? Semin. Oncol. **5:**450-464, 1978.
13. Bonadonna, G., et al.: CMF adjuvant chemotherapy in operable breast cancer. In Jones, S., and Salmon, F., editors: Adjuvant therapy of cancer II, New York, 1979, Grune & Stratton, pp. 227-235.
14. Fisher, B., Glass, A., Redmond, C., et al.: L-Phenylalanine mustard (L-PAM) in the management of primary breast cancer: an update of earlier findings and a comparison with those utilizing L-PAM plus 5-fluorouracil (5-FU), Cancer **39:** 2883-2903, 1977.

Section 3

CHEMOTHERAPEUTIC REGIMENS

This section outlines those chemotherapy programs considered to be the best treatments for specific cancers. For each regimen the general use, response rate, schedule and dose, precautions, and references are provided. It must be cautioned that considerable variation exists among investigators with regard to response criteria. The reader should refer to the specific reference for this information.

Once a particular regimen has been selected, the reader should refer to Section 5 for information on the suggested method of drug preparation and route of administration. Unless specified, the response rate quoted with each regimen indicates the objective response of the disease to the therapy. The objective response includes both complete and partial remissions unless the regimen is for a disease in which complete remissions are absent; then the objective response consists of partial remission rates only.

ACUTE LEUKEMIA
Vincristine and prednisone (VP)

GENERAL USE: Acute lymphocytic leukemia induction therapy
RESPONSE RATE: 80% to 90% complete remission
SCHEDULE AND DOSE:

	Day*															
	1	2	3	4	5	6	7	8	9	10	11	12	13	14	15	→
Vincristine†	X							X							X	
2.0 mg/m² BSA‡	Continue once weekly for total of 4 to 6 weeks															
IV, single dose (max. dose 2.0 mg)																
Prednisone	X	X	X	X	X	X	X	X	X	X	X	X	X	X	X	
60 mg/m² BSA‡	Continue daily, then taper over weeks 5 to 7															
Orally, *daily in divided doses*																

*X indicates day(s) to administer drug(s) indicated.
†Vincristine is given for a duration of 4 to 6 weeks.
‡BSA = body surface area.

REFERENCE:

Mauer, A. M., et al.: The current status of the treatment of childhood acute lymphoblastic leukemia, Cancer Treat. Rev. **3**:17-41, 1976.

Vincristine, prednisone, and daunorubicin (VP plus daunorubicin)

GENERAL USE: Acute lymphocytic leukemia induction therapy

RESPONSE RATE: 94% to 98% complete remission in previously untreated patients; 70% complete remission as secondary therapy

SCHEDULE AND DOSE:

	Day*														
	1	2	3	4	5	6	7	8	9	10	11	12	13	14	15 →
Vincristine†	X							X							X
2.0 mg/m² BSA‡	Continue once weekly for total of 4 to 6 weeks														
IV, single dose/week (max. dose 2.0 mg)															
Prednisone	X	X	X	X	X	X	X	X	X	X	X	X	X	X	X
60 mg/m² BSA‡	Continue daily, then taper over weeks 5 to 7														
Orally, *daily for 28 days*															
Daunorubicin§	X							X							X
25 mg/m² BSA‡	Continue once weekly for total of 4 weeks														
IV, single dose/week															

*X indicates day(s) to administer drug(s) indicated.

†Vincristine may be given for 4 to 6 weeks.

‡BSA = body surface area.

§NOTE: A dosage range of 25 to 60 mg/m² per dose of daunorubicin may be used. CAUTION: In pediatric patients with total cumulative doses of 450 mg/m² of daunorubicin (or 350 mg/m² in patients with previously irradiated heart tissue) there is a more common occurrence of cardiomyopathy or CHF or both.

REFERENCE:

Vietti, T. J., et al.: Vincristine, prednisone, and daunomycin in acute leukemia of childhood, Cancer **27**:602-607, 1971.

Vincristine, prednisone, and L-asparaginase (VP plus L-asparaginase)

GENERAL USE: Acute lymphocytic leukemia induction therapy

RESPONSE RATE: 97% complete remission in previously untreated patients; 77% complete remission when used as secondary therapy

SCHEDULE AND DOSE:

	Day*															
	1	2	3	4	5	6	7	8	9	10	11	12	13	14	15	→
Vincristine	X							X							X	
2.0 mg/m² BSA† IV (max. dose 2.0 mg)	Continue once weekly for total of 4 to 6 weeks															
Prednisone	X	X	X	X	X	X	X	X	X	X	X	X	X	X	X	
60 mg/m² BSA† Orally	Continue daily for total of 4 to 6 weeks, then taper															
L-Asparaginase 10,000 units/m² BSA† IV	X	X	X	X	X	X	X	X	X	X	X	X	X	X		

*X indicates day(s) to administer drug(s) indicated.

†BSA = body surface area.

REFERENCES:

Sutow, W. W., et al.: L-Asparaginase therapy in children with advanced leukemia, Cancer **28:**819-24, 1971.

Ortega, J. A., et al.: L-Asparaginase, vincristine, and prednisone for induction of first remission in acute lymphocytic leukemia, Cancer Res. **37:**535, 1977.

Intrathecal methotrexate and cranial irradiation

GENERAL USE: CNS prophylaxis for diffuse lymphoma (pediatrics), acute lymphocytic leukemia, and acute myelocytic leukemia

RESPONSE RATE: 50% long-term leukemia-free survival and possible cure

SCHEDULE AND DOSE:

	Day*														
	1	2	3	4	5	6	7	8	9	10	11	12	13	14	15 → 21
Methotrexate 12 mg/m² BSA,† IT (intrathecally)	X			X				X			X				X 7 day rest
Cranial irradiation															
2,400 rad (age > 2) over 2½ weeks															
2,000 rad (age 1 to 2) over 2½ weeks															
1,500 rad (age < 1) over 2½ weeks															

*X indicates day(s) to administer drug(s) indicated.
†BSA = body surface area.
NOTE: see Ancillary Therapy—Therapy of Central Nervous System Metastases, Section 7.

REFERENCES:

Aur, R. J. A., et al.: Central nervous system therapy and combination chemotherapy of childhood lymphocytic leukemia, Blood **37**:272-281, 1971.

Aur, R. J. A., et al.: Comparison of two methods of preventing central nervous system leukemia, Blood **42**:349-357, 1973.

Hustu, H. O., et al.: Prevention of central nervous system leukemia by irradiation, Cancer **32**:585-597, 1973.

Methotrexate and 6-mercaptopurine

GENERAL USE: Acute lymphocytic leukemia—maintenance therapy

SCHEDULE AND DOSE:

	Day*														
	1	2	3	4	5	6	7	8	9	10	11	12	13	14	15 →†
Methotrexate 20 mg/m² BSA‡ IV	X							X							X
	Continue weekly†														
6-Mercaptopurine 50 mg/m² BSA‡ Orally	X	X	X	X	X	X	X	X	X	X	X	X	X	X	X
	Continue daily†														

*X indicates day(s) to administer drug(s) indicated.

†Continue drug administration until relapse of disease or 3 years of remission has occurred.

‡BSA = body surface area.

CAUTION: Monitor blood count to maintain a leukocyte count of 2,000 to 3,000/cu mm.

REFERENCES:

Aur, R. J. A., et al.: A comparative study of central nervous system irradiation and intensive chemotherapy early in remission of childhood acute lymphocytic leukemia, Cancer **29**:381-391, 1972.

Simone, J.: Acute lymphocytic leukemia in childhood, Semin. Hematol. **11**:25-39, 1974.

Methotrexate, 6-mercaptopurine, and cyclophosphamide

GENERAL USE: Acute lymphocytic leukemia maintenance therapy

SCHEDULE AND DOSE:

	Day*															
	1	2	3	4	5	6	7	8	9	10	11	12	13	14	15	→†
Methotrexate 20 mg/m² BSA‡ IV	X							X							X	Continue weekly†
6-Mercaptopurine 50 mg/m² BSA‡ Orally	X	X	X	X	X	X	X	X	X	X	X	X	X	X	X	Continue daily†
Cyclophosphamide 200 mg/m² BSA‡ IV	X							X							X	Continue weekly†

*X indicates day(s) to administer drug(s) indicated.

†Continue drug administration until relapse of disease or 3 years of remission has occurred.

‡BSA = body surface area.

CAUTION: Monitor blood count to maintain a leukocyte count of 2,000 to 3,000/cu mm.

REFERENCE:

Simone, J. V., et al.: Combined modality therapy of acute lymphocytic leukemia, Cancer **35:**25-35, 1975.

Cytosine arabinoside (Ara-C) and doxorubicin (Adriamycin)

GENERAL USE: Induction remission of acute myelocytic leukemia (adult)
RESPONSE RATE: 80% complete remission
SCHEDULE AND DOSE: *One to 2 courses of therapy are usually all that is necessary.*

	Day*									
	1	2	3	4	5	6	7	8	9	10
Cytosine arabinoside 100 mg/m² BSA‡ Continuous 24-hour IV infusion	X	X	X	X	X	X	X	(X	X	X)†
Doxorubicin§ 30 mg/m² BSA‡ IV	X	X	X							

*X indicates day(s) to administer drug(s) indicated.
†Cytosine arabinoside is given 7 to 10 days.
‡BSA = body surface area.
§CAUTION: In adult patients with total cumulative doses of doxorubicin of 550 mg/m² (or 450 mg/m² in patients with previously irradiated heart tissue) there is a more common occurrence of cardiomyopathy or CHF or both.

REFERENCES:

Preisler, H. D., et al.: Adriamycin-cytosine arabinoside therapy for adult acute myelocytic leukemia, Cancer Treat. Rep. **61**:89-92, 1977.

Preisler, H. D., et al.: Treatment of acute nonlymphocytic leukemia (ANLL) using 3 doses of Adriamycin (Adr) and a 10-day infusion of cytosine arabinoside (Ara C), Proc. Am. Soc. Clin. Oncol. **20**:297, 1979.

Cortes, E. O., et al.: Adriamycin (NSC-123127) cardiotoxicity: a clinicopathologic correlation, Cancer Chemother. Rep. **6**:215-225, 1975.

Cytosine arabinoside and daunorubicin

GENERAL USE: Acute myelogenous leukemia induction therapy (adult)
RESPONSE RATE: 87% complete remission in patients less than 60 years old
SCHEDULE AND DOSE:

	Day*						
	1	2	3	4	5	6	7
Cytosine arabinoside 100 mg/m² BSA† IV infusion daily	X	X	X	X	X	X	X
Daunorubicin‡ 45 mg/m² BSA† IV	X	X	X				

*X indicates day(s) to administer drug(s) indicated.
†BSA = body surface area.
‡CAUTION: In adult patients with total cumulative doses of 550 mg/m² of daunorubicin (or 450 mg/m² in patients with previously irradiated heart tissue) there is a more common occurrence of cardiomyopathy or CHF or both.

REFERENCE:

Ellison, R. R.: Management of acute leukemia in adults, Med. Pediatr. Oncol. **1**:149-158, 1975.

Cytosine arabinoside (Ara-C) and 6-thioguanine (6-TG)

GENERAL USE: Acute myelogenous leukemia induction therapy (adult)
RESPONSE RATE: 50% complete remission
SCHEDULE AND DOSE: Repeat every 30 days until remission marrow is obtained.

	Day* 1	2	3	4	5	6	7	8	9	10 ⟶		30
Cytosine arabinoside 100 mg/m² BSA† IV every 12 hours	X	X	X	X	X	X	X	X	X	X	No therapy, 3 weeks	
6-Thioguanine 100 mg/m² BSA† Orally every 12 hours	X	X	X	X	X	X	X	X	X	X		

*X indicates day(s) to administer drug(s) indicated.
†BSA = body surface area.

REFERENCES:

Ellison, R. R., et al.: Management of acute leukemia in adults, Med. Pediatr. Oncol. **1:**149-158, 1975.

Gale, R. P.: Advances in the treatment of acute myelogenous leukemia, N. Engl. J. Med. **300:**1189-1199, 1979.

Cytosine arabinoside (Ara-C) and 6-thioguanine (6-TG) —open ended (Sloan-Kettering L-6 Protocol)

GENERAL USE: Acute myelocytic leukemia induction therapy (adult)
RESPONSE RATE: 65%
SCHEDULE AND DOSE:

	Day*										
	1	2	3	4	5	6	7	8	9	10† →	
Cytosine arabinoside‡ 3.0 mg/kg IV every 12 hours	X	X	X	X	X	X	X	X	X	X	Continue†
6-Thioguanine‡ 2.5 mg/kg Orally every 12 hours	X	X	X	X	X	X	X	X	X	X	Continue†

*X indicates day(s) to administer drug(s) indicated.
†Because of considerable variability among patients that cannot always be predicted on the basis of initial hematologic parameters, the duration of each course must be individualized depending on the rapidity of the patient's therapeutic response. The first course of Ara-C and 6-TG is continued until bone marrow biopsy is moderately to severely hypocellular. The number of doses required during the first course of treatment should not exceed 40. A rest period should follow each course to allow marrow cellularity to increase to normal or hypercellular. If the marrow is not in remission after the second course, the leukemic cells have probably developed resistance to the drugs, and further therapy with this combination will not succeed in inducing a remission.
‡Alternately, Ara-C 100 mg/m^2 IV push every 12 hours and 6-TG 100 mg/m^2 orally every 12 hours (Skeel, et al.: Proc. Am. Soc. Clin. Oncol. **17**:301, 1976).

REFERENCES:

Clarkson, B. D.: Acute myelocytic leukemia in adults, Cancer **30:**1572-1582, 1972.

Clarkson, B. D., et al.: Treatment of acute leukemia in adults, Cancer **36:**775-795, 1975.

Gale, R. P.: Advances in the treatment of acute myelogenous leukemia, N. Engl. J. Med. **300:**1189-1199, 1979.

6-Thioguanine (6-TG), cytosine arabinoside (Ara-C), daunorubicin (daunomycin), prednisone, and vincristine (Oncovin) (TADPO)

GENERAL USE: Adult myelocytic leukemia induction and consolidation therapy (adult)

RESPONSE RATE: 61%

INDUCTION SCHEDULE AND DOSE: Ordinarily no more than two induction courses will be given. If after two courses there has been no appreciable antitumor effect, then the patient's therapy is considered a failure.

	Day*															
		Course I								Course II						
	0	1	2	3	4	5	6	7	8 → 14	15	16	17	18	19	20	21
6-Thioguanine 2 mg/kg Orally every 12 hours for 14 doses		X	X	X	X	X	X	X	7-day rest, no therapy	X	X	X	X	X	X	X
Cytosine arabinoside 2 mg/kg IV push every 12 hours for 14 doses		X	X	X	X	X	X	X		X	X	X	X	X	X	X
Daunorubicin 1.5 mg/kg IV		X	X	X						X	X	X				
Prednisone 1 mg/kg Orally (divided doses)		X	X	X	X	X	X	X		X	X	X	X	X	X	X
Vincristine 1.0 mg/m² BSA‡ IV (max. dose 2.0 mg)		X						X		X						X
Marrow aspiration	X									X†						

*X indicates day(s) to administer drug(s) indicated or to take bone marrow aspiration.

†On day 15 (after 7-day rest) perform marrow aspirate and biopsy.

1. If aspirate or biopsy contains more than 5% leukemic cells (not including promyelocytes) and cellularity is 30% or greater, administer a second course at same doses and schedule.
2. If cellularity of marrow is 25% or less, wait 3 to 5 days and repeat aspiration and biopsy:
   a. If cellularity is still 25% or less, repeat again in 3 to 5 days.
   b. If cellularity is 30% or greater and there is greater than 5% leukemic cells, repeat course at *full* doses.

   NOTE: Normal myeloblasts, promyelocytes, and monocytes may appear in the bone marrow at a time of recovery from hypoplasia. This "reactive myeloblastosis" can be differentiated from leukemic repopulation by performing marrow aspirates at 3-day intervals and comparing to prior aspirations and with morphology of original leukemic population.
3. If there is less than 5% leukemic cells and cellularity is less than normal (40% to 60%), hold additional therapy and repeat aspirate and biopsy every 3 to 5 days until marrow reaches normal cellularity and then proceed to consolidation.

‡BSA = body surface area.

CONSOLIDATION SCHEDULE AND DOSE: Patients who receive a complete remission (M_1 marrow) will receive one course of consolidation therapy 14 days after the completion of the last course of induction therapy. It is not to be begun until the granulocyte count is greater than 1,500/cu mm and platelet count is greater than 100,000/cu mm. *Consolidation cycle is given one time only.*

	Day*				
	1	2	3	4	5
6-Thioguanine 2 mg/kg Orally every 12 hours for 10 doses	X	X	X	X	X
Cytosine arabinoside 2 mg/kg IV push every 12 hours for 10 doses	X	X	X	X	X
Daunorubicin† 1.5 mg/kg IV	X	X			
Prednisone 1 mg/kg Orally (divided doses)	X	X	X	X	X
Vincristine 1.0 mg/m² BSA‡ IV (max. dose 2.0 mg)	X				

*X indicates day(s) to administer drug(s) indicated.

†CAUTION: In adult patients with total cumulative doses of 550 mg/m² of daunorubicin (or 450 mg/m² in patients with previously irradiated heart tissue) there is a more common occurrence of cardiomyopathy or CHF or both.

‡BSA = body surface area.

REFERENCES:

Glucksberg, H.: Combination chemotherapy in adult non-lymphatic leukemia, Northwest Cooperative Group (WCSG) Protocol 122 (modified by Greenberg, B.), 1975.

Glucksberg, H., et al.: Combination chemotherapy for acute nonlymphoblastic leukemia in adults, Cancer Chemother. Rep. **59**(6):1131-1137, 1975.

Greenberg, B., Lewis, J., Burns, C., et al.: A re-evaluation of intensive induction therapy in adult acute nonlymphocytic leukemia, Proc. Am. Soc. Clin. Oncol. **17**:268, 1976.

Cyclophosphamide, vincristine (Oncovin), cytosine arabinoside, and prednisone (COAP)

GENERAL USE: Acute myelogenous leukemia (adult)

RESPONSE RATE: 55%

SCHEDULE AND DOSE: Continue at 2-week intervals until remission or progression of disease.

	Day* 1	2	3	4	5	→	14
Vincristine 2 mg IV (max. dose 2 mg)	X					1-week rest period, no therapy	
Prednisone 200 mg Orally in 4 divided doses	X	X	X	X	X		
Cytosine arabinoside 100 mg/m² BSA† IV push (given in divided doses every 8 hours)	X	X	X	X	X		
Cyclophosphamide 100 mg/m² BSA† IV push (given in divided doses every 8 hours)	X	X	X	X	X		

*X indicates day(s) to administer drug(s) indicated.

†BSA = body surface area.

NOTE: Maintenance therapy—continue with COAP at 3-week intervals rather than 2-week intervals.

REFERENCES:

Whitecar, J. P., et al.: Cyclophosphamide (NSC-26271), vincristine (NSC-67574), cytosine arabinoside (NSC-63878), and prednisone (NSC-10023) (COAP) combination chemotherapy for acute leukemia in adults, Cancer Chemother. Rep. **56:**543-550, 1972.

Gale, R. P.: Advances in the treatment of acute myelogenous leukemia, N. Engl. J. Med. **300:**1189-1199, 1979.

6-Mercaptopurine (Purinethol), vincristine (Oncovin), methotrexate, prednisone (POMP)

GENERAL USE: Induction therapy of previously treated acute myelogenous leukemia (adult)

RESPONSE RATE: 53%

SCHEDULE AND DOSE:

	Day*					
	0	1	2	3	4	5†
6-Mercaptopurine‡ 500 mg/m² BSA§ IV		X	X	X	X	X
Vincristine 2 mg IV (max. dose 2.0 mg)		X				
Methotrexate 7.5 mg/m² BSA§ IV		X	X	X	X	X
Prednisone 200 mg Orally		X	X	X	X	X
Bone marrow‖	X					

*X indicates day(s) to administer drug(s) or to take a bone marrow aspirate or biopsy.

†POMP may be repeated 9 days after completion of the previous course if marrow is not M_1 and if cellularity of marrow is 40% or greater. Patients will generally receive 4 to 5 courses unless there has been marked progression of disease or limiting toxicity such as hepatic toxicity or severe mouth sores. Vincristine can be deleted from first and subsequent courses if peripheral neuropathy with muscle weakness or autonomic nervous system toxicity is present or appears.

‡Dosage reduction of intravenous 6-mercaptopurine with the use of allopurinol is not required in this protocol.

§BSA = body surface area.

‖Bone marrow aspirations and biopsies will be performed before each course of chemotherapy.

REFERENCES:

Rodriquez, V., et al.: POMP combination chemotherapy of adult acute leukemia, Cancer **32:**69-72, 1973.

Gale, R. P.: Advances in the treatment of acute myelogenous leukemia, N. Engl. J. Med. **300:**1189-1199, 1979.

5-Azacitidine

GENERAL USE: Acute myelogenous leukemia induction therapy (adult)
RESPONSE RATE: 32% complete remission
SCHEDULE AND DOSE: Repeat every 14 to 28 days until remission.

	Day*							
	1	2	3	4	5	⟶	14-28	
5-Azacitidine 150-400 mg/m^2 BSA† Continuous IV infusion daily	X	X	X	X	X	No therapy		

*X indicates day(s) to administer drug(s) indicated.
†BSA = body surface area.

REFERENCES:

Vogler, W. R., et al.: Remission induction in refractory myeloblastic leukemia with continuous infusion of 5-azacytidine, Proc. Am. Assoc. Cancer Res. **16:**155, 1975.

Von Hoff, D. D., et al.: 5-Azacytidine, a new anticancer drug with effectiveness in acute myelogenous leukemia, Ann. Intern. Med. **85:**237-245, 1976.

Gale, R. P.: Advances in the treatment of acute myelogenous leukemia, N. Engl. J. Med. **300:**1189-1199, 1979.

Cytosine arabinoside (Ara-C) and 6-thioguanine (6-TG)

GENERAL USE: Maintenance of remission in acute myelogenous leukemia (adult)

RESPONSE RATE: 14-month median remission duration

SCHEDULE AND DOSE: Repeat cycle each month.

	Day* 1	2	3	4	5	→	28
Cytosine arabinoside 100 mg/m² BSA† IV every 12 hours for 5 days	X	X	X	X	X	No therapy, 3 weeks	
6-Thioguanine 100 mg/m² BSA† Orally every 12 hours for 5 days	X	X	X	X	X		

*X indicates day(s) to administer drug(s) indicated.
†BSA = body surface area.

REFERENCES:

Armitage, J. O., et al.: Maintenance of remission in adult acute nonlymphoblastic leukemia using intermittent courses of cytosine arabinoside (NSC-63878) and 6-thioguanine (NSC-752), Cancer Treat. Rep. **60:**585-589, May, 1976.

Gale, R. P.: Advances in the treatment of acute myelogenous leukemia, N. Engl. J. Med. **300:**1189-1199, 1979.

Cytosine arabinoside, daunorubicin, prednisolone, and 6-mercaptopurine

GENERAL USE: Acute myeloid leukemia induction and maintenance therapy (pediatric)

RESPONSE RATE: 93% (median survival 12½ months)

INDUCTION SCHEDULE AND DOSE: Repeat cycle weekly until remission.

	Day* 1	2	3	4	5	6	7 →
Daunorubicin† 25 mg/m² BSA‡ IV	X						
Cytosine arabinoside 80 mg/m² BSA‡ IV	X	X	X				
Prednisolone 40 mg/m² BSA‡ Orally	X	X	X	X	X	X	X
6-Mercaptopurine 100 mg/m² BSA‡ Orally	X	X	X	X	X	X	X

*X indicates day(s) to administer drug(s) indicated.
†CAUTION: In pediatric patients with total cumulative doses of 450 mg/m² of daunorubicin (or 350 mg/m² in patients with previously irradiated heart tissue) there is a more common occurrence of cardiomyopathy or CHF or both.
‡BSA = body surface area.

MAINTENANCE SCHEDULE AND DOSE: Repeat cycle every month or 28 days.

	Day* 1	2	3	4	5	6	7	——→	28
Daunorubicin† 25 mg/m² BSA‡ IV	X								
Cytosine arabinoside 80 mg/m² BSA‡ IV	X	X	X						
Prednisolone 40 mg/m² BSA‡ Orally	X	X	X	X	X	X	X		
6-Mercaptopurine 100 mg/m² BSA‡ Orally	X	X	X	X	X	X	X	Continue daily	

*X indicates day(s) to administer drug(s) indicated.
†CAUTION: In pediatric patients with total cumulative doses of 450 mg/m² of daunorubicin (or 350 mg/m² in patients with previously irradiated heart tissue) there is a more common occurrence of cardiomyopathy or CHF or both.
‡BSA = body surface area.

REFERENCE:

Evans, D. I. K., et al.: Treatment of acute myelogenous leukemia of childhood with cytosine arabinoside, daunorubicin, prednisolone and mercaptopurine or thioguanine, Cancer **36:**1547-1551, 1975.

Cytosine arabinoside (Ara-C), 6-thioguanine (6-TG), doxorubicin (Adriamycin), L-asparaginase (Sloan-Kettering)

GENERAL USE: Acute granulocytic leukemia (pediatric)

RESPONSE RATE: 74%

INDUCTION SCHEDULE AND DOSE:

	Day*										
	1	2	3	4	5	6	7	8	→	?	?
Cytosine arabinoside 100 mg/m² BSA‡ IV every 12 hours	X	X	X	X	X	X	X	†			
6-Thioguanine 75 mg/m² BSA‡ Orally every 12 hours	X	X	X	X	X	X	X	†			
Doxorubicin 30 mg/m² BSA‡ IV										X	X†

*X indicates day(s) to administer drug(s) indicated.
†Continue Ara-C and 6-TG therapy until bone marrow depression occurs (usually three courses); then give a dose of doxorubicin on two consecutive days after recovery from previous therapy. After remission is obtained, proceed to consolidation schedule.
‡BSA = body surface area.

CONSOLIDATION SCHEDULE AND DOSE:

	Day*											
	1	2	3	4	5	6	7	(8-21) 8-14	(22-28) 15-21	(29-42) 22-28	(43) 29	(44) 30
Cytosine arabinoside 100 mg/m² BSA‡ IV every 12 hours	X	X	X	X	X	(X	X)§	1-2 week rest	Repeat Ara-C and 6-TG cycle once	1-2 week rest		
6-Thioguanine 75 mg/m² BSA‡ Orally every 12 hours	X	X	X	X	X	(X	X)§					
L-Asparaginase 60,000 IU/m² BSA‡ IV											X	

	Day*											
	(45) 31	(46) 32	(47) 33	(48) 34	(49) 35	(50) 36	(51) 37	(52) 38	(53) 39	(54) 40	(55) 41	(56) 42†
Cytosine arabinoside 100 mg/m² BSA‡ IV every 12 hours												
6-Thioguanine 75 mg/m² BSA‡ Orally every 12 hours												
L-Asparaginase 60,000 IU/m² BSA‡ IV	X		X			X		X		X		

*X indicates day(s) to administer drug(s) indicated.

†Proceed to maintenance therapy of the LSA_2-L_2 protocol (pp. 63-64). Maintenance is continued 3 years provided the patient continues to remain in complete remission.

‡BSA = body surface area.

§Administration of drugs on days in parentheses is optional.

REFERENCE:

Haghbin, M., et al.: Treatment of acute nonlymphoblastic leukemia in children with a multiple-drug protocol, Cancer **40:**1417-1421, 1977.

Cyclophosphamide, vincristine (Oncovin), cytosine arabinoside, and prednisone (Mini-COAP)

GENERAL USE: Acute granulocytic leukemia (pediatric)

RESPONSE RATE: 41%

INDUCTION SCHEDULE AND DOSE: Repeat cycle after day 49.

	Day*																	
	1	2	3	4	5	→	8	→	15	→	22	→	28	29	→	35	→	49
Vincristine 2 mg/m² BSA† IV (max. dose 2.0 mg)	X						X		X		X			X			No therapy, 2 weeks	
Prednisone 60 mg/m² BSA† Orally in 4 divided doses (max. dose 60 mg)	X	Daily →												X	(Taper) →			
Cytosine arabinoside 40 mg/m² BSA† IV every 8 hours for 12 doses	X	X	X	X														
Cyclophosphamide 40 mg/m² BSA† Every 8 hours with cytosine arabinoside for 12 doses	X	X	X	X														

*X indicates day(s) to administer drug(s) indicated.

†BSA = body surface area.

MAINTENANCE SCHEDULE AND DOSE: Repeat at intervals of 2 weeks for 2 cycles, then at intervals of 3 weeks for 3 cycles, then every 4 weeks.

	Day*													
	1	2	3	4	5	6	7	8	9	10	11	12	13	14 →
Vincristine 2 mg/m² BSA† IV (max. dose 2.0 mg)	X													
Prednisone 120 mg/m² BSA†/day Orally in 4 divided doses	X	X	X	X										
Cytosine arabinoside 40 mg/m² BSA† IV every 8 hours for 12 doses	X	X	X	X										
Cyclophosphamide 40 mg/m² BSA† Every 8 hours with cytosine arabinoside for 12 doses	X	X	X	X										

*X indicates day(s) to administer drug(s) indicated.
†BSA = body surface area.

REFERENCE:

Madanat, F. F., et al.: Improved survival in young children with acute granulocytic leukemia treated with combination therapy using cyclophosphamide, Oncovin, cytosine arabinoside, and prednisone, Cancer **44:**819-823, 1979.

CHRONIC LEUKEMIA
Chlorambucil and prednisone (biweekly)

GENERAL USE: Chronic lymphocytic leukemia

RESPONSE RATE: 87%

SCHEDULE AND DOSE:

	Week*								
	1	2	3	4	5	6	7	8	→
Chlorambucil† 0.4 mg/kg Orally once biweekly	X		X		X		X		Continue biweekly
Prednisone 100 mg Orally 2 days biweekly	X		X		X		X		Continue biweekly

*X indicates *weeks* to administer drug(s) indicated.

†Initial dose of 0.4 mg/kg is increased by 0.1 mg/kg every 2 weeks until toxicity or disease control is achieved. *Dosage should be adjusted according to blood counts taken every 2 weeks prior to therapy.*

REFERENCES:

Knospe, W. H., et al.: Bi-weekly chlorambucil treatment of chronic lymphocytic leukemia, Cancer **33:**555-562, 1974.

Han, T., et al.: Chlorambucil vs. combined chlorambucil-corticosteroid therapy in chronic lymphocytic leukemia, Cancer **31:**502-508, 1973.

Chlorambucil and prednisone

GENERAL USE: Chronic lymphocytic leukemia

RESPONSE RATE: 87%

SCHEDULE AND DOSE:

	Day*							
	1	2	3	4	5	6	7	→
Chlorambucil† 6 mg Orally	X	X	X	X	X	X	X	Continue daily
Prednisone 30 mg Orally	X	X	X	X	X	X	X	Continue daily

*X indicates day(s) to administer drug(s) indicated.
†Take blood counts every 1 to 2 weeks. Adjust chlorambucil dose according to blood counts.

REFERENCE:

Han, T., et al.: Chlorambucil vs. combined chlorambucil-corticosteroid therapy in chronic lymphocytic leukemia, Cancer **31**:502-508, 1973.

Busulfan (chronic intermittent therapy)

GENERAL USE: Chronic myelocytic leukemia
RESPONSE RATE: 90%
SCHEDULE AND DOSE:

	Day*							
	1	**2**	**3**	**4**	**5**	**6**	**7**	**→†**
Busulfan† 4 to 6 mg Orally	X	X	X	X	X	X	X	Continue daily

*X indicates day(s) to administer drug(s) indicated.
†Continue busulfan until leukocytes fall to 15,000/cu mm and platelets to 150,000/cu mm. *Reinstitute* busulfan when leukocyte count is ≥50,000/cu mm.

REFERENCES:

Haut, A., et al.: Busulfan in the treatment of chronic myelocytic leukemia. The effect of long term intermittent therapy, Blood **17**:1-19, 1961.

Huguley, C. M.: Chronic myelocytic and chronic lymphocytic leukemia, Cancer **30**:1583-1587, 1972.

Busulfan (chronic continuous therapy)

GENERAL USE: Chronic myelocytic leukemia

RESPONSE RATE: 90%

SCHEDULE AND DOSE:

	Day*							
	1	2	3	4	5	6	7	→†
Busulfan† 0.06 mg/kg (max. dose 4 mg) Orally	X	X	X	X	X	X	X	Continue daily

*X indicates day(s) to administer drug(s) indicated.

†Continue busulfan until leukocytes (WBC) drop to 15,000 to 20,000/cu mm and platelets drop to 150,000/cu mm. Then after a period of no drug begin daily maintenance at reduced dosage to maintain WBC at this level.

REFERENCES:

Galton, D. A. G.: Chemotherapy of chronic myelocytic leukemia, Semin. Hematol. **6:**323-343, 1969.

Huguley, C. M.: Chronic myelocytic and chronic lymphocytic leukemia, Cancer **30:**1583-1587, 1972.

Hydroxyurea

GENERAL USE: Chronic myelogenous leukemia

RESPONSE RATE: 90%

SCHEDULE AND DOSE:

	Day*							
	1	2	3	4	5	6	7	→†
Hydroxyurea 50 mg/kg Orally in two divided doses/day	X	X	X	X	X	X	X	Continue daily†

*X indicates day(s) to administer drug(s) indicated.

†Continue hydroxyurea until leukocytes (WBC) drop to 15,000 to 20,000/cu mm and platelets drop to 150,000/cu mm. Then titrate to a daily maintenance to maintain WBC at this level.

REFERENCE:

Kennedy, B. J., et al.: Metabolic and therapeutic effects of hydroxyurea in chronic myeloid leukemia, J.A.M.A. **195:**1038-43, 1966.

Dibromomannitol

GENERAL USE: Chronic myelogenous leukemia

RESPONSE RATE: 70% complete remission

SCHEDULE AND DOSE:

	Day* 1	2	3	4	5	6	7	→†
Dibromomannitol 250 mg/m² BSA‡ Orally	X	X	X					
Dibromomannitol 150 mg/m² BSA‡ Orally				X	X	X	X	Continue daily until remission†

*X indicates day(s) to administer drug(s) indicated.
†MAINTENANCE THERAPY: continue with 150 mg/m² to keep leukocyte count between 10,000/cu mm and 15,000/cu mm. Hemoglobin and platelet counts should be ≥12 g/100 ml and ≥100,000/cm mm respectively.
‡BSA = body surface area.

REFERENCE:

Canellos, G. P., et al.: Dibromomannitol in the treatment of chronic granulocytic leukemia: a prospective randomized comparison with busulfan, Blood **45:**197-203, 1975.

BLAST CRISIS
Daunorubicin and cytarabine

GENERAL USE: Blast crisis in chronic myelogenous leukemia or acute leukemia

RESPONSE RATE: 30%

SCHEDULE AND DOSE:

	Day*				
	1	2	3	4	5
Daunorubicin† 45 mg/m² BSA‡ IV push	X	X	X		
Cytarabine 100 mg/m² BSA‡ IV push twice a day	X	X	X	X	X

*X indicates day(s) to administer drug(s) indicated.

†CAUTION: In adult patients with total cumulative doses of daunorubicin of 550 mg/m² (or 450 mg/m² in patients with previously irradiated heart tissue) there is a more common occurrence of cardiomyopathy or CHF or both.

‡BSA = body surface area.

REFERENCE:

Hoagland, H. C., et al.: Blast cell crisis in acute or chronic leukemia, J.A.M.A. **235:**1888-1889, 1976.

Vincristine (Oncovin) and prednisone

GENERAL USE: Blast crisis in chronic myelocytic leukemia or acute leukemia

RESPONSE RATE: 30%

SCHEDULE AND DOSE:

	Day*															
	1	2	3	4	5	6	7	8	9	10	11	12	13	14	15†	⟶
Vincristine† 2 mg/m² BSA‡ IV (max. dose 2.0 mg)	X							X							X Continue weekly	
Prednisone 60 mg/m² BSA‡ Orally	X	X	X	X	X	X	X	X	X	X	X	X	X	X	(X)§ Taper →	

*X indicates day(s) to administer drug(s) indicated.

†Generally patients receive at least three doses of vincristine, at which time they can be reevaluated. Therapy should be discontinued in the event of progression of disease or failure to achieve an improvement in marrow morphology and peripheral counts. Treatment should be continued in patients with hematologic improvement.

‡BSA = body surface area.

§Begin tapering prednisone gradually after the patient has received 2 weeks of full doses.

REFERENCE:

Canellos, G. P., et al.: Hematologic and cytogenetic remission of blastic transformation in chronic granulocytic leukemia, Blood **38:**671-679, 1971.

Hydroxyurea

GENERAL USE: Blast crisis in chronic myelogenous leukemia or acute leukemia

RESPONSE RATE: 30%

SCHEDULE AND DOSE:

	Day*	
	1	2†
Hydroxyurea 80 mg/kg Orally in divided doses every 6 hours	X	X

*X indicates day(s) to administer drug(s) indicated.
†Usually two doses bring blood counts down so other therapy can be initiated.

REFERENCE:

Hoagland, H. C., et al.: Blast cell crisis in acute or chronic leukemia, J.A.M.A. **235:**1888-1889, 1976.

HODGKIN'S DISEASE AND NON-HODGKIN'S LYMPHOMA
Nitrogen mustard, vincristine (Oncovin), procarbazine, and prednisone (MOPP)

GENERAL USE: Hodgkin's disease (adult and pediatric) and non-Hodgkin's lymphoma (adult)

RESPONSE RATE: 95% (81% complete remission)

SCHEDULE AND DOSE: Repeat cycle every 28 days.

	Day*															
	1	2	3	4	5	6	7	8	9	10	11	12	13	14	⟶	28†
Nitrogen mustard 6 mg/m^2 BSA‡ IV	X							X								
Vincristine 2 mg/m^2 BSA‡ IV (max. dose 2.0 mg)	X							X							2-week rest period	
Procarbazine 100 mg/m^2 BSA‡ Orally	X	X	X	X	X	X	X	X	X	X	X	X	X	X		
Prednisone 40 mg/m^2 BSA‡ Orally	X	X	X	X	X	X	X	X	X	X	X	X	X	X		

*X indicates day(s) to administer drug(s) indicated.

†May be delayed 1 week if recovery of the granulocytes and platelets is not complete by day 28.

1. MOPP is repeated for 6 cycles and the patient is then thoroughly reevaluated.
2. Prednisone is rarely restricted to cycles 1 and 4 only, as reported by original investigators, but is given with each cycle.

‡BSA = body surface area.

REFERENCES:

Lowenbraun, S., et al.: Combination chemotherapy with nitrogen mustard, vincristine, procarbazine, and prednisone in lymphosarcoma and reticulum cell sarcoma, Cancer **25:**1018-1025, 1970.

Devita, V., et al.: Combination chemotherapy in the treatment of advanced Hodgkin's disease, Ann. Intern. Med. **73:**881-895, 1970.

Frei, M., et al.: Combination chemotherapy in advanced Hodgkin's disease, Ann. Int. Med. **79:**376-382, 1973.

Donaldson, S. S., et al.: Pediatric Hodgkin's disease. II. Results of therapy, Cancer **37:**2436-2447, 1976.

Nitrogen mustard, vincristine (Oncovin), procarbazine, prednisone, and bleomycin (MOPP-LO BLEO)

GENERAL USE: Hodgkin's disease (adult and pediatric)
RESPONSE RATE: 94% complete remission
SCHEDULE AND DOSE: Repeat every 4 weeks.

	Day*													
	1	2	3	4	5	6	7	8	9	10	11	12	→	28‡
Nitrogen mustard 6 mg/m² BSA† IV	X							X					No therapy, 2 weeks	
Vincristine 1.5 mg/m² BSA† IV (max. dose 2.0 mg)	X							X						
Procarbazine 100 mg/m² BSA† Orally		X	X	X	X	X	X		X	X	X	X		
Prednisone 40 mg/m² BSA† Orally in divided doses		X	X	X	X	X	X		X	X	X	X		
Bleomycin 2 mg/m² BSA† IV	X							X						

*X indicates day(s) to administer drug(s) indicated.
†BSA = body surface area.
‡MOPP-LO BLEO is repeated for 6 cycles and the patient is then thoroughly reevaluated.

REFERENCE:

Coltman, C. A.: Bleomycin in malignant lymphoma combinations. In Soper, W. T., et al.: New drug seminar on bleomycin, National Cancer Institute, Silver Spring, Md., 1977, Automation Industries, pp. 97-107.

Doxorubicin (Adriamycin), bleomycin, vinblastine, and dacarbazine (DTIC) (ABVD)

GENERAL USE: Hodgkin's disease resistant to MOPP (adult and pediatric)
RESPONSE RATE: 90% (75% complete remission)
SCHEDULE AND DOSE: Repeat cycle every 28 days.

	Day*														
	1	2	3	4	5	6	7	8	9	10	11	12	13	14	15 → 28†
Doxorubicin‡ 25 mg/m^2 BSA§ IV	X													X	No therapy, two weeks
Bleomycin‖ 10 mg/m^2 BSA§ IV	X													X	
Vinblastine 6 mg/m^2 BSA§ IV	X													X	
Dacarbazine 375 mg/m^2 BSA§ IV	X													X	

*X indicates day(s) to administer drug(s) indicated.
†May be delayed one week if recovery of the granulocytes and platelets is not complete by day 28.

1. ABVD is repeated for six cycles and the patient is then thoroughly reevaluated. The number of cycles of doxorubicin and bleomycin is limited to maximum total cumulative doses at which their respective toxicities appear.
2. Alternate Schedule: Dacarbazine may be given 150 mg/m^2 on days 1 to 5 rather than 375 mg/m^2 on days 1 and 14.

‡CAUTION: In adult patients with total cumulative doses of doxorubicin of 550 mg/m^2 (or 450 mg/m^2 in patients with previously irradiated heart tissue) there is a more common occurrence of cardiomyopathy or CHF or both. In pediatric patients with total cumulative doses of doxorubicin of 450 mg/m^2 (or 350 mg/m^2 in patients with previously irradiated heart tissue) there is a more common occurrence of cardiomyopathy or CHF or both.
§BSA = body surface area.
‖CAUTION: In patients with total cumulative doses of bleomycin of 400 units or more there is a more common occurrence of pulmonary fibrosis. It can be exacerbated by prior irradiation or pulmonary disease in patients over 60 years of age. Bleomycin, 1 mg = 1 unit.

REFERENCE:

Bonadonna, G., et al.: Combination chemotherapy of Hodgkin's disease with Adriamycin, bleomycin, vinblastine, and imidazole carboxamide versus MOPP, Cancer **36:**252-259, 1975.

Carmustine (BCNU), cyclophosphamide, vinblastine, procarbazine, and prednisone (BCVPP)

GENERAL USE: Hodgkin's lymphoma

RESPONSE RATE: 75% complete remission (equivalent to MOPP with less toxicity)

SCHEDULE: Repeat cycle every 28 days.

	Day*										
	1	2	3	4	5	6	7	8	9	10 →	28†
Carmustine‡ 100 mg/m² BSA§ IV	X										
Cyclophosphamide 600 mg/m² BSA§ IV	X									2-week rest period	
Vinblastine 5 mg/m² BSA§ IV	X										
Procarbazine 100 mg/m² BSA§ Orally	X	X	X	X	X	X	X	X	X	X	
Prednisone 60 mg/m² BSA§ Orally	X	X	X	X	X	X	X	X	X	X	

*X indicates day(s) to administer drug(s) indicated.

†NOTE: BCVPP is repeated for 6 cycles and the patient is then thoroughly reevaluated.

‡CAUTION: The nadir of carmustine may be *delayed* 6 weeks after drug administration.

§BSA = body surface area.

REFERENCE:

Costello, W. G., et al.: "Chemoimmunotherapy of Hodgkin's disease (HD), Proc. Am. Soc. Clin. Oncol. **20**:392, 1979.

Nitrogen mustard, vinblastine, procarbazine, and prednisolone (MVPP)

GENERAL USE: Hodgkin's disease (adult and pediatric)
RESPONSE RATE: 81% complete remission
SCHEDULE AND DOSE: Repeat cycle every 6 weeks.

	Day*															
	1	**2**	**3**	**4**	**5**	**6**	**7**	**8**	**9**	**10**	**11**	**12**	**13**	**14**	**15**	**→ 42†**
Nitrogen mustard 6 mg/m² BSA‡ IV	X							X								4-week rest period
Vinblastine 10 mg IV	X							X							X	
Procarbazine 100 mg/m² BSA‡ Orally	X	X	X	X	X	X	X	X	X	X	X	X	X	X	X	
Prednisolone 40 mg Orally	X	X	X	X	X	X	X	X	X	X	X	X	X	X	X	

*X indicates day(s) to administer drug(s) indicated.
†NOTE: MVPP is repeated for 6 cycles and the patient is then thoroughly reevaluated.
‡BSA = body surface area.
Alternatively: vinblastine 6 mg/m² BSA IV on days 1 and 8 only and prednisone 40 mg/m² BSA orally on days 1-14.

REFERENCES:

Nicholson, W. M., et al.: Combination chemotherapy in generalized Hodgkin's disease, Br. Med. J. **3**:7-10, 1970.

McElwain, T. J., et al.: Combination chemotherapy in advanced and recurrent Hodgkin's disease, National Cancer Institute monograph **36**:395-402, 1973.

Doxorubicin (Adriamycin), prednisone, vincristine, procarbazine, and cyclophosphamide (MAC) (Memorial Sloan-Kettering Program)

GENERAL USE: Hodgkin's disease (pediatric)

RESPONSE RATE: 92% (74% complete remission)

SCHEDULE AND DOSE: Repeat cycle every 90 days for 1 to 2 years.

	Day*												
	1	2	3	→	28	→	35	→	42	→	63	→	90
Doxorubicin† 20 mg/m² BSA‡ IV	X	X	X	No therapy, 3½-weeks rest period								No therapy, 4 weeks	
Prednisone 1 mg/kg Orally					X Daily →	→	→	→	→				
Vincristine 1-2.0 mg/m² BSA‡ IV (max. dose 2.0 mg)					X		X		X				
Procarbazine 50-100 mg/m² BSA‡ Orally					X Daily →	→	→	→	→				
Cyclophosphamide† 40 mg/m² BSA‡ IV											X		

*X indicates day(s) to administer drug(s) indicated.

†CAUTION: In pediatric patients with total cumulative dose of doxorubicin of 350 mg/m² when given concurrently with cyclophosphamide, there is a more common occurrence of cardiomyopathy or CHF or both.

‡BSA = body surface area.

REFERENCE:

Tan, C., et al.: The changing management of childhood Hodgkin's disease, Cancer **35**:808-816, 1975.

Doxorubicin (Adriamycin), cyclophosphamide, vincristine (Oncovin), procarbazine, and prednisone (A-COPP)

GENERAL USE: Hodgkin's disease (pediatrics)

RESPONSE RATE: 80% (survival 5 years), 74% (survival 10 years)

SCHEDULE AND DOSE: Repeat every 42 days for 6 cycles.

	Day* 1	→	14	→	20	→	27	28	→	42
Doxorubicin† 60 mg/m² BSA‡ IV	X								No therapy, 2 weeks	
Cyclophosphamide† 300 mg/m² BSA‡ IV			X		X					
Vincristine 1.5 mg/m² BSA‡ IV (max. dose 2.0 mg)			X		X					
Procarbazine 100 mg/m² BSA‡ Orally			X → Daily →							
Prednisone 40 mg/m² BSA‡ Orally										
Cycles 1 and 4:	X → Daily →									
Cycles 2, 3, 5, 6:			X → Daily →							

*X indicates day(s) to administer drug(s) indicated.

†CAUTION: In pediatric patients with total cumulative dose of doxorubicin of 350 mg/m² when given concurrently with cyclophosphamide, there is a more common occurrence of cardiomyopathy or CHF or both.

‡BSA = body surface area.

REFERENCE:

Sullivan, M. P., et al.: Hodgkin's disease in children. In Sutow, W., Vietti, T., and Fernbach, D., editors: Clinical pediatric oncology, ed. 2, St. Louis, 1977, The C. V. Mosby Co., pp. 408-443.

Lomustine (CCNU), doxorubicin (Adriamycin), and vinblastine (CAVe)

GENERAL USE: Hodgkin's disease resistant to MOPP

RESPONSE RATE: 50%

SCHEDULE AND DOSE: Repeat cycle every 6 weeks.

	Day* 1	→	42†
Lomustine‡ 100 mg/m² BSA§ Orally	X	6-week rest period	
Doxorubicin‖ 60 mg/m² BSA§ IV	X		
Vinblastine 5 mg/m² BSA§ IV	X		

*X indicates day(s) to administer drug(s) indicated.

†Repeat cycle for 9 courses of therapy if blood counts permit.

‡CAUTION: The nadir of lomustine may be *delayed* 6 weeks after drug administration.

§BSA = body surface area.

‖CAUTION: In adult patients with total cumulative doses of doxorubicin of 550 mg/m² (or 450 mg/m² in patients with previously irradiated heart tissue) there is a more common occurrence of cardiomyopathy or CHF or both.

REFERENCE:

Kaplan, H. S., et al.: The management of Hodgkin's disease, Cancer **36:** 796-803, 1975.

Chlorambucil

GENERAL USE: Hodgkin's disease
RESPONSE RATE: 61% (16% complete remission) (adult)
SCHEDULE AND DOSE:

	Day*							
	1	2	3	4	5	6	7	⟶†
Chlorambucil 0.1 to 0.2 mg/kg	X	X	X	X	X	X	X	Continue daily†

*X indicates day(s) to administer drug(s) indicated.
†Continue daily until toxic reactions in the bone marrow or improvement occurs.

REFERENCE:

Carter, S. K., et al.: Single-agent therapy for Hodgkin's disease, Arch. Intern. Med. **131**:377-387, 1973.

Cyclophosphamide, vincristine (Oncovin), and prednisone (CVP)

GENERAL USE: Favorable histologic types (nodular non-Hodgkin's lymphoma except histiocytic lymphoma)

RESPONSE RATE: 41% complete remission of lymphocytic lymphomas

SCHEDULE AND DOSE: Repeat cycle every 21 or 28 days.

	Day*						
	1	2	3	4	5	6 →	21†
Cyclophosphamide 400 mg/m^2 BSA‡ Orally		X	X	X	X	X	No therapy, 2-week rest period	
Vincristine 1.4 mg/m^2 BSA‡ IV (max. dose 2.0 mg)	X							
Prednisone 100 mg/m^2 BSA‡ Orally		X	X	X	X	X		

*X indicates day(s) to administer drug(s) indicated.

†May be delayed 1 week if recovery of the granulocytes and platelets is not complete by day 21 or 28.

NOTE: CVP is usually repeated for 6 cycles, and the patient is then thoroughly reevaluated.

‡BSA = body surface area

REFERENCES:

Bagley, C. M., et al.: Advanced lymphosarcoma: intensive cyclical combination chemotherapy with cyclophosphamide, vincristine, and prednisone, Ann. Intern. Med. **76:**227-234, 1972.

Razek, A., et al.: Optimum time sequence for the administration of vincristine and cyclophosphamide in vivo, Cancer Res. **34:**1857-1861, 1974.

Poullart, Proc. Am. Assoc. Cancer Res. **458:**115, 1973.

Cyclophosphamide, vincristine (Oncovin), and prednisone (COP)

GENERAL USE: Favorable histologic types (nodular non-Hodgkin's lymphoma except histiocytic lymphoma)

RESPONSE RATE: 50% complete remission, lymphosarcoma; 39% complete remission, reticulum cell sarcoma; remission duration shorter than CVP

SCHEDULE AND DOSE: Repeat cycle every 21 or 28 days.

	Day*						
	1	2	3	4	5	→	21†
Cyclophosphamide 1000 mg/m² BSA‡ IV	X					No therapy, 2 weeks	
Vincristine 1.4 mg/m² BSA‡ IV (max. dose 2.0 mg)	X						
Prednisone 60 mg/m² BSA‡ Orally	X	X	X	X	X		

*X indicates day(s) to administer drug(s) indicated.

†May be delayed 1 week if recovery of the granulocytes and platelets is not complete by day 21 or 28.

NOTE: COP is usually repeated for 6 cycles, and then the patient is thoroughly reevaluated.

‡BSA = body surface area.

REFERENCES:

Luce, J. K., et al.: Combined cyclophosphamide, vincristine and prednisone therapy of malignant lymphoma, Cancer **28**:306-317, 1971.

Skarin, A. T., et al.: Combination chemotherapy of advanced lymphocytic lymphoma: importance of histiologic classification in evaluating response, Cancer **34**:1023-1029, 1974.

Chlorambucil

GENERAL USE: Favorable histologic types (nodular non-Hodgkin's lymphomas except histiocytic lymphoma)

RESPONSE RATE: 74% (13% complete remission)

SCHEDULE AND DOSE:

	Day*								
	1	2	3	4	5	6	7	8	9 ⟶ †
Chlorambucil 8 to 12 mg Orally	X	X	X	X	X	X	X	X	X Continue daily†

*X indicates day(s) to administer drug(s) indicated.
†Titrate dose against the clinical response and marrow suppressive effects.

ALTERNATE SCHEDULE: Give chlorambucil daily continuously for 6 weeks. Stop for 2 weeks and resume with three 15-day courses with 15-day treatment-free intervals between each course. Then stop all treatment after the third course.

REFERENCES:

Jones, S. E., et al.: Non-Hodgkin's lymphomas. II. Single agent chemotherapy, Cancer **30:**31-38, 1972.

Lister, T. A., et al.: Comparison of combined and single-agent chemotherapy in non-Hodgkin's lymphoma of favourable histologic type, Br. Med. J. **1:**533-537, 1978.

Monfardini, S., et al.: Single agent sequential chemotherapy in non-Hodgkin's lymphomas, Tumori **59:**219, 1973.

Cyclophosphamide, doxorubicin (hydroxydaunorubicin; Adriamycin), vincristine (Oncovin), and prednisone (CHOP)

GENERAL USE: Unfavorable histologic types (diffuse non-Hodgkin's lymphoma)

RESPONSE RATE: 60% complete remission

SCHEDULE AND DOSE: Repeat cycle every 21 or 28 days.

	Day*					
	1	2	3	4	5 ⟶	21†
Cyclophosphamide 750 mg/m² BSA‡ IV	X				No therapy, 2- to 3-week rest period	
Doxorubicin§ 50 mg/m² BSA‡ IV	X					
Vincristine (Oncovin) 1.4 mg/m² BSA‡ IV (max. dose 2.0 mg)	X					
Prednisone 100 mg/day Orally	X	X	X	X	X	

*X indicates day(s) to administer drug(s) indicated.

†May be delayed 1 week if recovery of the granulocytes and platelets is not complete by day 21 or 28.

NOTE: CHOP is usually repeated for 6 cycles and the patient is then thoroughly reevaluated.

‡BSA = body surface area.

§CAUTION: Discontinue doxorubicin after total cumulative dose reaches 450 mg/m². In adult patients with total cumulative doses greater than 450 mg/m² of doxorubicin when given concurrently with cyclophosphamide, there is a more common occurrence of cardiomyopathy or CHF or both.

REFERENCES:

McKelvey, E. M., et al.: Hydroxyldaunomycin (Adriamycin) combination chemotherapy in malignant lymphoma, Cancer **38:**1484-1493, 1976.

Jones, S.: Non-Hodgkin's lymphomas, J.A.M.A. **234**(6):633-638, 1975.

Cyclophosphamide, doxorubicin (hydroxydaunorubicin; Adriamycin), vincristine (Oncovin), prednisone, and bleomycin (CHOP-BLEO)

GENERAL USE: Unfavorable histologic types (advanced diffuse non-Hodgkin's lymphoma)

RESPONSE RATE: 94% complete remission

SCHEDULE AND DOSE: Repeat cycle every 21 or 28 days.

	Day* 1	2	3	4	5	6	7	8	→	21
Cyclophosphamide 750 mg/m² BSA† IV	X								No therapy, 2-week rest period	
Doxorubicin‡ 50 mg/m² BSA† IV	X									
Vincristine 1 mg/m² BSA† IV (max. dose 2 mg)	X							X		
Prednisone 100 mg Orally	X	X	X	X	X					
Bleomycin§ 8 units/m² BSA† IV	X							X		

*X indicates day(s) to administer drug(s) indicated.

†BSA = body surface area.

‡Discontinue doxorubicin after total cumulative dose reaches 450 mg/m². CAUTION: In adult patients with total cumulative doses of doxorubicin greater than 450 mg/m² when given concurrently with cyclophosphamide, there is a more common occurrence of cardiomyopathy or CHF or both.

§CAUTION: In patients with total cumulative doses of bleomycin of 400 units or more there is a more common occurrence of pulmonary fibrosis. It can be exacerbated by prior irradiation or pulmonary disease or in patients over 60 years of age.

NOTE: Repeat CHOP-BLEO for 12 cycles, then thoroughly reevaluate the patient.

REFERENCE:

Case, D. C., et al.: Combination chemotherapy ("CHOP-BLEO") in advanced diffuse non-Hodgkin's lymphoma, Proc. Am. Soc. Clin. Oncol. **20:**303, 1979.

Doxorubicin (Adriamycin), cyclophosphamide, vincristine (Oncovin), methotrexate, cytosine arabinoside (Ara-C), and leucovorin (ACOMA)

GENERAL USE: Unfavorable histologic types (advanced diffuse histiocytic lymphoma)

RESPONSE RATE: 69% complete remission (remission 30+ months)

SCHEDULE AND DOSE:

	Day*: 1	→	8	→	15	→	21	22	→
Doxorubicin† 40 mg/m² BSA‡ IV	X								
Cyclophosphamide 1 g/m² BSA‡ IV	X								
Vincristine 2 mg IV (max. dose 2 mg)	X		X		X				
Methotrexate 120 mg/m² BSA‡ IV							X	Continue once every week for 8 doses	
Cytosine arabinoside 300 mg/m² BSA‡ IV 1 hour after methotrexate							X	Continue once every week for 8 doses	
Leucovorin 25 mg Orally every 6 hours for 6 doses; begin 24 hours after methotrexate								X	Continue every week for 8 weeks

*X indicates day(s) to administer drug(s) indicated.

†CAUTION: In adult patients with total cumulative doses of doxorubicin greater than 450 mg/m² when given concurrently with cyclophosphamide, there is a more common occurrence of cardiomyopathy or CHF or both.

‡BSA = body surface area.

REFERENCE:

Cadman, E. C., et al.: An improved treatment program for advanced diffuse histiocytic lymphoma (DHL), Proc. Am. Soc. Clin. Oncol. **20:** 396, 1979.

Cyclophosphamide, vincristine (Oncovin), procarbazine, and prednisone (COPP) (C MOPP)

GENERAL USE: Unfavorable histologic types (diffuse histiocytic and mixed non-Hodgkin's lymphoma), Hodgkin's disease (adult) or Hodgkin's disease (pediatric)

RESPONSE RATE: 43% complete remission

SCHEDULE AND DOSE: Repeat cycle every 28 days.

	Day*															
	1	2	3	4	5	6	7	8	9	10	11	12	13	14	→	28†
Cyclophosphamide 650 mg/m² BSA‡ IV	X							X							No therapy, 2-week rest period	
Vincristine (Oncovin) 1.4 mg/m² BSA‡ IV (max. dose 2.0 mg)	X							X								
Procarbazine 100 mg/m² BSA‡ Orally	X	X	X	X	X	X	X	X	X	X	X	X	X	X		
Prednisone 40 mg/m² BSA‡ Orally	X	X	X	X	X	X	X	X	X	X	X	X	X	X		

*X indicates day(s) to administer drug(s) indicated.

†May be delayed 1 week if recovery of the granulocytes and platelets is not complete by day 28.

1. C MOPP is usually repeated 6 cycles and then the patient is thoroughly reevaluated.
2. Prednisone is rarely restricted to cycles 1 and 4 only as reported by original investigators but is given with each cycle.

‡BSA = body surface area.

REFERENCES:

Schein, P. S., et al.: Potential for prolonged disease-free survival following combination chemotherapy of non-Hodgkin's lymphoma, Blood **43:**181-189, 1974.

Mukherji, B., et al.: Cyclic chemotherapy in lymphoma, Cancer **28:**886-893, 1971.

Schein, P. S., et al.: Results of combination chemotherapy of non-Hodgkin's lymphoma, Br. J. Cancer **31**(suppl. 2):465-473, 1975.

Bleomycin, doxorubicin (Adriamycin), cyclophosphamide, vincristine (Oncovin), and prednisone (BACOP)

GENERAL USE: Unfavorable histologic types (diffuse non-Hodgkin's lymphoma)

RESPONSE RATE: 43% complete remission of diffuse histiocytic and diffuse mixed lymphomas

SCHEDULE AND DOSE: Repeat every 28 days.

	Day*												
	1	2	3	4	5	6	7	8	→	15	→	22	→ 28†
Bleomycin 5 mg/m² BSA‡ IV, day 15 *and* 22 only										X		X	
Doxorubicin§ 25 mg/m² BSA‡ IV	X							X					
Cyclophosphamide 650 mg/m² BSA‡ IV	X							X					
Vincristine 1.4 mg/m² BSA‡ IV (max. dose 2 mg)	X							X					
Prednisone 60 mg/m² BSA‡ Orally										X Daily →			

*X indicates day(s) to administer drug(s) indicated.
†May be delayed 1 week if recovery of the granulocytes and platelets is not complete by day 28.
NOTE: BACOP is usually repeated for 6 cycles and the patient is then thoroughly evaluated. Bleomycin, 1 mg = 1 unit.
‡BSA = body surface area.
§CAUTION: In adult patients who have received both doxorubicin and cyclophosphamide with total cumulative doses of 450 mg/m² of doxorubicin there is a more common occurrence of cardiomyopathy or CHF or both.

REFERENCE:

Schein, P., et al.: A new combination chemotherapy program for diffuse and mixed non-Hodgkin's lymphoma, Proc. Am. Assoc. Cancer Res. **16:**248, 1975.

PEDIATRIC NON-HODGKIN'S LYMPHOMA
LSA_2-L_2 Protocol

GENERAL USE: Remission induction of childhood non-Hodgkin's lymphoma

RESPONSE RATE: 90% to 96% complete remissions (88% alive 3 to 4 years after diagnosis)

INDUCTION SCHEDULE AND DOSE: A 3- to 5-day rest period follows day 31.

	Day*																		
	1	2	3	4	5	→	10	11	12	13	→	17	→	24	→	27	→	30	31
Cyclophosphamide 1,200 mg/m² BSA† IV push	X																		
Vincristine 1.5 to 2.5 mg/m² BSA† IV (max. dose 2 mg)			X				X					X		X					
Daunorubicin 60 mg/m² BSA† IV									X	X									
Prednisone 60 mg/m² BSA† Orally in 4 divided doses			X Daily →																
Methotrexate 6.25 mg/m² BSA† IT					X											X		X	

±Radiation therapy to single or multiple bulky disease areas (3,000 rads beginning week 3 or 4)‡

*X indicates day(s) to administer drug(s) indicated.

†BSA = body surface area.

‡Whether to give radiation therapy or time to give it is dependent on site and state of the disease and prior therapy.

CONSOLIDATION SCHEDULE AND DOSE: Beginning day 34 or 36

Phase I	**Day*** 1 → 5	→ 8 → 12	→ 15 → 19	→ 30	→ 35†
Cytosine arabinoside 150 mg/m² BSA‡ IV	X Daily →	X Daily →	X Daily →		
6-Thioguanine 75 mg/m² BSA‡ Orally, 8 to 12 hours after each cytosine arabinoside injection	X Daily →	X Daily →	X Daily →		

Phase II	36 → 40	→ 43 → 47	→ 50	51	→ 54	→ 57	→ 61
L-Asparaginase 6,000 IU/m² BSA‡ IV	X Daily →	X Daily →	X	X			
Methotrexate 6.25 mg/m² BSA‡ IT Give 2-3 days after last dose of L-asparaginase					X	X	
Carmustine 60 mg/m² BSA‡ IV							X

*X indicates day(s) to administer drug(s) indicated.
†Phase 1—6-thioguanine is given through the weekends if leukocytes are more than 1,500/cu mm and platelets are more than 150,000/cu mm, which will result in more than 15 doses of 6-thioguanine. Phase I's usual duration is from 30 to 35 days. It is completed when dose 15 of cytosine arabinoside is given. NOTE: Average duration of induction plus consolidation is 85 to 120 days.
‡BSA = body surface area.

MAINTENANCE SCHEDULE AND DOSE: Maintenance begins 3 to 4 days after consolidation therapy is completed. It consists of 5-day treatment cycles separated by intervals of 7 to 10 days. On completion of cycle 5, maintenance is continued following a 7- to 10-day rest period by repeating cycles 1 through 5. See note below chart for cycle 5.

CYCLE 1, WEEKS 15 AND 16

	Day* 1	2	3	4	5	6 →
6-Thioguanine 300 mg/m² BSA† Orally	X	X	X	X		7- to 10-day rest, no therapy
Cyclophosphamide 600 mg/m² BSA† IV					X	

CYCLE 2, WEEKS 17 AND 18

	Day* 1	2	3	4	5	6 →
Hydroxyurea 2,400 mg/m² BSA† Orally	X	X	X	X		7- to 10-day rest, no therapy
Daunorubicin‡ 45 mg/m² BSA† IV					X	

CYCLE 3, WEEKS 19 AND 20

	Day* 1	2	3	4	5	6 →
Methotrexate 10 mg/m² BSA† Orally	X	X	X	X		7- to 10-day rest, no therapy
Carmustine§ 60 mg/m² BSA† IV					X	

*X indicates day(s) to administer drug(s) indicated.

†BSA = body surface area.

‡In pediatric patients with total cumulative doses of daunorubicin of 450 mg/m² (350 mg/m² in patients with previously irradiated heart tissue) there is a more common occurrence of cardiomyopathy or CHF or both.

§CAUTION: The nadir of carmustine (BCNU) may be *delayed* 6 weeks after drug administration.

CYCLE 4, WEEKS 21 AND 22

	Day*					
	1	2	3	4	5	6→
Cytosine arabinoside 150 mg/m² BSA† IV	X	X	X	X		7- to 10-day rest, no therapy
Vincristine 2.0 mg/m² BSA† IV (max. dose 2.0 mg)					X	

CYCLE 5, WEEKS 23 AND 24

	Day*					
	1	2	3	4	5	6→
Methotrexate 6.25 mg/m² BSA† IT	X				X	7- to 10-day rest

*X indicates day(s) to administer drug(s).

†BSA = body surface area.

NOTE: Continue to repeat maintenance therapy (cycles 1 to 5) for 2 years for Stages I, II, and III disease. For Stage IV disease continue repeating for 3 years; then discontinue unless there is a recurrence of disease.

REFERENCES:

Murphy, S. B.: Management of childhood non-Hodgkin's lymphoma, Cancer Treat. Rep. **61:**1161-1173, 1977.

Wollner, N., et al.: Non-Hodgkin's lymphoma in children: a comparative study of two modalities of therapy, Cancer **37:**123-134, 1976.

Cyclophosphamide, vincristine (Oncovin), methotrexate, and prednisone (COMP)

GENERAL USE: Remission induction in childhood non-Hodgkin's lymphoma
RESPONSE RATE: 96% complete remission (18-month duration).
INDUCTION SCHEDULE AND DOSE:

	Day*																		
	1	2	3	4	5	→	10	11	12	→	17	→	24	→	28	→	31	→	34†
Cyclophosphamide 1.2 g/m² BSA‡ IV	X																		
Vincristine 2.0 mg/m² BSA‡ IV (max. dose 2 mg)			X				X				X		X						
Methotrexate 200 mg/m² BSA‡ IV push									X										
Methotrexate 100 mg/m² BSA‡ IV infusion over 4 hours immediately after IV push									X										
Prednisone 60 mg/m² BSA‡ Orally	X	Daily →													→				
Methotrexate 6.25 mg/m² BSA‡ IT					X												X		X

*X indicates day(s) to administer drug(s) indicated.
†Radiotherapy is given for 1 month to all sites grossly involved at diagnosis.
‡BSA = body surface area.

NOTE: Maintenance consists of drug cycles COMP + intrathecal methotrexate essentially as above, repeated monthly.

CAUTION: Leucovorin rescue usually accompanies methotrexate doses of more than 100 mg/m² to prevent possible severe toxicity. See Section 7, Leucovorin Rescue, and Section 5, Leucovorin.

Procedures of allopurinol administration, alkalinization of the urine, and taking 24-, 48-, and 72-hour methotrexate serum blood levels should be done to prevent severe methotrexate toxicity. If abnormally high 24-hour methotrexate serum levels are obtained, continue citrovorum factor past 72 hours until it is clear that the patient will not develop severe methotrexate toxicity, which usually occurs 5 days after MTX infusion. (See Section 6, Renal Dysfunction, and Table 6-15 and Table 6-17.)

REFERENCES:

Murphy, S. B., et al.: Management of childhood non-Hodgkin's lymphoma, Cancer Treat. Rep. **61:**1161-1173, 1977.

Meadows, A. T., et al.: Remission induction in childhood non-Hodgkin's lymphoma (NHL) with cyclophosphamide (CPM), vincristine (VCR), prednisone and intravenous methotrexate (MTX), Proc. Am. Soc. Clin. Oncol. **19:**365, 1978.

Jenkin, R., et al.: Grossly localized childhood non-Hodgkin's lymphoma (NHL). Response to irradiation and effective 4 or 10 drug combination chemotherapy, Proc. Am. Soc. Clin. Oncol. **20:**354, 1979.

Doxorubicin (Adriamycin), prednisone, and vincristine (Oncovin) (APO)

GENERAL USE: Childhood non-Hodgkin's lymphoma

RESPONSE RATE: 90% complete remission (86% disease free at 41 months)

INDUCTION SCHEDULE AND DOSE:

	Day*											
	1	→	8	→	15	→	21	22	→	29	→	35
Doxorubicin† 75 mg/m^2 BSA‡ IV	X							X			1-week rest period	
Vincristine 1.5 mg/m^2 BSA‡ IV (max. dose 2.0 mg)	X		X		X			X		X		
Prednisone 40 mg/m^2 BSA‡ Orally	X	Daily →						X	(Taper) →			

*X indicates day(s) to administer drug(s) indicated.

†CAUTION: In pediatric patients with total cumulative doses of 450 mg/m^2 of doxorubicin (or 350 mg/m^2 in patients with previously irradiated heart tissue) there is a more common occurrence of cardiomyopathy or CHF or both.

‡BSA = body surface area.

CONSOLIDATION SCHEDULE AND DOSE: (beginning the sixth week of therapy):

	Day* (Week 6)							
	1	2	3	4	5	6	7	→
Doxorubicin 30 mg/m^2 BSA† IV	X							
Vincristine 2.0 mg/m^2 BSA† IV (max. dose 2 mg)	X							
Prednisone 120 mg/m^2 BSA† Orally	X	X	X	X	X			
6-Mercaptopurine 225 mg/m^2 BSA† Orally	X	X	X	X	X			

*X indicates day(s) to administer drug(s) indicated.

†BSA = body surface area.

CONSOLIDATION SCHEDULE AND DOSE—cont'd

	Day*													
	←Week 7→							←Week 8→						
	1	2	3	4	5	6	7	1	2	3	4	5	6	7
Doxorubicin 22.5 mg/m² BSA† IV														
Vincristine 2.0 mg/m² BSA† IV (max. dose 2.0 mg)														
Prednisone 120 mg/m² BSA† Orally														
L-Asparaginase ≤6 years; 56,000 IU/m² BSA† IV ≥6 years; 28,000 IU/m² BSA† IV	X		X		X		X		X					
Methotrexate 12 mg/m² BSA† IT (max. dose 12 mg)									X					X
Cranial radiation 2400 rads/13 fractions/17 days									X		X	X	X	X

*X indicates day(s) to administer drug(s) indicated.
†BSA = body surface area.

	Day*														
	←Week 9→							←Week 10→							
	1	**2**	**3**	**4**	**5**	**6**	**7**	**1**	**2**	**3**	**4**	**5**	**6**	**7**	→
Doxorubicin 22.5 mg/m² BSA† IV	X														Week 11, no therapy
Vincristine 2.0 mg/m² BSA† IV (max. dose 2.0 mg)	X														
Prednisone 120 mg/m² BSA† Orally	X	X	X	X	X										
L-Asparaginase ≤6 year; 56,000 IU/m² BSA† IV ≥6 years; 28,000 IU/m² BSA† IV															
Methotrexate 12 mg/m² BSA† IT (max. dose 12 mg)				X				X				X			
Cranial radiation 2400 rads/13 fractions/ 17 days	X	X	X	X	X	X	X	X	X	X	X	X			

*X indicates day(s) to administer drug(s) indicated.
†BSA = body surface area.

MAINTENANCE SCHEDULE AND DOSE (beginning week 12 of therapy):

	Day* (Week 12) 1	2	3	4	5	6	7	→	
Doxorubicin† 30 mg/m² BSA‡ IV	X							No therapy, 2 weeks	Repeat every 3 weeks†
Vincristine 2.0 mg/m² BSA‡ IV (max. dose 2.0 mg)	X								
Prednisone 120 mg/m² BSA‡ Orally	X	X	X	X	X				
6-Mercaptopurine 225 mg/m² BSA‡ Orally	X	X	X	X	X				

*X indicates day(s) to administer drug(s) indicated.
†Continue every 3 weeks until a total cumulative dose of 450 mg/m² of doxorubicin is achieved; then replace it by parenteral methotrexate 7.5 mg/m² daily for 5 days (IV, day 1; IM, days 2 to 5) as shown for week 18. Usually the total cumulative dose of doxorubicin is achieved around week 15, and methotrexate is begun about week 18.
‡BSA = body surface area.

MAINTENANCE SCHEDULE AND DOSE—cont'd: beginning week 18 and continuing every 3 weeks for 2 years.

	Day* (Week 18)							
	1	**2**	**3**	**4**	**5**	**6**	**7**	**→**
Methotrexate† 7.5 mg/m² BSA‡ IV	X							No therapy, 2 weeks
Methotrexate† 7.5 mg/m² BSA‡ IM		X	X	X	X			
Vincristine 2.0 mg/m² BSA‡ IV (max. dose 2.0 mg)	X							
Prednisone 120 mg/m² BSA‡ Orally	X	X	X	X	X			
6-Mercaptopurine 225 mg/m² BSA‡ Orally	X	X	X	X	X			
Methotrexate§ 12 mg/m² BSA‡ IT (max. dose 12 mg)	X							

*X indicates day(s) to administer drug(s) indicated.

†NOTE: IV and IM methotrexate should not be given in week 18 in place of doxorubicin until a total cumulative dose of 450 mg/m² of doxorubicin has been achieved.

‡BSA = body surface area.

§Give intrathecal methotrexate every 18th week of maintenance therapy for 2 years.

REFERENCES:

Weinstein, H. J., et al.: Improved prognosis for patients with mediastinal lymphoblastic lymphoma, Blood **53:**687-694, 1979.

Jaffe, N., et al.: Role of staging in childhood non-Hodgkin's lymphoma, Cancer Treat. Rep. **61:**1001-1007, 1977.

BREAST CANCER
Cyclophosphamide, methotrexate, and 5-fluorouracil (CMF)

GENERAL USE: Breast cancer—metastatic or recurrent disease
REPONSE RATE: 53% in previously untreated patients
SCHEDULE AND DOSE: Repeat cycle every 28 days.

	Day*														
	1	**2**	**3**	**4**	**5**	**6**	**7**	**8**	**9**	**10**	**11**	**12**	**13**	**14**	**→ 28†**
Cyclophosphamide 100 mg/m^2 BSA‡ Orally	X	X	X	X	X	X	X	X	X	X	X	X	X	X	2-week rest period
Methotrexate 40 to 60 mg/m^2 BSA‡ IV	X							X							
5-Fluorouracil 600 mg/m^2 BSA‡ IV	X							X							

*X indicates day(s) to administer drug(s) indicated.
†May delay 1 week if recovery of the granulocytes and platelets is not complete by day 28.
‡BSA = body surface area.

REFERENCES:

Canellos, G. P., et al.: Combination chemotherapy for metastatic breast carcinoma: prospective comparison of multiple drug therapy with L-phenylalanine mustard, Cancer **38:**1882-1886, 1976.

Davis, T. E., et al.: Drug treatment of breast cancer, Drugs **16:**441-464, 1978.

Cyclophosphamide, doxorubicin (Adriamycin), and 5-fluorouracil (CAF)

GENERAL USE: Metastatic breast cancer

RESPONSE RATE: 82%

SCHEDULE AND DOSE: Repeat cycle every 28 days.

	Day*															
	1	2	3	4	5	6	7	8	9	10	11	12	13	14	→	28†
Cyclophosphamide 100 mg/m² BSA‡ Orally	X	X	X	X	X	X	X	X	X	X	X	X	X	X	2-week rest period	
Doxorubicin§ 30 mg/m² BSA‡ IV	X							X								
5-Fluorouracil 500 mg/m² BSA‡ IV	X							X								

*X indicates day(s) to administer drug(s) indicated.

†May delay 1 week if recovery of granulocytes and platelets is not completely by day 28.

‡BSA = body surface area.

§NOTE: Repeat the 28-day cycle until a total cumulative dose of 450 mg/m² of doxorubicin occurs; then discontinue doxorubicin and substitute it with methotrexate 40 mg/m² IV and increase the 5-fluorouracil dose to 600 mg/m² IV.

REFERENCE:

Bull, J. M., et al.: A randomized comparative trial of adriamycin versus methotrexate in combination drug therapy, Cancer **41**:1649-1657, 1978.

5-Fluorouracil, doxorubicin (Adriamycin), and cyclophosphamide (FAC)

GENERAL USE: Metastatic breast carcinoma

RESPONSE RATE: 72%

SCHEDULE AND DOSE: Repeat cycle every 21 days.

	Day*								
	1	2	3	4	5	6	7	8	9 → 21†
5-Fluorouracil 500 mg/m² BSA‡ IV	X							X	2-week rest period, no therapy
Doxorubicin§ 50 mg/m² BSA‡ IV	X								
Cyclophosphamide 500 mg/m² BSA‡ IV	X								

*X indicates day(s) to administer drug(s) indicated.

†May be delayed 1 week if recovery of the granulocytes and platelets is not complete by day 21.

‡BSA = body surface area.

§CAUTION: In adult patients with total cumulative doses of 450 mg/m² of doxorubicin who have received both doxorubicin and cyclophsophamide there is a more common occurrence of cardiomyopathy or CHF or both.

REFERENCES:

Blumenschein, G. R., et al.: FAC chemotherapy for breast cancer, Proc. Am. Soc. Clin. Oncol. **15:**193, 1974.

Legha, S. S., et al.: Complete remissions in metastatic breast cancer treated with combination drug therapy, Ann. Intern. Med. **91:**847-852, 1979.

Doxorubicin (Adriamycin) and cyclophosphamide (ACe)

GENERAL USE: Metastatic or recurrent breast cancer
RESPONSE RATE: 70% in previously untreated patients
SCHEDULE AND DOSE: Repeat cycle every 21 or 28 days.

	Day*						
	1	2	3	4	5	6	→	21†
Cyclophosphamide 200 mg/m² BSA‡ Orally			X	X	X	X	3- to 4- week rest period, no therapy	
Doxorubicin§ 40 mg/m² BSA‡ IV	X							

*X indicates day(s) to administer drug(s) indicated.
†May delay 1 week if recovery of the granulocytes and platelets is not complete by day 21 or 28.
‡BSA = body surface area.
§CAUTION: In adult patients with total cumulative doses of 450 mg/m² of doxorubicin who have received both doxorubicin and cyclophosphamide there is a more common occurrence of cardiomyopathy or CHF or both.

REFERENCES:

Jones, et al.: Combination chemotherapy with Adriamycin and cyclophosphamide for advanced breast cancer, Cancer **36:**90-97, 1975.
Salmon, S. E., et al.: Chemotherapy of advanced breast cancer with a combination of Adriamycin and cyclophosphamide, Proc. Am. Assoc. Cancer Res. **15:**90 (abstract), 1974.

Cyclophosphamide, methotrexate, 5-fluorouracil, and prednisone (CMF-P)

GENERAL USE: Metastatic breast cancer

RESPONSE RATE: 68%

SCHEDULE AND DOSE: Repeat cycle every 28 days.

	Day*															
	1	**2**	**3**	**4**	**5**	**6**	**7**	**8**	**9**	**10**	**11**	**12**	**13**	**14**	**→**	**28†**
Cyclophosphamide 100 mg/m² BSA‡ Orally	X	X	X	X	X	X	X	X	X	X	X	X	X	X	2-week rest period	
Methotrexate 60 mg/m² BSA‡ IV	X							X								
5-Fluorouracil 700 mg/m² BSA‡ IV	X							X								
Prednisone§ 40 mg/m² BSA‡ Orally	X	X	X	X	X	X	X	X	X	X	X	X	X	X		

*X indicates day(s) to administer drug(s) indicated.

†May delay 1 week if recovery of the granulocytes and platelets is not complete by day 28.

‡BSA = body surface area.

§Omit prednisone in estrogen receptor (ER) negative patients.

REFERENCE:

Canellos, G. P., et al.: Combination chemotherapy for advanced breast cancer: response and effect on survival, Ann. Intern. Med. **84**:389-392, 1976.

Cyclophosphamide, methotrexate, 5-fluorouracil, vincristine, and prednisone (CMFVP)

GENERAL USE: Metastatic or recurrent breast cancer
RESPONSE RATE: 47%
SCHEDULE AND DOSE:

	Day* 1	→	8	→	15	→	21	→
Cyclophosphamide 2.0 mg/kg Orally	X	Daily →						Continue daily
Methotrexate 0.75 mg/kg IV	X		X		X		X	Continue weekly
5-Fluorouracil 12 mg/kg IV	X		X		X		X	Continue weekly
Vincristine 0.025 mg/kg IV (max. dose 2.0 mg)	X		X		X		X	Continue weekly
Prednisone† 0.75 mg/kg Orally	X	Daily →						Taper

*X indicates day(s) to administer drug(s) indicated.
†Omit prednisone in estrogen receptor (ER) negative patients.

REFERENCES:

Carter, S. K.: Integration of chemotherapy into combined modality treatment of solid tumors. VII. Adenocarcinoma of the breast, Cancer Treat. Rev. **3**:141-174, 1976.

Cooper, R.: Combination chemotherapy in hormone-resistant breast cancer, Proc. Am. Assoc. Cancer Res. **10**:15 (abstract), 1969.

Cyclophosphamide, methotrexate, 5-fluorouracil and tamoxifen (CMF plus tamoxifen)

GENERAL USE: Metastatic breast cancer

RESPONSE RATE: 72%

SCHEDULE AND DOSE: Repeat cycle every 28 days.

	Day*															
	1	2	3	4	5	6	7	8	9	10	11	12	13	14	15	→ 28
Cyclophosphamide 100 mg/m^2 BSA† Orally	X							Daily						→		
Methotrexate 40 mg/m^2 BSA† IV	X							X								
5-Fluorouracil 600 mg/m^2 BSA† IV	X							X								
Tamoxifen 10 mg Orally, twice daily (20 mg/day)	X								Twice daily							→

*X indicates day(s) to administer drug(s) indicated.

†BSA = body surface area.

REFERENCE:

Cocconi, G., et al.: Chemotherapy (CMF) vs. combination of hormonal and chemotherapy (CMF plus Tamoxifen) in metastatic breast cancer, Proc. Am. Soc. Clin. Oncol. **20**:302, 1979.

Doxorubicin (Adriamycin) and vincristine

GENERAL USE: Metastatic breast cancer

RESPONSE RATE: 53%

SCHEDULE AND DOSE: Repeat cycle every 21 or 28 days.

	Day*			
	1	⟶	21†	
Doxorubicin‡ 60 mg/m² BSA§ IV	X	No therapy, 3-week rest period		
Vincristine 1.4 mg/m² BSA§ IV (max. dose 2.0 mg)	X			

*X indicates day(s) to administer drug(s) indicated.

†May be delayed 1 week if recovery of the granulocytes is not complete by day 21.

‡CAUTION: In adult patients with total cumulative doses of 550 mg/m² of doxorubicin (or 450 mg/m² in patients with previously irradiated heart tissue) there is a more common occurrence of cardiomyopathy or CHF or both.

§BSA = body surface area.

REFERENCES:

Band, P. R., et al.: Induction chemotherapy and maintenance chemo-hormonotherapy in metastatic breast cancer, Proc. Am. Assoc. Cancer Res. **18:**228, 1977.

Brambilla, C., et al.: Response and survival in advanced breast cancer after two non-cross-resistant combinations, Br. Med. J. **1:**801-804, 1976.

DeLena, M., et al.: Adriamycin plus vincristine compared to and combined with CMF for advanced breast cancer, Cancer **35:**1108-1115, 1975.

5-Fluorouracil, vincristine (Oncovin), doxorubicin (Adriamycin), and mitomycin-C (FOAM)

GENERAL USE: Metastatic breast cancer
RESPONSE RATE: 62% in CMF failures
SCHEDULE AND DOSE: Repeat cycle every 8 weeks.

	Week* 1	2	3	4	5	6	→	8
5-Fluorouracil 400 mg/m² BSA† IV, single dose	X	X			X	X	2-week rest period	
Vincristine 1.0 mg/m² BSA† IV, single dose (max. dose 2.0 mg)	X				X			
Doxorubicin‡ 40 mg/m² BSA† IV, single dose	X				X			
Mitomycin C§ 10 mg/m² BSA† IV, single dose	X							

*X indicates week(s) to administer drug(s) indicated.
†BSA = body surface area.
‡CAUTION: In adult patients with total cumulative dose of doxorubicin of 550 mg/m² (or 450 mg/m² in previously irradiated heart tissue) there is a more common occurrence of cardiomyopathy or CHF or both.
§CAUTION: The nadir of mitomycin C may be *delayed* 6 weeks after administration.

REFERENCE:

Marcus, F., et al.: 5 FU + Oncovin + Adriamycin + mitomycin C (FOAM): an effective new therapy for metastatic breast cancer patients—even those who have failed CMF, Proc. Am. Soc. Clin. Oncol. **20**:306, 1979.

Doxorubicin (Adriamycin)

GENERAL USE: Metastatic or recurrent breast cancer

RESPONSE RATE: 40% with no prior chemotherapy, 30% with prior chemotherapy

SCHEDULE AND DOSE: Repeat cycle every 21 or 28 days.

	Day*			
	1	→	21†	
Doxorubicin‡ Patients with prior chemotherapy: 75 mg/m² BSA§ IV Patients with no prior chemotherapy: 20 to 25 mg/m² BSA§ IV for 3 days	X	3- to 4-week rest period		

*X indicates day(s) to administer drug(s) indicated.

†May be delayed 1 week if recovery of the granulocytes and platelets is not complete by day 21 or 28.

‡CAUTION: In adult patients with total cumulative doses of doxorubicin of 550 mg/m² (or 450 mg/m² in patients with previously irradiated heart tissue) there is a more common occurrence of cardiomyopathy or CHF or both.

§BSA = body surface area.

REFERENCE:

Hoogstraten, B.: Adriamycin (NSC-123127) in the treatment of advanced breast cancer: studies by the Southwest Oncology Group, Cancer Chemother. Rep. **6**:329-334, 1975.

Diethylstilbestrol (DES)

GENERAL USE: Metastatic breast carcinoma—more than 5 years postmenopausal (estrogen-"poor")

RESPONSE RATE: 30%. May approach 50% in women older than 70 years with predominant cutaneous or lymph node metastases (estrogen receptor positive, 63%)

SCHEDULE AND DOSE:

	Day*										
	1	2	3	4	5	6	7	8	9	10	→†
Diethylstilbestrol 5 to 10 mg, 3 times daily Orally	X	X	X	X	X	X	X	X	X	X	Continue daily†

*X indicates day(s) to administer drug(s) indicated.

†Generally 6 weeks is required to assess effectiveness of estrogens. Continue daily until relapse of disease. See Chapter 4, Hormone Therapy in Breast Cancer.

REFERENCES:

Kennedy, B. J.: Hormonal therapies in breast cancer, Semin. Oncol. **1:** 119-130, 1974.

Carbone, P. P., et al.: Medical treatment for advanced breast cancer, Semin. Oncol. **4:**417-427, 1978.

Tamoxifen

GENERAL USE: Breast cancer

RESPONSE RATE: 33% (estrogen receptor positive, 53%)

SCHEDULE AND DOSE:

	Day*										
	1	2	3	4	5	6	7	8	9	10	→†
Tamoxifen 20 mg Orally	X	X	X	X	X	X	X	X	X	X	Continue daily†

*X indicates day(s) to administer drug(s) indicated.

†Generally 6 weeks is required to assess effectiveness of antiestrogens. Continue daily until relapse of disease. See Chapter 4, Hormone Therapy in Breast Cancer.

REFERENCES:

Legha, S. S., et al.: Hormonal therapy of breast cancer: new approaches and concepts, Ann. Intern. Med. **88**:69-77, 1978.

Carbone, P. P., et al.: Medical treatment for advanced breast cancer, Semin. Oncol. **4**:417-427, 1978.

Fluoxymesterone (Halotestin, Ora-testryl, Ultandren)

GENERAL USE: Metastatic breast carcinoma—more than 5 years postmenopausal (estrogen "poor"); hormone therapy of choice in patients with bone metastasis and estrogen failures

RESPONSE RATE: 15% (ER positive—36%)

SCHEDULE AND DOSE:

	Day*										
	1	2	3	4	5	6	7	8	9	10	→†
Fluoxymesterone 10 to 20 mg Orally	X	X	X	X	X	X	X	X	X	X	Continue daily†

*X indicates day(s) to administer drug(s) indicated.

†Generally 6 weeks is required to assess effectiveness of androgens. Continue daily until relapse of disease. See Chapter 4, Hormone Therapy in Breast Cancer.

REFERENCES:

Kennedy, B. J.: Hormonal therapies in breast cancer, Semin. Oncol. **1:** 119-130, 1974.

Carbone, P. P., et al.: Medical treatment for advanced breast cancer, Semin. Oncol. **4:**417-427, 1978.

LUNG CANCER

Cyclophosphamide, doxorubicin (Adriamycin) and vincristine (CAV)

GENERAL USE: Small cell lung carcinoma

RESPONSE RATE: 100% limited disease (75% alive at 19 months); 100% extensive disease (30% alive at 16 months)

SCHEDULE AND DOSE: Repeat every 3 weeks for 6 cycles.

	Day*										
	1	2	3	4	5	6	7	8	9	10	→ 21†
Cyclophosphamide 1,000 mg/m² BSA‡ IV	X										
Doxorubicin§ 40 mg/m² BSA‡ IV	X										
Vincristine 1 mg/m² BSA‡ IV (max. dose 2.0 mg)	X										
Radiation therapy‖ 3,000 rads in 10 fractions	X	X	X	X	X	X	X	X	X	X	

*X indicates day(s) to administer drug(s) indicated.

†May be delayed 1 week if recovery of granulocytes or platelets is not complete by day 21.

‡BSA = body surface area.

§CAUTION: In adult patients with total cumulative doses of doxorubicin of 450 mg/m² when given concurrently with cyclophosphamide there is a more common occurrence of cardiomyopathy or CHF or both.

‖Radiation therapy is given to the primary tumor concurrently with CAV during the first cycle only.

REFERENCE:

Oldham, R. K., et al.: Small cell lung cancer: a potentially curable neoplasm, Proc. Am. Soc. Clin. Oncol. **19**:361, 1978.

Cyclophosphamide, methotrexate, and lomustine (CCNU) (CMC standard dose)

GENERAL USE: Small cell bronchogenic carcinoma of the lung

RESPONSE RATE: 56% (median survival time 36 weeks)

SCHEDULE AND DOSE:

	Week*							
	1	2	3	4	5	6	7	†
Cyclophosphamide 500 mg/m^2 BSA‡ IV, single dose	X			X			X	Continue once every 3 weeks†
Lomustine§ 50 mg/m^2 BSA‡ Orally, single dose	X						X	Continue once every 6 weeks†
Methotrexate 10 mg/m^2 BSA‡ Orally *twice* weekly	X	Twice weekly →						Continue twice weekly†

*X indicates week(s) to administer drug(s) indicated.

†May be delayed 1 week if recovery of the granulocytes and platelets is not complete by the week indicated for next dose to be given.

‡BSA = body surface area.

§CAUTION: The nadir of lomustine (CCNU) may be *delayed* 6 weeks after administration.

REFERENCES:

Edmonson, J. H., et al.: Combination chemotherapy for metastatic lung cancer, Proc. Am. Assoc. Cancer. Res. **15:**180 (abstract), 1974.

Hansen, H. H., et al.: Combination chemotherapy of advanced lung cancer: a randomized trial, Cancer **38:**2201-2207, 1976.

Cyclophosphamide, methotrexate, and lomustine (CCNU) (CMC high dose)

GENERAL USE: Small cell bronchogenic carcinoma

RESPONSE RATE: 96% (30% complete remission with median survival 16+ months)

SCHEDULE AND DOSE:

	Week*						
	1	2	3	4	5	6	†
Cyclophosphamide 1,000 mg/m² BSA‡ IV, one dose	X			X			
Methotrexate 15 mg/m² BSA‡ IV *twice* weekly	X	Twice weekly →					
Lomustine§ 100 mg/m² BSA‡ Orally, one dose	X						

*X indicated week(s) to administer drug(s) indicated.

†NOTE: If response, proceed to maintenance therapy. For maintenance, see preceding CMC standard dose regimen.

‡BSA = body surface area.

§CAUTION: The nadir of lomustine may be *delayed* 6 weeks after administration.

REFERENCE:

Cohen, M. H., et al.: Intensive chemotherapy of small cell bronchogenic carcinoma, Cancer Treat. Rep. **61**:349-354, 1977.

Cyclophosphamide, doxorubicin (hydroxydaunorubicin; Adriamycin), vincristine (Oncovin), and radiation (CHOR)

GENERAL USE: Small cell bronchogenic carcinoma of the lung

RESPONSE RATE: 75% (median survival for extensive disease, 26 weeks; for limited disease, 52 weeks)

SCHEDULE AND DOSE:

	Days* 1	→	8	→	15	→	22	→ 36†
Cyclophosphamide 750 mg/m² BSA‡ IV	X						X	Discontinue for 8 weeks
Doxorubicin§ 50 mg/m² BSA‡ IV	X						X	Discontinue for 8 weeks
Vincristine 1 mg IV	X		X		X		X	Continue weekly for total of 12 weeks
Radiation‖ 3,000 rad in 10 daily fractions over a 2-week period beginning day 36‖								Day 36—Begin 10 daily fractions‖

*X indicates day(s) to administer drug(s) indicated.

†Resume chemotherapy week 12 with doxorubicin 50 mg/m² IV every 3 weeks (until a total cumulative dose of 450 mg/m² [usually 9 courses], then discontinue), cyclophosphamide 1,000 mg/m² IV every 4 weeks, and methotrexate, 30 mg/m² IV 3 weeks after each dose of cyclophosphamide for 2 years. In patients with limited disease a second radiation treatment is given during week 15 with 1,500 rads over 5 days to the primary tumor. Chemotherapy is withheld until week 18.

‡BSA = body surface area.

§CAUTION: In adult patients with total cumulative doses of doxorubicin of 450 mg/m² who have received both doxorubicin and cyclophosphamide there is a more common occurrence of cardiomyopathy or CHF or both.

‖A 2-week rest period follows the 2-week 3,000-rad radiation treatment.

REFERENCE:

Livingstone, R. B., et al.: Small cell carcinoma of the lung: combined chemotherapy and radiation, Ann. Intern. Med. **88:**194-99, 1978.

Procarbazine, vincristine (Oncovin), cyclophosphamide, and lomustine (CCNU) (POCC)

GENERAL USE: Oat cell carcinoma of the lung

RESPONSE RATE: 68% (median survival 14 months)

SCHEDULE AND DOSE: Repeat cycle every 28 days.

	Day*														
	1	2	3	4	5	6	7	8	9	10	11	12	13	14 →	28
Procarbazine 100 mg/m² BSA† Orally	X	X	X	X	X	X	X	X	X	X	X	X	X	X	2-week rest period
Vincristine 2 mg IV (max. dose 2.0 mg)	X							X							
Cyclophosphamide 600 mg/m² BSA† IV	X							X							
Lomustine‡ 60 mg/m² BSA† Orally	X														

*X indicates day(s) to administer drug(s) indicated.

†BSA = body surface area.

‡CAUTION: The nadir of lomustine (CCNU) may be *delayed* 6 weeks after administration.

REFERENCE:

Alexander, M., et al.: Combined modality treatment for oat cell carcinoma of the lung: a randomized trial, Cancer Treat. Rep. **61**:1-6, 1977.

Cyclophosphamide, vincristine (Oncovin), and methotrexate (COM) (Eagan Program)

GENERAL USE: Small cell (oat cell) carcinoma of the lung

RESPONSE RATE: 89%

SCHEDULE AND DOSE: Repeat cycle every 28 days.

	Day*				
	1	→	21†	→	28†
Cyclophosphamide *Cycles 1-2‡:* 2000 mg/m² BSA§ IV *Cycles 3-6:* 1500 mg/m² BSA§ IV	X	No therapy, 3-week rest period		No therapy, 1-week rest period	
Vincristine 1.5 mg/m² BSA§ IV (max. dose 2.0 mg)	X	No therapy, 3-week rest period		No therapy, 1-week rest period	
Methotrexate 30 mg/m² BSA§ IV		No therapy, 3-week rest period	X	No therapy, 1-week rest period	

*X indicates day(s) to administer drug(s) indicated.

†May be delayed 1 week if recovery of the granulocytes and platelets is not complete by day 21 or 28.

‡1. A break in chemotherapy is generally made after 2 cycles for irradiation to the chest primary.

2. Alternate schedule: cyclophosphamide can be given 400 mg/m² BSA§ orally on days 2 to 6.

§BSA = body surface area.

REFERENCES:

Eagan, R. T., et al.: Combination chemotherapy and radiation therapy in small cell carcinoma of the lung, Cancer **32:**371-379, 1973.

Eagan, R. T., et al.: Small cell carcinoma of the lung: staging paraneoplastic syndromes, treatment, and survival, Cancer **33:**527-532, 1974.

Methotrexate, doxorubicin (Adriamycin), cyclophosphamide, and lomustine (CCNU) (MACC)

GENERAL USE: Non–oat cell carcinoma of the lung
RESPONSE RATE: 46% (median survival 9 months)
SCHEDULE AND DOSE: Repeat cycle every 21 days.

	Day*		
	1	→	21†
Methotrexate‡ 40 mg/m² BSA§ IV	X	3-week rest period, no therapy	
Doxorubicin‡ 40 mg/m² BSA§ IV	X		
Cyclophosphamide 400 mg/m² BSA§ IV	X		
Lomustine‖ 30 mg/m² BSA§ Orally	X		

*X indicates day(s) to administer drug(s) indicated.
†May be delayed 1 week if recovery of granulocytes is not complete by day 21.
‡NOTE: Vincristine may be added to the above regimen. Administer 2 mg IV 30 minutes prior to the other drugs. *Reduce doses* of doxorubicin and methotrexate by 25% if vincristine is added. CAUTION: In adult patients with total cumulative doses of 450 mg/m² of doxorubicin who have received both doxorubicin and cyclophosphamide there is a more common occurrence of cardiomyopathy or CHF or both.
§BSA = body surface area.
‖CAUTION: The nadir of lomustine (CCNU) may be *delayed* 6 weeks after drug administration.

REFERENCE:

Chahinian, A. P., et al.: Chemotherapy for bronchogenic carcinoma, J.A.M.A. **237**:2392-2396, 1977.

5-Fluorouracil, doxorubicin (Adriamycin), and mitomycin C (FAM)

GENERAL USE: Advanced adenocarcinoma of the lung
RESPONSE RATE: 36% (median duration 8.5+ months)
SCHEDULE AND DOSE: Repeat cycle every 56 days.

	Day* 1	→	8	→	28	→	36	→	56
5-Fluorouracil 600 mg/m² BSA† IV	X		X		X		X	3-week rest period	
Doxorubicin‡ 30 mg/m² BSA† IV	X				X				
Mitomycin C§ 10 mg/m² BSA† IV	X								

*X indicates day(s) to administer drug(s) indicated.
†BSA = body surface area.
‡CAUTION: In adult patients with total cumulative doses of doxorubicin of 550 mg/m² (or 450 mg/m² in patients with previously irradiated heart tissue) there is a more common occurrence of cardiomyopathy or CHF or both.
§CAUTION: The nadir of mitomycin C may be *delayed* 6 weeks after drug administration.

REFERENCES:

Macdonald, J., et al.: 5-Fluorouracil (5-FU), Adriamycin (ADR), and mitomycin-C (MMC), FAM, for advanced adenocarcinoma of the lung, Proc. Am. Soc. Clin. Oncol. **18**:306, 1977.

Butler, T. P., et al.: Fluorouracil, Adriamycin, and mitomycin C (FAM) chemotherapy for adenocarcinoma of the lung, Cancer **43**:1183-1188, 1979.

Cyclophosphamide, doxorubicin (Adriamycin), methotrexate, and procarbazine (CAMP)

GENERAL USE: Non–oat cell carcinoma of the lung

RESPONSE RATE: 20% (5-month median survival)

SCHEDULE AND DOSE: Repeat cycle every 4 weeks.

	Day* 1	2	3	4	5	6	7	8	9	10	→	28
Cyclophosphamide 300 mg/m² BSA† IV	X							X			2½-week rest period	
Doxorubicin‡ 20 mg/m² BSA† IV	X							X				
Methotrexate 15 mg/m² BSA† IV	X							X				
Procarbazine 100 mg/m² BSA† Orally	X	X	X	X	X	X	X	X	X	X		

*X indicates day(s) to administer drug(s) indicated.

†BSA = body surface area.

‡CAUTION: In adult patients who have received both doxorubicin and cyclophosphamide with total cumulative dose of 450 mg/m² of doxorubicin there is a more common occurrence of cardiomyopathy or CHF or both.

REFERENCE:

Opfell, R. W., et al.: Combination chemotherapy for non–oat cell carcinoma of the lung: a randomized study, Proc. Am. Soc. Clin. Oncol. **20:**356, 1979.

BONE TUMORS
Melphalan (L-PAM) and prednisone

GENERAL USE: Multiple myeloma

RESPONSE RATE: 50%

SCHEDULE AND DOSE: Repeat cycle every 28 days.

	Day* 1	2	3	4	5	6	7	→	28†
Melphalan 8 mg/m² BSA‡ Orally	X	X	X	X				No therapy, 3 weeks	
Prednisone 75 mg/m² BSA‡ Orally	X	X	X	X	X	X	X		

*X indicates day(s) to administer drug(s) indicated.

†May be delayed 1 week if recovery of the granulocytes and platelets is not complete by day 28. If granulocytes or platelets are not reversed after a course of therapy with an additional waiting period of 1 week, a bone marrow aspiration or biopsy may be indicated. Regimen is to be repeated for six courses. For those patients who receive a response, the regimen is continued every 4 weeks as maintenace therapy.

‡BSA = body surface area.

REFERENCES:

Hammack, W. J., Schilling, A., et al.: Phase III study of intermittent BCNU, cyclophosphamide and prednisone versus intermittent melphalan and prednisone in myeloma and of the addition of fluoxymesterone, sodium flouride and calcium gluconate versus placebo, EST 4472, SEG #343, pp. 1-13, April, 1972.

Alexanian, R., et al.: Treatment for multiple myeloma: combination chemotherapy with different melphalan dose regimens, J.A.M.A. **208:** 1680-1685, 1969.

Melphalan (L-PAM) and prednisone

GENERAL USE: Multiple myeloma

RESPONSE RATE: 50%

SCHEDULE AND DOSE: Repeat cycle every 6 weeks.

	Day* 1	2	3	4	→	42†
Melphalan 0.25 mg/kg Orally	X	X	X	X	No therapy, 5 weeks	
Prednisone 2.0 mg/kg	X	X	X	X		

*X indicates day(s) to administer drug(s) indicated.

†May be delayed 1 week if recovery of the granulocytes and platelets is not complete by day 42. If granulocytes or platelets are not reversed after a course of therapy with an additional waiting period of 1 week, a bone marrow aspiration or biopsy may be indicated.

REFERENCE:

Alexanian, R., et al.: Treatment for multiple myeloma, J.A.M.A. **208:** 1680-1685, 1969.

Carmustine (BCNU), melphalan, cyclophosphamide, vincristine, and prednisone (M-2 Protocol)

GENERAL USE: Multiple myeloma

RESPONSE RATE: 87% (median duration of response is 20+ months); 50% in previously treated patients

SCHEDULE AND DOSE: Repeat every 35 days until progression of disease.

	Day*										
	1	2	3	4	5	6	7	→	21†	→	35
Vincristine 0.03 mg/kg IV (max. dose 2.0 mg)	X										
Carmustine‡ 0.5 mg/kg IV	X										
Cyclophosphamide 10 mg/kg IV	X										
Melphalan§ 0.25 mg/kg Orally	X	X	X	X							
Prednisone† 1.0 mg/kg Orally	X	X	X	X	X	X	X	(Taper to day 21)†			

*X indicates day(s) to administer drug(s) indicated.

†Continue prednisone after day 21 if hypercalcemia or bony disease remain symptomatic.

‡CAUTION: The nadir of BCNU (carmustine) may be *delayed* 6 weeks after administration.

§Melphalan may be given 0.1 mg/kg for 7 to 10 days rather than schedule presented.

REFERENCE:

Case, D. C., et al.: Improved survival times in multiple myeloma treated with melphalan, prednisone, cyclophosphamide, vincristine, and BCNU: M-2 Protocol, Am. J. Med. **63:**897-903, 1977.

Vincristine, melphalan, cyclophosphamide, and prednisone (VMCP)

GENERAL USE: Multiple myeloma

RESPONSE RATE: 62%

SCHEDULE AND DOSE: Repeat cycle every 21 days.

	Day*								
	1	**2**	**3**	**4**	**5**	**6**	**7**	**→**	**21†**
Vincristine 1.0 mg IV	X							2½-week rest, no therapy	
Melphalan 5 mg/m² BSA‡ Orally	X	X	X	X					
Cyclophosphamide 100 mg/m² BSA‡ Orally	X	X	X	X					
Prednisone 60 mg/m² BSA‡ Orally	X	X	X	X					

*X indicates day(s) to administer drug(s) indicated.
†May be delayed 1 week if recovery of granulocytes and platelets is not complete by day 21.
‡BSA = body surface area.

REFERENCE:

Alexanian, R., et al.: Combination therapy for multiple myeloma, Cancer **40:**2765-2771, 1977.

Vincristine, cyclophosphamide, doxorubicin (Adriamycin), and prednisone (VCAP)

GENERAL USE: Multiple myeloma

RESPONSE RATE: 57%

SCHEDULE AND DOSE: Repeat cycle every 21 days.

	Day* 1	2	3	4	→	21†
Vincristine 1.0 mg IV	X				2-week rest period, no therapy	
Cyclophosphamide 100 mg/m² BSA‡ Orally	X	X	X	X		
Doxorubicin§ 25 mg/m² BSA‡ IV		X				
Prednisone 60 mg/m² BSA‡ Orally	X	X	X	X		

*X indicates day(s) to administer drug(s) indicated.

†May be delayed 1 week if recovery of the granulocytes and platelets is not complete by day 21.

‡BSA = body surface area.

§CAUTION: In adult patients with total cumulative doses of doxorubicin of 450 mg/m² who have received both doxorubicin and cyclophosphamide there is a more common occurrence of cardiomyopathy or CHF or both.

REFERENCE:

Alexanian, R., et al.: Combination therapy for multiple myeloma, Cancer **40**:2765-2771, 1977.

Cyclophosphamide and prednisone

GENERAL USE: Multiple myeloma

RESPONSE RATE: 50%

SCHEDULE AND DOSE: Repeat cycle every 3 weeks.

	Day*					
	1	2	3	4	→	21†
Cyclophosphamide‡ 1.0 g/m² BSA§ IV	X				2-week rest period, no therapy	
Prednisone‡ 60 mg/m² BSA§ Orally	X	X	X	X		

*X indicates day(s) to administer drug(s) indicated.

†May be delayed 1 week if recovery of the granulocytes and platelets is not complete by day 21. If granulocytes or platelets are not reversed after a course of therapy with additional waiting period of 1 week, a bone marrow aspiration or biopsy may be indicated.

‡NOTE: Cyclophosphamide may be given orally in doses of 0.25 g/m²/day for 4 days. Prednisone may be given in doses of 100 to 200 mg/day for 4 days.

§BSA = body surface area.

REFERENCES:

Bergsagel, D. E., et al.: Plasma cell myeloma: response of melphalan-resistant patients to high-dose intermittent cyclophosphamide, Can. Med. Assoc. J. **107:**851-855, 1972.

Alexanian, R., et al.: Treatment for multiple myeloma: combination chemotherapy with different melphalan dose regimens, J.A.M.A. **208:** 1680-1685, 1969.

Doxorubicin (Adriamycin) and carmustine (BCNU)

GENERAL USE: Multiple myeloma in relapse (alkylating agent resistant)
RESPONSE RATE: 54%
SCHEDULE AND DOSE: Repeat cycle every 21 or 28 days.

	Day* 1	→	21 or 28†	
Doxorubicin‡ 30 mg/m² BSA§ IV	X	No therapy, 3 or 4 weeks		
Carmustine‖ 30 mg/m² BSA§ IV	X			

*X indicates day(s) to administer drug(s) indicated.
†May be delayed 1 week if recovery of the granulocytes and platelets is not complete by day 21 or 28.
‡CAUTION: In adult patients with total cumulative doses of doxorubicin of 550 mg/m² (or 450 mg/m² in patients with previously irradiated heart tissue) there is a more common occurrence of cardiomyopathy or CHF or both.
§BSA = body surface area.
‖NOTE: The nadir of carmustine may be *delayed* 6 weeks after drug administration.

REFERENCE:

Alberts, D. S., et al.: Doxorubicin/BCNU chemotherapy for multiple myeloma in relapse, Lancet **1**(7966):926-928, 1976.

Carmustine (BCNU) and prednisone

GENERAL USE: Multiple myeloma secondary

RESPONSE RATE: 40% in previously untreated patients; 5% to 10% in previously treated patients

SCHEDULE AND DOSE: Repeat cycle every 6 weeks.

	Day* 1	2	3	4	→	42†
Carmustine‡ 150 mg/m² BSA§ IV				X	5-week rest period, no therapy	
Prednisone 60 mg/m² BSA§ Orally	X	X	X	X		

*X indicates day(s) to administer drug(s) indicated.

†May be delayed 1 week if recovery of the granulocytes and platelets is not complete by day 42. If granulocytes or platelets are not reversed after a course of therapy with an additional waiting period of 1 week, a bone marrow aspiration or biopsy may be indicated.

‡CAUTION: The nadir related to Carmustine may be *delayed* 6 weeks after administration.

§BSA = body surface area.

REFERENCES:

Salmon, S. E.: Nitrosoureas in multiple myeloma, Cancer Treat. Rep. **60:**789-794, 1976.

Alexanian, R., et al.: Remission maintenance therapy for multiple myeloma, Arch. Intern. Med. **135:**147-152, 1975.

T-6 Protocol

GENERAL USE: Ewing's sarcoma

RESPONSE RATE: Expected to supersede T-2 Protocol; preliminary results, 85% disease free at 26+ months.

INDUCTION SCHEDULE AND DOSE: Before use of T-6 Protocol consult references for timetable of surgery and radiation.

Day*	1	→	5	→	8	→	15	→	22	23	→	26	→	29	→	36	→	43†
Dactinomycin 300 $\mu g/m^2$ BSA‡ IV	X	Daily →		¶														
Cyclophosphamide 300 mg/m^2 BSA‡ IV	X	Daily →							X									X
Bleomycin 6 mg/m^2 BSA‡ IV	X	Daily →																
Vincristine 1.5 mg/m^2 BSA‡ IV (max. dose 2.0 mg)	X				X		X		X					X		X		
Methotrexate 10 mg/m^2 BSA‡ IV										X	Daily →							
Doxorubicin 12 mg/m^2 BSA‡ IV									X	Daily →								
Carmustine§ 90 mg/m^2 BSA‡ IV																		X

*X indicates day(s) to administer drug(s) indicated.

†After a rest period from day 44 to 70, repeat the first 63 days of induction schedule once, then proceed to maintenance schedule.

‡BSA = body surface area.

§CAUTION: The nadir of carmustine may be delayed 6 weeks after drug administration.

¶It is optional to administer dactinomycin on days 6 and 7.

MAINTENANCE SCHEDULE AND DOSE: Begin 3 weeks following second course of carmustine and cyclophosphamide of T-6 induction—day 64 of cycle 2.

	Day*																
	1	**2**	**3**	**4**	**5**	**→**	**14**	**15**	**16**	**→**	**28**	**→**	**35**	**→**	**42**	**→**	**49†**
Dactinomycin *Cycle 1:* 300 μg/m² BSA‡ IV *Remaining cycles:* 450 μg/m² BSA‡ IV	X	X	X	X	X												
Doxorubicin§ 20 mg/m² BSA‡ IV							X	X	X								
Vincristine 1.5 to 2.0 mg/m² BSA‡ IV (max. dose 2.0 mg)											X		X		X		X
Cyclophosphamide 1,200 mg/m² BSA‡ IV											X				X		

*X indicates day(s) to administer drug(s) indicated.
†Repeat the 49-day cycle 5 times.
‡BSA = body surface area.
§CAUTION: In adult patients with total cumulative doses of dosorubicin of 450 mg/m² who have received both doxorubicin and cyclophosphamide there is a more common occurrence of cardiomyopathy or CHF or both. In pediatric patients with total cumulative doses of 350 mg/m² who have received both doxorubicin and cyclophosphamide there is a more likely occurrence of cardiomyopathy or CHF or both.

REFERENCES:

Rosen, G., et al.: Curability of Ewing's sarcoma and considerations for future therapeutic trials, Cancer **41**:888-899, 1978.

Rosen, G., et al.: Malignant small-cell sarcomas of bone, Pediatr. Ann. **7**:30-51, 1978.

T-2 Protocol

GENERAL USE: Ewing's sarcoma

RESPONSE RATE: 100% complete remission (75% 5-year disease-free survival rate)

SCHEDULE AND DOSE: Cycle 1 consists of 3 months of therapy. For cycle 2 repeat cycle 1 but exclude radiation therapy. Cycles 3 to 8 consist of cycle 3 (3 months of therapy) repeated five times for a total of 6 cycles (18 months).

CYCLE 1, MONTH 1

	Day* 1	→	5	→	20	21	22	→	28
Actinomycin D 450 μg/m² BSA† IV	X Daily →							No therapy, 1 week	
Doxorubicin 20 mg/m² BSA† IV					X	X	X		
Radiation§ Total dose over 21 days 3,000-4,000 rads	X Daily →								

CYCLE 1, MONTH 2

	Day* 1	→	8	9	10	→	24	→	28
Doxorubicin 20 mg/m² BSA† IV			X	X	X				
Vincristine 1.5 to 2.0 mg/m² BSA† IV (max. dose 2.0 mg)							X		
Cyclophosphamide 1,200 mg/m² BSA† IV							X		
Radiation§ Total dose over 21 days 2,000-3,000 rads			X Daily →						

*X indicates day(s) to administer drug(s) indicated.

†BSA = body surface area.

§See Chabora, B. M., for methods to employ irradiation to the primary tumor.

CYCLE 1, MONTH 3

Drug	Day* 1	→	3	→	9	→	15	⟶	28†
Vincristine 1.5 to 2.0 mg/m² BSA‡ IV (max. dose 2.0 mg)			X		X		X	No therapy, 2 weeks	
Cyclophosphamide 1,200 mg/m² BSA‡ IV					X				

*X indicates day(s) to administer drug(s) indicated.
†CYCLE 2—*Repeat cycle 1 excluding radiation therapy;* then proceed to cycle 3.
‡BSA = body surface area.

SCHEDULE AND DOSE—cont'd: Repeat cycle 3 (3 months therapy) five times for a total of 6 cycles (18 months of therapy).

CYCLE 3, MONTH 1

Drug	Day* 1	→	5	→	20	21	22	→	28
Actinomycin D 450 μg/m² BSA† IV	X	Daily →	Daily →						
Doxorubicin‡ 20 mg/m² BSA† IV					X	X	X		

CYCLE 3, MONTH 2

Drug	Day* 1	→	8	→	15	→	22	→	28§
Vincristine 1.5 to 2.0 mg/m² BSA† IV (max. dose 2.0 mg/m²)			X		X		X		X
Cyclophosphamide 1,200 mg/m² BSA† IV			X				X		

*X indicates day(s) to administer drug(s) indicated.
†BSA = body surface area.
‡CAUTION: In pediatric and adult patients who have received both doxorubicin and cyclophosphamide with a total cumulative dose of doxorubicin of 350 mg/m² and 450 mg/m² respectively there is a more common occurrence of cardiomyopathy or CHF or both.
§CYCLE 3, MONTH 3—*no drugs are given for 28 days.* In the next month begin cycle 4 (repeating cycle 3).

REFERENCE:

Chabora, B. M., et al.: Radiotherapy of Ewing's sarcoma: local control with and without intensive chemotherapy, Ther. Radiol. **120:**667-671, 1976.

Rosen, G., et al.: Disease-free survival in children with Ewing's sarcoma treated with radiation therapy and adjuvant four-drug sequential chemotherapy, Cancer **33:**384-393, 1974.

Rosen, G., et al.: Curability of Ewing's sarcoma and considerations for future therapeutic trials, Cancer **41:**888-899, 1978.

Rosen, G.: Malignant small-cell sarcomas of bone, Pediatr. Ann. **7:**30-51, 1978.

Actinomycin D, doxorubicin (Adriamycin), vincristine, and cyclophosphamide

GENERAL USE: Ewing's sarcoma (pediatric)

RESPONSE RATE: 100% (10- to 37-month duration disease free)

SCHEDULE AND DOSE: Repeat 90-day cycle for 2 years. (Radiation is only given during cycle 1.)

	Day*													
	1	→	5	→	20	21	22	→	37	38	39	→	45	→
Actinomycin D 0.45 mg/m² BSA† IV	X	Daily	→											
Doxorubicin‡ 20 mg/m² BSA† IV					X	X	X		X	X	X			
Cyclophosphamide 1200 mg/m² BSA† 30-minute IV infusion														
Vincristine 1.5 mg/m² BSA† IV (escalation to 2.5 mg) (max. dose 2.5 mg)														
Radiation (first 90-day cycle only)§ 7,000 rads in divided doses over 45 days	X						Daily						→	

*X indicates day(s) to administer drug(s) indicated.

†BSA = body surface area.

‡Doxorubicin is stopped at a total cumulative dose of 720 mg/m² or 500 mg/m² if radiation therapy to the lungs or mediastinum has been employed. CAUTION: In pediatric patients with total cumulation doses of 350 mg/m² of doxorubicin when given concurrently with cyclophosphamide there is a more common occurrence of cardiomyopathy or CHF or both.

§NOTE: A 3-week rest period is taken halfway through the course of radiation therapy depending on local skin toxicity. Radiation is given only during the first cycle and not during subsequent cycles over the next two years.

	Day*								
	54	→	61	→	68	→	75	→	90
Actinomycin D 0.45 mg/m² BSA† IV								No therapy, 2-week rest period	
Doxorubicin‡ 20 mg/m² BSA† IV									
Cyclophosphamide 1200 mg/m² BSA† 30-minute IV infusion	X				X				
Vincristine 1.5 mg/m² BSA† IV (escalation to 2.5 mg) (max. dose 2.5 mg)	X		X		X		X		
Radiation (first 90-day cycle only)§ 7,000 rads in divided doses over 45 days									

*X indicates day(s) to administer drug(s) indicated.
†BSA = body surface area.
‡Doxorubicin is stopped at a total cumulative dose of 720 mg/m² or 500 mg/m² if radiation therapy to the lungs or mediastinum has been employed. CAUTION: In pediatric patients with total cumulation doses of 350 mg/m² of doxorubicin when given concurrently with cyclophosphamide there is a more common occurrence of cardiomyopathy or CHF or both.
§NOTE: A 3-week rest period is taken halfway through the course of radiation therapy depending on local skin toxicity. Radiation is given only during the first cycle and not during subsequent cycles over the next two years.

REFERENCE:

Rosen, G., et al.: Disease-free survival in children with Ewing's sarcoma treated with radiation therapy and adjuvant four-drug sequential chemotherapy, Cancer **33**:384-393, 1974.

Cyclophosphamide, vincristine (Oncovin), and doxorubicin (Adriamycin)

GENERAL USE: Ewing's sarcoma

RESPONSE RATE: 56% 2-year survival and 35% 5-year survival

SCHEDULE AND DOSE: Repeat cycle every 7 weeks.

	Day*				
	1	→	21†	→	49†
Doxorubicin‡ 75 mg/m² BSA§ IV	X	No therapy, 3 weeks		No therapy, 4 weeks	
Cyclophosphamide 40 mg/kg IV (with hydration)			X		
Vincristine 0.04 mg/kg IV (max. dose 2.0 mg)			X		

*X indicates day(s) to administer drug(s) indicated.

†May be delayed 1 week if recovery of the granulocytes and platelets is not complete by day 21 or 49.

‡With total cumulative doses of doxorubicin of 450 mg/m² in patients who have received both doxorubicin and cyclophosphamide there is a more common occurrence of cardiomyopathy or CHF or both.

§BSA = body surface area.

REFERENCE:

Pomeroy, T. C., et al.: Combined modality therapy of Ewing's sarcoma, Cancer **35**:36-47, 1975.

Vincristine, methotrexate, citrovorum factor, doxorubicin (Adriamycin), and cyclophosphamide

GENERAL USE: Nonmetastatic osteogenic sarcoma—adjuvant chemotherapy (pediatric)

RESPONSE RATE: 64% disease free in three years

SCHEDULE AND DOSE: Preoperative chemotherapy

	Day*													
	1	2	3	4	→	12	13	→	23	24	25	26	→	30†
Vincristine 1.5 mg/m^2 BSA‡ IV (max. dose 2.0 mg)	X								X					
Methotrexate§ 200 mg/kg IV 4-hour infusion		X			No therapy, 10 to 14 days			No therapy, 10 to 14 days		X			No therapy, 10 to 14 days	
Citrovorum factor 9-12 mg Orally every 6 hours for 12 doses Begin 2 hours after methotrexate		X	X	X						X	X	X		
Doxorubicin§ 45 mg/m^2 BSA‡ IV						X	X							

*X indicates day(s) to administer drug(s) indicated.

†Continue to alternate doxorubicin on day 34 with vincristine, methotrexate, and citrovorum factor every 10 to 14 days for 2 to 3 months prior to surgery as long as there is no severe manifestation of bone marrow depression and oropharyngeal mucositis. Some patients receive as many as 4 cycles depending upon the time to acquire the prosthetic bone replacement.

‡BSA = body surface area.

§CAUTION: Procedures of allopurinol administration, hydration, alkalinization of the urine, and taking 24-, 48-, and 72-hour methotrexate (MTX) blood levels should be done after MTX administration to prevent severe MTX toxicity. *If abnormally high 24-hour MTX serum levels are obtained, continue citrovorum factor past 72 hours* until it is clear that the patient will not develop severe MTX toxicity which usually occurs 5 days after the MTX infusion. If after 10 days from methotrexate administration the *platelet count is ≤ 100,000/mm³ and the total white count is ≤2,000/mm³, doxorubicin should not be given.* (See Section 6, Renal Dysfunction, Table 6-15, and Section 7, Leucovorin Rescue).

SCHEDULE AND DOSE: Postoperative adjuvant chemotherapy.* Begin therapy 4 to 8 weeks after surgery. Repeat cycle every 60 days.

	Day†												
	1	**→**	**15**	**16**	**17**	**18**	**→**	**30**	**→**	**44**	**45**	**→**	**60‡**
Cyclophosphamide§ 1200 mg/m² BSA‖ IV	X	No therapy, 14 days					No therapy, 12 days	X	No therapy, 14 days			No therapy, 15 days	
Vincristine 1.5 mg/m² BSA‖ IV (max. dose 2.0 mg)			X										
Methotrexate¶ 200 mg/kg IV 4-hour infusion				X									
Citrovorum factor 9 to 12 mg Orally every 6 hours for 12 doses Begin 2 hours after methotrexate infusion				X	X	X							
Doxorubicin# 45 mg/m² BSA‖ IV										X	X		

*CAUTION: Postoperative adjuvant chemotherapy should not be given until the wound is completely healed with no evidence of infection or drainage.

†X indicates days to administer drug(s) indicated.

‡Chemotherapy is continued until the patient has received a total cumulative dose of doxorubicin of 550 mg/m², usually 6 cycles. Then it is discontinued. Patients who have received more preoperative chemotherapy will receive less adjuvant chemotherapy after surgery.

§NOTE: Cyclophosphamide may be given in doses of 1,800 mg/m² IV in patients with metastatic disease if bone marrow depression is not a limiting factor.

‖BSA = body surface area.

¶CAUTION: Procedures of allopurinol administration, hydration, alkalinization of the urine, and taking 24-, 48-, and 72-hour methotrexate (MTX) blood levels should be resumed after MTX administration to prevent severe MTX toxicity. *If abnormally high 24-hour MTX serum levels are obtained, continue citrovorum factor past 72 hours until it is clear that the patient will not develop severe MTX toxicity,* which usually occurs 5 days after the MTX infusion. (See Section 6, Renal Dysfunction, Table 6-15, and Section 7, Leucovorin Rescue.)

#CAUTION: In adult patients who have received both doxorubicin and cyclophosphamide with a total cumulative dose of 450 mg/m² of doxorubicin, there is a more common occurrence of cardiomyopathy or CHF or both. In pediatric patients who have received both doxorubicin and cyclophosphamide with a total cumulative dose of 350 mg/m² of doxorubicin there is a more common occurrence of cardiomyopathy or CHF or both.

REFERENCE:

Rosen, G., et al.: Chemotherapy, en bloc resection, and prosthetic bone replacement in the treatment of osteogenic sarcoma, Cancer **37:**1-11, 1976.

Cyclophosphamide, vincristine (Oncovin), phenylalanine mustard (L-PAM), and doxorubicin (Adriamycin) (CONPADRI-I)

GENERAL USE: Adjuvant chemotherapy for nonmetastatic osteosarcoma (pediatric)

RESPONSE RATE: 55% disease free at 2 years, 59% disease free at 1 year

SCHEDULE AND DOSE: This regimen consists of 73 weeks of chemotherapy. Therapy for weeks 33 to 73 is continued on the next page.

	Week*																	
	1	→	4	5	6	7	→	13	14	→	19	→	22	→	25	→	31	32
Cyclophosphamide 10 mg/kg PO or IV daily for 7 days (max. dose 500 mg)								X†										
Vincristine 0.05 mg/kg IV for 1 day (max. dose 2.0 mg)	X	Weekly →						X	X								X	X
Doxorubicin‡ 1.5 mg/kg IV for 1 day	X		X			X					X		X		X			
Doxorubicin‡ 1.0 mg/kg IV for 1 day																		
Phenylalanine mustard 0.3 mg/kg Orally for 1 day																	X	

*X indicates week(s) to administer drug(s) indicated.

†NOTE: Cyclophosphamide is given daily for 7 days during weeks indicated.

‡CAUTION: Note decrease in doxorubicin dose to 1.0 mg/kg IV at week 37. In adult patients who have received both doxorubicin and cyclophosphamide with a total cumulative dose of 450 mg/m^2 of doxorubicin there is a more common occurrence of cardiomyopathy or CHF or both. In pediatric patients who have received doxorubicin and cyclophosphamide with a total cumulative dose of 350 mg/m^2 of doxorubicin there is a more common occurrence of cardiomyopathy or CHF or both.

	Week*																
	→	37	38	→	43	44	→	49	→	55	56	→	61	→	67	→	73§
Cyclophosphamide 10 mg/kg PO or IV daily for 7 days (max. dose 500 mg)								X†							X†		
Vincristine 0.05 mg/kg IV for 1 day (max. dose 2.0 mg)					X	X											
Doxorubicin‡ 1.5 mg/kg IV for 1 day																	
Doxorubicin‡ 1.0 mg/kg IV for 1 day		X	X							X	X						
Phenylalanine mustard 0.3 mg/kg Orally for 1 day					X								X				X

*X indicates week(s) to administer drug(s) indicated.

†NOTE: Cyclophosphamide is given daily for 7 days during weeks indicated.

‡CAUTION: Note decrease in doxorubicin dose to 1.0 mg/kg IV at week 37. In adult patients who have received both doxorubicin and cyclophosphamide with a total cumulative dose of 450 mg/m² of doxorubicin there is a more common occurrence of cardiomyopathy or CHF or both. In pediatric patients who have received doxorubicin and cyclophosphamide with a total cumulative dose of 350 mg/m² of doxorubicin there is a more common occurrence of cardiomyopathy or CHF or both.

§NOTE: After the completion of 73 weeks of chemotherapy, observe the patient without further treatment.

CONPADRI-II and CONPADRI-III are 5-drug regimens more toxic than CONPADRI-I with similar response rates. Methotrexate is added to the CONPADRI-I regimen with 75 mg/kg (dose 1), 100 mg/kg (dose 2), and 150 mg/kg (dose 3). CONPADRI-I is thus far the regimen of choice among the three.

REFERENCES:

Sutow, W. W., et al.: Adjuvant chemotherapy in primary treatment of osteogenic sarcoma, Cancer **36:**1598-1602, 1975.

Sutow, W. W., et al.: Multidrug adjuvant chemotherapy for osteosarcoma: interim report of the Southwest Oncology Group Studies, Cancer Treat. Rep. **62:**265-269, 1978.

Bleomycin, cyclophosphamide, and dactinomycin (BCD)

GENERAL USE: Metastatic osteogenic sarcoma
RESPONSE RATE: 61.5%
SCHEDULE AND DOSE: Repeat cycle every 2 weeks.

	Day* 1	2	⟶	14
Bleomycin† 12 mg/m² BSA‡ IV	X	X	No therapy, 2-week rest period	
Cyclophosphamide 600 mg/m² BSA‡ IV	X	X		
Dactinomycin 450 μg/m² BSA‡ IV	X	X		

*X indicates day(s) to administer drug(s) indicated.
†CAUTION: In patients with total cumulative doses of bleomycin of 400 units or more there is a more common occurrence of pulmonary fibrosis. It can be exacerbated by prior irradiation or pulmonary disease or in patients over 60 years of age.
‡BSA = body surface area.
NOTE: Adequate intravenous hydration is important because of severe nausea and vomiting during this regimen.

REFERENCE:

Mosende, C., et al.: Combination chemotherapy with bleomycin, cyclophosphamide and dactinomycin for the treatment of osteogenic sarcoma, Cancer **40:**2779-2787, 1977.

Vincristine, methotrexate, and citrovorum factor (VCR-MTX-CF) (every-7-day protocol)

GENERAL USE: Metastatic osteogenic sarcoma

RESPONSE RATE: 56%

SCHEDULE AND DOSE:

	Week*													
	1	2	3	4	5	6	7	8	9	10	11	12	13	14
Vincristine 2 mg/m² BSA† IV, 30 minutes before methotrexate (max. dose 2.0 mg)	X	X	X	X	X	X	X	X			X			X
Methotrexate‡ 3 g/m² BSA† IV infusion over 6 hours	X													
Methotrexate‡ 6 g/m² BSA† IV infusion over 6 hours		X												
Methotrexate‡ 7.5 g/m² BSA† IV infusion over 6 hours			X	(X	X	X	X	X‡)			X			X
Citrovorum factor 15 mg IV every 3 hours for 24 hours beginning 2 hours after methotrexate infusion	X	X	X	(X	X	X	X	X‡)			X			X
Citrovorum factor 15 mg Orally every 6 hours for 48 hours beginning 3 hours after IV citrovorum factor	X	X	X	(X	X	X	X	X‡)			X			X

*X indicates week(s) to administer drug(s) indicated.

†BSA = body surface area

‡Methotrexate is escalated from 3 g/m² to 7.5 g/m² at weekly intervals. Three to eight weekly administrations may occur before response. *After response,* patients are to continue the vincristine, methotrexate, and citrovorum factor with dosage intervals of 2 to 3 weeks. CAUTION: Patient should be hospitalized the first 3 days before initiation of the treatment. Procedures of allopurinol administration, hydration, alkalinization of the urine, and taking 24-, 48-, and 72-hour methotrexate (MTX) serum blood levels should be done to prevent severe MTX toxicity. *If abnormally high 24-hour MTX serum levels are obtained, continue citrovorum factor past 72 hours until it is clear that the patient will not develop severe MTX toxicity,* which usually occurs 5 days after the MTX infusion. See Section 6, Renal Dysfunction, Table 6-15, and Section 7, Hyperuricemia and Leucovorin Rescue.

REFERENCE:

Jaffe, N., et al.: Weekly high-dose methotrexate-citrovorum factor in osteogenic sarcoma, Cancer **39:**45-50, 1977.

High-dose methotrexate, citrovorum factor, and doxorubicin (Adriamycin)

GENERAL USE: Metastatic osteogenic sarcoma (pediatric)

RESPONSE RATE: 54%

SCHEDULE AND DOSE: Repeat cycle every 32 days.

	Day*								
	1	2	3	→	16	17	18	→	32
Methotrexate† 100 to 300 mg/kg IV infusion over 4 hours	X							No therapy, 2-week rest period	
Citrovorum factor 9 mg *orally* every 6 hours for 12 doses Begin 2 hours after methotrexate	X	X	X						
Doxorubicin‡ 1.0 mg/kg IV					X	X			
Doxorubicin‡ 0.5 mg/kg IV							X		

*X indicates day(s) to administer drug(s) indicated.

†Escalate methotrexate by 100 mg/kg each subsequent cycle until a response occurs. Usually a response occurs between 300 to 500 mg/kg. CAUTION: Procedures of allopurinol administration, hydration, alkalinization of the urine, and taking 24-, 48-, and 72-hour methotrexate (MTX) serum blood levels should be done to prevent severe MTX toxicity. *If abnormally high 24-hour MTX serum levels are obtained, continue citrovorum factor past 72 hours until it is clear that the patient will not develop severe MTX toxicity,* which usually occurs 5 days after the MTX infusion. (See Section 6, Renal Dysfunction, Table 6-15; Section 7, Leucovorin Rescue and Hyperuricemia.)

‡CAUTION: In pediatric patients with total cumulative doses of doxorubicin of 450 mg/m² (350 mg/m² in patients with previously irradiated heart tissue) there is a more likely occurrence of cardiomyopathy or CHF or both.

REFERENCE:

Rosen, G., et al.: High-dose methotrexate with citrovorum factor rescue and Adriamycin in childhood osteogenic sarcoma, Cancer **33:**1151-1163, 1974.

Doxorubicin (Adriamycin)

GENERAL USE: Metastatic osteosarcoma—adjuvant therapy
RESPONSE RATE: 45% disease free in 18 months
SCHEDULE AND DOSE: Repeat cycle every 4 to 6 weeks. Six courses are given to the patient.

	Day*					
	1	2	3	→	28 or 42†	
Doxorubicin‡ 30 mg/m² BSA§ IV	X	X	X	No therapy, 3 to 5 weeks		

*X indicates day(s) to administer drug(s) indicated.
†May be delayed one week if recovery of the granulocytes and platelets is not complete by day 28 or 42.
‡CAUTION: In adult patients with total cumulative doses of 550 mg/m² (or 450 mg/m² in patients with previously irradiated heart tissue) there is a more common occurrence of cardiomyopathy or CHF or both. In pediatric patients with total cumulative doses of 450 mg/m² (or 350 mg/m² in patients with previously irradiated heart tissue) there is a more common occurrence of cardiomyopathy or CHF or both.
§BSA = body surface area.

REFERENCES:

Cortes, E. P., et al.: Amputation and Adriamycin in primary osteosarcoma, N. Engl. J. Med. **291**:998-1000, 1974.

Tan, C., et al.: Adriamycin (NSC-123127) in pediatric malignancies, Cancer Chemother. Rep. **6**:259-266, 1975.

MELANOMA
Dacarbazine (DTIC)

GENERAL USE: Metastatic malignant melanoma

RESPONSE RATE: 19%

SCHEDULE AND DOSE: Repeat cycle every 21 or 28 days. Adequate trial of therapy is 2 treatment cycles. If there is no response, discontinue.

	Day*						
	1	2	3	4	5	→	21†
Dacarbazine 250 mg/m² BSA‡ IV	X	X	X	X	X	No therapy, 2 to 3 weeks	

*X indicates day(s) to administer drug(s) indicated.

†May be delayed 1 week if recovery of the granulocytes and platelets is not complete by day 21 or 28.

‡BSA = body surface area.

REFERENCES:

Luce, J. K., et al.: Clinical trials with the antitumor agent 5-(3,3-dimethyl-1-triazeno) imidazole-4-carboxamide (NSC-45388), Cancer Chemother. Rep. **54:**119-124, 1970.

Comis, R. L., and Carter, S. K.: Integration of chemotherapy into combined modality treatment of solid tumors. IV. Malignant melanoma, Cancer Treat. Rev. **1:**285-304, 1974.

Semustine (MeCCNU)

GENERAL USE: Metastatic malignant melanoma
RESPONSE RATE: 18%
SCHEDULE AND DOSE: Repeat cycle every 6 weeks.

	Week*			
	1	→	6†	
Semustine‡ 250 mg/m² BSA§ Orally	X	No therapy, 6 weeks		

*X indicates week(s) to administer drug(s) indicated.
†May be delayed 1 week if recovery of the granulocytes and platelets is not complete by the sixth week.
‡NOTE: Semustine given 150 mg/m² PO every 3 weeks yields less toxicity and possibly superior rate and duration of response when compared with 250 mg/m² PO every 6 weeks.
CAUTION: The nadir of semustine may be *delayed* 6 weeks after administration.
§BSA = body surface area.

REFERENCES:

Ahmann, D. L.: Nitrosoureas in the management of disseminated malignant melanoma, Cancer Treat. Rep. **60:**747-751, 1976.

Nathanson, T., et al.: Combination chemoimmunotherapy of malignant melanoma, Proc. Am. Soc. Clin. Oncol. **20:**314, 1979.

Carmustine (BCNU), vincristine, and dacarbazine (DTIC) (BVD)

GENERAL USE: Metastatic malignant melanoma

RESPONSE RATE: 42.5%

SCHEDULE AND DOSE: Repeat 6-week cycle one time.

	Day*															
	1	2	3	4	5	6	7	8	9	10	11	12	13	14	15	→ 42†
Carmustine‡ 65 mg/m^2 BSA§ IV	X	X	X	(X)												
Vincristine‖ 1.0-1.5 mg IV	X							X							X‖	
Dacarbazine 250 mg/m^2 BSA§ IV	X	X	X	(X)												

*X indicates day(s) to administer drug(s) indicated.

†Responding patients are placed on maintenance therapy of dacarbazine 125 mg/m^2 IV biweekly, and carmustine 65 mg/m^2 IV monthly, and vincristine 1 mg biweekly (if tolerated) after cycle 2. Carmustine and dacarbazine can be given in one total dose on day 1 of each cycle.

‡CAUTION: The nadir of carmustine may be *delayed* 6 weeks after drug administration.

§BSA = body surface area.

‖Continue vincristine 1.0 to 1.5 mg IV weekly until toxicity.

NOTE: There have been no conclusive studies to reveal that the BVD regimen is better than dacarbazine alone.

REFERENCE:

Cohen, S. M., et al.: Combination chemotherapy of malignant melanoma with imidazole carboxamide, BCNU and vincristine, Cancer **39:**41-44, 1977.

GASTROINTESTINAL CANCER
5-Fluorouracil

GENERAL USE: Colorectal carcinoma

RESPONSE RATE: 21%

INDUCTION SCHEDULE AND DOSE:

	Day*								
	1	2	3	4	5	6	7	8	→ 26
5-Fluorouracil 12 mg/kg IV push	X	X	X	X	X				
5-Fluorouracil† 6 mg/kg IV push						X		X	Continue every other day through day 26

MAINTENANCE SCHEDULE AND DOSE: Begin 1 week after induction schedule. Adequate trial of therapy is 6 weeks. If there is response (greater than 50% shrinkage), continue maintenance therapy until there is progression of disease. If there is no response in 6 weeks, a change in therapy is indicated.

	Day*														
	1	2	3	4	5	6	7	8‡	9	10	11	12	13	14	15‡	→
5-Fluorouracil 15 mg/kg IV	X							X							X	Continue weekly‡

*X indicates day(s) to administer drug(s) indicated.

†CAUTION: Stop at earliest sign of mouth sores, diarrhea, proctitis, or granulocytes less than 2000/mm³ or platelet count less than 125,000/mm³.

‡May be delayed 1 week if recovery of granulocytes and platelets is not complete after a week.

REFERENCE:

Ansfield, F., et al.: A phase III study comparing the clinical utility of four regimens of 5-fluorouracil, Cancer **39:**34-40, 1977.

5-Fluorouracil and semustine (MeCCNU)

GENERAL USE: Large-bowel carcinoma

RESPONSE RATE: 30%

SCHEDULE AND DOSE:

	Week*									
	1	2	3	4	5	6	7	8	9	→
5-Fluorouracil 400 mg/m² BSA† IV, single dose	X	X	X	X	X	X	X	X	X	Continue once weekly
Semustine‡ 175 mg/m² BSA† Orally, single dose	X						X			Continue once every 6 weeks

*X indicates week(s) to administer drug(s) indicated.
†BSA = body surface area.
‡CAUTION: The nadir of semustine may be *delayed* 6 weeks after administration.

REFERENCE:

Baker, L. H., et al.: 5-FU versus 5-FU and MeCCNU in gastrointestinal cancers. A phase III study of the Southwest Oncology Group, Proc. Am. Assoc. Cancer Res. **16**:229, 1975.

5-Fluorouracil, semustine (MeCCNU), and vincristine

GENERAL USE: Advanced colorectal carcinoma

RESPONSE RATE: Greater than 30%

SCHEDULE AND DOSE:

	Day*													
	1	2	3	4	5	6	7	8	9	10	11	12	13	14 →
5-Fluorouracil 10 mg/kg IV bolus	X	X	X	X	X									X
		Continue with a single dose every 7 days												
Semustine† 100 mg/m² BSA‡ Orally	X	Continue every 6 weeks												
Vincristine 1.4 mg/m² BSA‡ IV (max. dose 2.0 mg)	X	Continue every 3 weeks												

*X indicates day(s) to administer drug(s) indicated.

†CAUTION: The nadir of semustine may be *delayed* 6 weeks after administration.

‡BSA = body surface area.

REFERENCES:

Carter, S. K., et al.: Chemotherapy of cancer, New York, 1977, John Wiley & Sons, pp. 116-122.

Carter, S. K., et al.: Current protocol approaches in large bowel cancer, Semin. Oncol. **3**:433-443, 1976.

Moertel, C. G., et al.: Therapy of advanced colorectal cancer with a combination of 5-fluorouracil, methyl-1,3-cis(2-chloroethyl)-1-nitrosourea, and vincristine, J. Natl. Cancer Inst. **54**:69-71, 1975.

Mitomycin C and floxuridine (hepatic arterial infusion)

GENERAL USE: Metastatic colorectal carcinoma to the liver

RESPONSE RATE: 83%

SCHEDULE AND DOSE: Repeat cycle every 30 days.

	Day*						
	1	2	3	4	5	→	30
Mitomycin C† 15 mg/m² BSA‡ Hepatic arterial infusion	X					No therapy, 3-week rest period	
Floxuridine 100 mg/m² BSA‡ Continuous hepatic arterial infusion	X	X	X	X	X		

*X indicates day(s) to administer drug(s) indicated.
†CAUTION: The nadir of mitomycin C may be *delayed* 6 weeks after drug administration.
‡BSA = body surface area.

REFERENCE:

Patt, Y. Z., et al.: Hepatic arterial infusion (HAI) of mitomycin C (MTC) and floxuridine (FUDR)—an effective treatment for metastatic colorectal carcinoma to the liver, Proc. Am. Soc. Clin. Oncol. **20**:316, 1979.

5-Fluorouracil, doxorubicin (Adriamycin), and mitomycin C (FAM)

GENERAL USE: Advanced gastric carcinoma

RESPONSE RATE: 50%

SCHEDULE AND DOSE: Repeat 56-day cycle every 8 weeks.

	Day* 1	→	8	→	29	→	36	→	56
5-Fluorouracil 600 mg/m² BSA† IV	X		X		X		X		2-week rest period
Doxorubicin‡ 30 mg/m² BSA† IV	X				X				
Mitomycin C§ 10 mg/m² BSA† IV	X								

*X indicates day(s) to administer drug(s) indicated.

†BSA = body surface area.

‡CAUTION: In adult patients with total cumulative doses of doxorubicin of 550 mg/m² (or 450 mg/m² in patients with previously irradiated heart tissue) there is a more common occurrence of cardiomyopathy or CHF or both.

§CAUTION: The nadir of mitomycin C may be *delayed* 6 weeks after drug administration.

REFERENCES:

Macdonald, J. S., et al.: 5-Fluorouracil (5-FU), Mitomycin-C (MMC) and Adriamycin (ADR)-FAM: a new combination chemotherapy program for advanced gastric carcinoma, Proc. Am. Soc. Clin. Oncol., p. 264, 1976.

Macdonald, J. S., et al.: 5-Fluorouracil, Adriamycin, and mitomycin-C (FAM) combination chemotherapy in the treatment of advanced gastric cancer, Cancer **44**:42-47, 1979.

5-Fluorouracil and semustine (MeCCNU)

GENERAL USE: Gastric adenocarcinoma

RESPONSE RATE: 40%

SCHEDULE AND DOSE: Repeat cycle every 7 weeks.

	Day* 1	2	3	4	5	→	49†
5-Fluorouracil 300 mg/m² BSA‡ IV	X	X	X	X	X	No therapy, 6-week rest period	
Semustine§ 175 mg/m² BSA‡ Orally	X						

*X indicates day(s) to administer drug(s) indicated.

†Leukocyte and platelet counts are recommended twice weekly following therapy.

‡BSA = body surface area.

§CAUTION: The nadir of semustine may be *delayed* 6 weeks after administration.

REFERENCES:

Baker, L. H., et al.: 5-FU and Me-CCNU in gastrointestinal cancers. A phase III study of the Southwest Oncology Group, Proc. Am. Assoc. Cancer Res. **16**:220 (abstract), 1975.

Moertel, C. G., et al.: Sequential and combination chemotherapy of advanced gastric cancer, Cancer **38**:678-682, 1976.

5-Fluorouracil and carmustine (BCNU)

GENERAL USE: Gastric adenocarcinoma

RESPONSE RATE: 41%

SCHEDULE AND DOSE: Repeat cycle every 8 weeks.

	Day*						
	1	2	3	4	5†	→	56‡
5-Fluorouracil 10 mg/kg IV	X	X	X	X	X	No therapy, 7-week rest period	
Carmustine§ 40 mg/m² BSA‖ IV	X	X	X	X	X		

*X indicates day(s) to administer drug(s) indicated.

†NOTE: Therapy should be discontinued if the patient develops stomatitis or diarrhea during the 5-day treatment period.

‡May be delayed 1 week if recovery of the granulocytes and platelets is not complete by day 56.

§CAUTION: The nadir of Carmustine may be *delayed* 6 weeks after drug administration.

‖BSA = body surface area.

REFERENCE:

Kovach, J. S., et al.: A controlled study of combined 1,3-bis(2-chloroethyl)-1-nitrosourea and 5-fluorouracil therapy for advanced gastric and pancreatic cancer, Cancer **33:**563-567, 1974.

Mitomycin C

GENERAL USE: Gastric adenocarcinoma

RESPONSE RATE: 30%

SCHEDULE AND DOSE: Repeat every 6 to 8 weeks.

	Day*												
	1	2	3	4	5	6	7	8	9	10	11	12	→	42 or 56†
Mitomycin C‡ 2 mg/m² BSA§ IV	X	X	X	X	X			X	X	X	X	X	No therapy, 4- to 6-week rest period	

*X indicates day(s) to administer drug(s) indicated.
†NOTE: Alternate schedule—mitomycin C 20 mg/m² BSA IV once every 6 to 8 weeks.
‡CAUTION: The nadir related to mitomycin C may be *delayed* to 6 weeks after administration.
§BSA = body surface area.

REFERENCES:

Baker, C. E., et al.: Physicians' desk reference, Oradell, N.J., 1979, Medical Economics Company, p. 709.

Comis, R. L., et al.: Integration of chemotherapy into combined modality treatment of solid tumors. III. Gastric cancer, Cancer Treat. Rev. **1:** 221-238, 1974.

Streptozocin, mitomycin C and 5-fluorouracil (SMF)

GENERAL USE: Advanced pancreatic cancer

RESPONSE RATE: 43%

SCHEDULE AND DOSE: Repeat cycle every 8 weeks.

	Week*							
	1	2	3	4	5	6	7	8
Streptozocin† 1 g/m² BSA‡ IV, single dose	X	X			X	X	No therapy, 2-week rest period	
Mitomycin C§ 10 mg/m² BSA‡ IV, single dose	X							
5-Fluorouracil 600 mg/m² BSA‡ IV, single dose	X	X			X	X		

*X indicates week(s) to administer drug(s) indicated.

†CAUTION: Discontinue streptozocin if proteinuria >1 g/24 hours, renal glycosuria, renal tubular acidosis, Fanconi's syndrome, serum creatinine above 2 mg/100 ml, or creatinine clearance is less than 70 ml/minute.

‡BSA = body surface area.

§CAUTION: The nadir of mitomycin C may be delayed 6 weeks.

REFERENCE:

Wiggans, R. G., et al.: Phase II trial of streptozotocin, mitomycin-C, and 5-fluorouracil (SMF) in the treatment of advanced pancreatic cancer, Cancer **41**:397-391, 1978.

5-Fluorouracil, doxorubicin (Adriamycin), and mitomycin C (FAM)

GENERAL USE: Advanced pancreatic cancer
RESPONSE RATE: 40% (median survival, 8+ months)
SCHEDULE AND DOSE:

	Week*								
	1	2	3	4	5	6	7	8	9
5-Fluorouracil 600 mg/m² BSA† IV, single dose	X	X			X	X			X
Doxorubicin‡ 30 mg/m² BSA† IV, single dose	X				X				X
Mitomycin C§ 10 mg/m² BSA† IV, single dose	X								X

*X indicates week(s) to administer drug(s) indicated.
†BSA = body surface area.
‡CAUTION: In adult patients with total cumulative doses of doxorubicin of 550 mg/m² (or 450 mg/m² in patients with previously irradiated heart tissue) there is a more common occurrence of cardiomyopathy or CHF or both.
§CAUTION: The nadir of mitomycin C may be *delayed* 6 weeks after drug administration.

REFERENCE:

Smith, F. P., et al.: Phase II evaluation of FAM, 5-fluorouracil (F), Adriamycin (A) and mitomycin-C (M) in advanced pancreatic cancer (PC), Proc. Am. Soc. Clin. Oncol. **20:**415, 1979.

GYNECOLOGIC CANCER
Melphalan

GENERAL USE: Ovarian carcinoma

RESPONSE RATE: 47%

SCHEDULE AND DOSE: Repeat cycle every 3 to 5 weeks.

	Day*					
	1	2	3	4	5	→ 21 or 35
Melphalan 0.2 mg/kg Orally or IV	X	X	X	X	X	No therapy, 2- to 4-week rest period

*X indicates day to administer drug indicated.

REFERENCES:

Smith, J. P., et al.: Chemotherapy in the treatment of cancer of the ovary, Am. J. Obstet. Gynecol. **107**:691-703, 1970.

Young, R. C.: Chemotherapy of ovarian cancer: Past and present, Semin. Oncol. **2**:267-276, 1975.

Doxorubicin (Adriamycin) and cyclophosphamide (ACe)

GENERAL USE: Ovarian carcinoma

RESPONSE RATE: 73%

SCHEDULE AND DOSE: Repeat cycle every 4 weeks.

	Day* 1	2	3	4	→	28
Adriamycin† 50 mg/m² BSA‡ IV	X				No therapy, 3-week rest period	
Cyclophosphamide 250 mg/m² BSA‡ Orally	X	X	X	X		

*X indicates day(s) to administer drug(s) indicated.

†NOTE: Patients with a cumulative dose of doxorubicin of 450 mg/m² are continued on single-agent chemotherapy other than doxorubicin.

‡BSA = body surface area.

REFERENCE:

Turbow, M. M., et al.: Chemotherapy of ovarian carcinoma: randomization between melphalan and adriamycin-cyclophosphamide, Proc. Am. Soc. Clin. Oncol. **19**:394, 1978.

Hexamethylmelamine, cyclophosphamide, methotrexate (amethopterin), and 5-fluorouracil (Hexa-CAF)

GENERAL USE: Advanced ovarian adenocarcinoma

RESPONSE RATE: 76% (survival, 29 months)

SCHEDULE AND DOSE:

	Day*													
	1	2	3	4	5	6	7	8	9	10	11	12	13	14
Hexamethylmelamine 150 mg Orally	X	X	X	X	X	X	X	X	X	X	X	X	X	X
Cyclophosphamide 150 mg Orally	X	X	X	X	X	X	X	X	X	X	X	X	X	X
Methotrexate 40 mg/m² BSA† IV	X							X						
5-Fluorouracil 600 mg/m² BSA† IV	X							X						

*X indicates day(s) to administer drug(s) indicated.
†BSA = body surface area.

REFERENCES:

Young, R. C., et al.: Advanced ovarian adenocarcinoma: melphalan (PAM) vs. combination chemotherapy (Hexa-CAF), Proc. Am. Soc. Clin. Oncol. **19:**393, 1978.

Young, R. C., et al.: Advanced ovarian adenocarcinoma—a prospective trial of melphalan (L-PAM) versus combination chemotherapy, N. Engl. J. Med. **299:**1261-1266, 1978.

Cyclophosphamide, hexamethylmelamine, doxorubicin (Adriamycin), and cisplatin (cis-diamminedichloroplatinum) (CHAD)

GENERAL USE: Advanced ovarian carcinoma (ECOG pilot study)

RESPONSE RATE: 91.3% (disease free 7 to 17 months)

SCHEDULE AND DOSE: Repeat cycle every 28 days.

	Day*														
	1	**2**	**3**	**4**	**5**	**6**	**7**	**8**	**9**	**10**	**→**	**19**	**20**	**21**	**→**	**28**
Cyclophosphamide 600 mg/m² BSA† IV	X														1-week rest period, no therapy	
Doxorubicin‡ 25 mg/m² BSA† IV	X															
Cisplatin§ 50 mg/m² BSA† IV with hydration	X															
Hexamethylmelamine 150 mg/m² BSA† Orally								X	Daily →	→	→	→	→	→		

*X indicates day(s) to administer drug(s) indicated.

†BSA = body surface area.

‡CAUTION: In adult patients who have received both doxorubicin and cyclophosphamide with a total cumulative dose of 450 mg/m² of doxorubicin there is a more common occurrence of cardiomyopathy or CHF or both.

§CAUTION: Prehydration and a sustained mannitol diuresis is necessary to prevent kidney damage with cisplatin infusions. (See Section 6, Renal Dysfunction, and Table 6-18.)

REFERENCE:

Vogl, S. E., et al.: The 'CHAD' regimen (cyclophosphamide [C], hexamethylmelamine [H], Adriamycin [A], and diamminedichloroplatinum [D]) in advanced ovarian cancer, Proc. Am. Soc. Clin. Oncol. **20**:384, 1979.

Cyclophosphamide, hexamethylmelamine, and 5-fluorouracil (CHF)

GENERAL USE: Advanced ovarian cancer

RESPONSE RATE: 83%, no prior chemotherapy; 46%, prior chemotherapy; median survival, 14 months

SCHEDULE AND DOSE: Repeat cycle every 28 days.

	Day*														
	1	2	3	4	5	6	7	8	9	10	11	12	13	14	→28
Cyclophosphamide 100 mg/m² BSA† Orally	X	X	X	X	X	X	X	X	X	X	X	X	X	X	2-week rest period, no therapy
Hexamethylmelamine 150 mg/m² BSA† Orally	X	X	X	X	X	X	X	X	X	X	X	X	X	X	
5-Fluorouracil 600 mg/m² BSA† IV	X							X							

*X indicates day(s) to administer drug(s) indicated.
†BSA = body surface area.

REFERENCE:

Delgado, G., et al.: L-PAM vs. cyclophosphamide, hexamethylmelamine and 5-fluorouracil (CHF) for advanced ovarian cancer, Proc. Am. Soc. Clin. Oncol. **20:**434, 1979.

Cyclophosphamide

GENERAL USE: Ovarian carcinoma

RESPONSE RATE: 44%

I. SCHEDULE AND DOSE:

	Day*									
	1	2	3	4	5	6	7	8	9	→
Cyclophosphamide 50 to 150 mg Orally	X	X	X	X	X	X	X	X	X	Continue daily

*X indicates day(s) to administer drug(s) indicated.

II. ALTERNATE SCHEDULE AND DOSE:

	Day*											
	1	2	3	4	5	6	7	8	9	10	11	12 →
Cyclophosphamide 400 mg IV	X	X	X	X								
Cyclophosphamide 50 to 150 mg Orally					X	X	X	X	X	X	X	Continue daily

*X indicates day(s) to administer drug(s) indicated.

REFERENCES:

Beck, R. E., et al.: Treatment of 126 cases of advanced ovarian carcinoma with cyclophosphamide, Can. Med. Assoc. J. **98:**539-541, 1968.

Young, R. C.: Chemotherapy of ovarian cancer: past and present, Semin. Oncol. **2:**267-276, 1975.

Mitomycin C, vincristine (Oncovin), and bleomycin (MOBI)

GENERAL USE: Squamous cell carcinoma of the uterine cervix
RESPONSE RATE: 48%
SCHEDULE AND DOSE:

	Week* 1	2	3	4	5	6	7	8	9	10	11	12	
Vincristine† 0.5 mg/m² BSA‡ IV *twice weekly,* day 1, 4 (max. dose 2.0 mg)	X	X	X	X	X	X	X	X	X	X	X	X	Discontinue
Bleomycin† 6 mg/m² BSA‡ IM *twice weekly* 6 hours after vincristine day 1, 4	X	X	X	X	X	X	X	X	X	X	X	X	Discontinue
Mitomycin C§ 20 mg/m² BSA‡ IV, *single dose,* day 2	X						X	Repeat every 6 weeks					

*X indicates week(s) to administer drug(s) indicated.
†CAUTION: Vincristine and bleomycin should be discontinued if significant toxicity results from either.
‡BSA = body surface area.
§CAUTION: Mitomycin C nadir may be delayed to 6 weeks.

REFERENCE:

Baker, L. H., et al.: Phase II study of mitomycin-C, vincristine, and bleomycin in advanced squamous cell carcinoma of the uterine cervix, Cancer **38**:2222-2224, 1976.

Cisplatin

GENERAL USE: Advanced squamous cell carcinoma of the cervix

RESPONSE RATE: 50% (median survival, 9 months)

SCHEDULE AND DOSE:

	Week*										
	1	2	3	4	5	6	7	8	9	10	→
Cisplatin† 50 mg/m² BSA‡ IV, single dose	X			X			X			X	Continue every 3 weeks

*X indicates week(s) to administer drug(s) indicated.
†CAUTION: Prehydration and a sustained mannitol diuresis is necessary to prevent kidney damage with cisplatin infusions. (See Section 6, Renal Dysfunction, and Table 6-18.)
‡BSA = body surface area.

REFERENCE:

Thigpen, T., et al.: Phase II trial of cis-platinum as first or second line treatment for advanced squamous cell carcinoma of the cervix, Am. Soc. Clin. Oncol. **20:**388, 1979.

Doxorubicin (Adriamycin)

GENERAL USE: Advanced carcinoma of the cervix

RESPONSE RATE: 32%

SCHEDULE AND DOSE: Repeat every 3 weeks.

	Day*			
	1	→	21	→
Doxorubicin† 60 mg/m² BSA‡ IV	X	No therapy, 3 weeks		

*X indicates day(s) to administer drug indicated.
†CAUTION: In adult patients with total cumulative doses of doxorubicin of 550 mg/m² (or 450 mg/m² in patients with previously irradiated heart tissue) there is a more common occurrence of cardiomyopathy or CHF or both.
‡BSA = body surface area.

REFERENCES:

Blum, R. H., et al.: Adriamycin: a new anticancer drug with significant clinical activity, Ann. Intern. Med. **80:**249-259, 1974.

O'Bryan, R. M., et al.: Phase II evaluation of Adriamycin human neoplasia, Cancer **32:**1-8, 1973.

UROLOGIC CANCER
Vinblastine, bleomycin, and cisplatin (VBP)

GENERAL USE: Disseminated testicular cancer primary treatment

RESPONSE RATE: 100% (74% complete)

SCHEDULE AND DOSE:

	Day* 1	2	3	4	5	6	7	8	9	→
Vinblastine† 0.2 mg/kg IV	X	X								Repeat every 3 weeks for 5 courses†
Cisplatin‡ 20 mg/m² BSA§ IV infusion over 15 minutes 6 hours after vinblastine	X	X	X	X	X					Repeat every 3 weeks for 3 courses
Bleomycin‖ 30 mg IV 6 hours after vinblastine		X							X	Continue to give on day 2 of each week for total of 12 weeks

*X indicates day(s) to administer drug(s) indicated.

†After 5 courses of vinblastine continue single injections in a dosage of 0.3 mg/kg every 4 weeks for a total of 2 years. NOTE: Vinblastine dose should be reduced 25% in patients who have had previous radiotherapy.

‡CAUTION: Prehydration and a sustained mannitol diuresis is necessary to prevent kidney damage with cisplatin infusions (see Section 6, Renal Dysfunction, and Table 6-18).

§BSA = body surface area.

‖Give bleomycin on day 2 of each week for a total of 12 weeks and discontinue after total cumulative dose of 360 mg (1 mg = 1 unit).

REFERENCES:

Einhorn, L. H., et al.: Cis-diamminedichloroplatinum, vinblastine, and bleomycin and combination chemotherapy in disseminated testicular cancer, Ann. Intern. Med. **87:**293-298, 1977.

Einhorn, L. H., et al.: Combination chemotherapy of disseminated testicular carcinoma with cis-diamminedichloroplatinum, vinblastine and bleomycin (DVB): an update, Proc. Am. Soc. Clin. Oncol. **19:**308, 1978.

Anderson, T., et al.: Testicular germ-cell neoplasms: recent advances in diagnosis and therapy, Ann. Intern. Med. **90:**373-385, 1979.

Cisplatin, bleomycin, vinblastine, vincristine, and actinomycin D

GENERAL USE: Advanced testicular tumor
RESPONSE RATE: 100% (67.5% complete)
INDUCTION SCHEDULE AND DOSE:

	Day*														
	1	2	3	4	5	6	7	8	9	10	11	12	13	14	→	28†
Cisplatin‡ 4 mg/kg IV	X														2-week rest period, no therapy	
Bleomycin 420 mg IV	X															
Vinblastine 2 mg/kg IV	X															
Prednisone 20 mg/kg Orally	X	X	X	X	X	X	X	X	X	X	X	X	X	X		

*X indicates day(s) to administer drug(s) indicated.
†Proceed to consolidation schedule.
‡CAUTION: Prehydration and a sustained mannitol diuresis is necessary to prevent kidney damage with cisplatin infusions (see Section 6, Renal Dysfunction, and Table 6-18).

CONSOLIDATION SCHEDULE AND DOSE: 6 weeks

	Week*		
	1	→	6†
Actinomycin D 5 mg IV, single dose	X	5-week rest period, no therapy	
Vincristine ~~6 mg~~ 2 mg IV, single dose	X		
Cisplatin‡ 6 mg/kg IV infusion, single dose	X		

*X indicates week(s) to administer drug(s) indicated.
†Proceed to maintenance schedule.
‡CAUTION: Prehydration and a sustained mannitol diuresis is necessary to prevent kidney damage with cisplatin infusions (see Section 6, Renal Dysfunction, and Table 6-18).

MAINTENANCE SCHEDULE AND DOSE:

	Week*							
	1	2	3	4	5	6	7	→
Actinomycin D 2.5 mg IV	X						X	Continue once every 6 weeks
Cisplatin† 1 mg/kg IV	X			X			X	Continue once every 3 weeks

*X indicates week(s) to administer drug(s) indicated.
†CAUTION: Prehydration and a sustained mannitol diuresis is necessary to prevent kidney damage with cisplatin infusions (see Section 6, Renal Dysfunction, and Table 6-18).

REFERENCES:

Merrin, C., et al.: Multimodal treatment of advanced testicular tumor with cis-diaminedichloroplatinum (CPDD), bleomycin (BLEO), vinblastine (VBL), vincristine (VCR) and actinomycin D (ACT D), Proc. Am. Soc. Clin. Oncol. **18:**298, 1977.

Anderson, T., et al.: Testicular germ-cell neoplasms: recent advances in diagnosis and therapy, Ann. Intern. Med. **90:**373-385, 1979.

Vinblastine, actinomycin D, bleomycin, cyclophosphamide, and cisplatin (VAB III)

GENERAL USE: Metastatic or unresectable germ cell tumors
RESPONSE RATE: 86% (60% complete)
INDUCTION SCHEDULE AND DOSE:

	Day*												
	1	**2**	**3**	**4**	**5**	**6**	**7**	**8**	**9**	**10**	**11**	**12**	**→**	**21†**
Vinblastine 4 mg/m² BSA‡ IV	X												1-week rest period	
Actinomycin D 1.0 mg/m² BSA‡ IV	X													
Bleomycin 20 mg/m² BSA‡ IV, continuous infusion	X	X	X	X	X	X	X							
Cyclophosphamide 600 mg/m² BSA‡ IV	X													
Cisplatin 120 mg/m² BSA‡ IV								X						

*X indicates day(s) to administer drugs indicated.
†Proceed to consolidation schedule. CAUTION: Prehydration and a sustained mannitol diuresis is necessary to prevent kidney damage with cisplatin infusions (see Section 6, Renal Dysfunction, and Table 6-18).
‡BSA = body surface area.

CONSOLIDATION SCHEDULE AND DOSE:

	Week*																	
	1	2	3	4	5	6	7	8	9	10	11	12	13	14	15	16	17	18†
Vinblastine 4 mg/m² BSA‡ IV, single dose	X			X			X			X			X			X		
Chlorambucil 4 mg/m² BSA‡ Orally, *daily for 14 days*	X	X		X	X		X	X		X	X		X	X		X	X	
Doxorubicin§ 45 mg/m² BSA‡ IV, single dose	X									X								
Actinomycin 1.0 mg/m² BSA‡ IV, single dose				X									X					
Cisplatin‖ 50 mg/m² BSA‡ IV, single dose							X									X		

*X indicates week(s) to administer drug(s) indicated.
†Repeat induction schedule, then proceed to maintenance schedule.
‡BSA = body surface area.
§CAUTION: In adult patients with total cumulative doses of doxorubicin of 550 mg/m² (or 450 mg/m² in patients with previously irradiated heart tissue) there is a more common occurrence of cardiomyopathy or CHF or both.
‖CAUTION: Prehydration and a sustained mannitol diuresis is necessary to prevent kidney damage with cisplatin infusions (see Section 6, Renal Dysfunction, and Table 6-18).

MAINTENANCE SCHEDULE AND DOSE: Continue cycle every 3 weeks for 2 years. Intermittently give the induction schedule every 4 to 5 months.

	Week*														
	1	2	3	4	5	6	7	8	9	10	11	12	13	14	→
Vinblastine 4 mg/m² BSA† IV, single dose	X			X			X			X			X		
Actinomycin D 1.0 mg/m² BSA† IV, single dose	X			X			X			X			X		
Chlorambucil 4 mg/m² BSA† Orally, *daily for 14 days*	X	X		X	X		X	X		X	X		X	X	

*X indicates week(s) to administer drug(s) indicated.
†BSA = body surface area.

REFERENCES:

Cvitkovic, E., et al.: Primary combination chemotherapy (VAB III) for metastatic or unresectable germ cell tumors, Proc. Am. Assoc. Cancer Res. **17:**296, 1976.

Golbey, R. B., et al.: Chemotherapy of metastatic germ cell tumors, Semin. Oncol. **6:**82-86, 1979.

Anderson, T., et al.: Testicular germ-cell neoplasms: recent advances in diagnosis and therapy, Ann. Intern. Med. **90:**373-385, 1979.

Vinblastine, actinomycin D, bleomycin, cyclophosphamide, cisplatin, chlorambucil, and doxorubicin (Adriamycin) (VAB IV)

GENERAL USE: Metastatic germ cell tumors

RESPONSE RATE: 86% (59% complete)

INDUCTION AND REINDUCTION II SCHEDULE AND DOSE:

	Day*								
	1	2	3	4	5	6	7	→	21†
Cyclophosphamide 600 mg/m^2 BSA‡ IV	X							No therapy, 2-week rest period	
Vinblastine 4 mg/m^2 BSA‡ IV	X								
Actinomycin D 1.0 mg/m^2 BSA‡ IV	X								
Bleomycin 30 mg/m^2 BSA‡ IV	X								
Bleomycin 20 mg/m^2 BSA‡ Continuous IV infusion	X	X	X	X	X	X			
Cisplatin§ 120 mg/m^2 BSA‡ IV							X		

*X indicates day(s) to administer drug(s) indicated.

†After induction proceed to consolidation I schedule given below. After reinduction II proceed to maintenance schedule (p. 146).

‡BSA = body surface area.

§Prehydration and mannitol diuresis is necessary to prevent kidney damage with cisplatin infusions (see Section 6, Renal Dysfunction, and Table 6-18).

CONSOLIDATION I AND II SCHEDULE AND DOSE:

	Week*											
	1	2	3	4	5	6	7	8	9	10	11	12†
Vinblastine 4 mg/m^2 BSA‡ IV, single dose	X			X			X			X		
Chlorambucil 4 mg/m^2 BSA‡ Orally, *daily for 7 days*	X			X			X			X		
Doxorubicin 30 mg/m^2 BSA‡ IV, single dose	X						X					
Actinomycin D 1.0 mg/m^2 BSA‡ IV, single dose				X						X		

*X indicates the week(s) to administer drug(s) indicated.

†After consolidation I proceed to reinduction I schedule (p. 146). After consolidation II proceed to reinduction II (same as induction schedule given above).

‡BSA = body surface area.

REINDUCTION I (WEEK 16) SCHEDULE AND DOSE:

	Day*							
	1	2	3	4	5	6	7	→ 21†
Cyclophosphamide 600 mg/m² BSA‡ IV	X							No therapy, 2-week rest period
Vinblastine 4 mg/m² BSA‡ IV	X							
Actinomycin D 1.0 mg/m² BSA‡ IV	X							
Cisplatin§ 120 mg/m² BSA‡ IV							X	

*X indicates day(s) to administer drug(s) indicated.
†Repeat previous consolidation schedule to complete consolidation II (p. 145).
‡BSA = body surface area.
§CAUTION: Prehydration and mannitol diuresis is necessary to prevent kidney damage with cisplatin infusions (see Section 6, Renal Dysfunction, and Table 6-18).

MAINTENANCE SCHEDULE AND DOSE: Continue cycle every 3 weeks for 2 years.

	Week*														
	1	2	3	4	5	6	7	8	9	10	11	12	13	14	→
Vinblastine 4 mg/m² BSA† IV, single dose	X			X			X			X			X		
Actinomycin D 1.0 mg/m² BSA† IV, single dose	X			X			X			X			X		
Chlorambucil 4 mg/m² BSA† Orally, *daily for 14 days*	X	X		X	X		X	X		X	X		X	X	

*X indicates week(s) to administer drug(s) indicated.
†BSA = body surface area.

REFERENCES:

Vugrin, D., et al.: Chemotherapy of testicular carcinoma with VAB IV, Proc. Am. Soc. Clin. Oncol. **20:**338, 1979.

Golbey, R. B., et al.: Chemotherapy of metastatic germ cell tumors, Semin. Oncol. **6:**82-86, 1979.

Anderson, T., et al.: Testicular germ-cell neoplasms: recent advances in diagnosis and therapy, Ann. Intern. Med. **90:**373-385, 1979.

Diethylstilbestrol (DES)

GENERAL USE: Metastatic prostatic carcinoma
RESPONSE RATE: 80%
SCHEDULE AND DOSE:

	Day*										
	1	2	3	4	5	6	7	8	9	10	→
Diethylstilbestrol† 1 to 3 mg Orally, *three times daily*	X	X	X	X	X	X	X	X	X	X	Continue daily

*X indicates day(s) to administer drug(s) indicated.
†See Section 4, Hormone Therapy—Prostate Cancer.

REFERENCES:

Bailar, J. C., et al.: Veterans Administration Cooperative Urological Research Group: estrogen treatment for cancer of the prostate—early results with 3 doses of diethylstilbestrol and placebo, Cancer **26:**257-261, 1970.

Prout, G. R.: Prostate gland. In Holland, J. F., editor: Cancer medicine, Philadelphia, 1973, Lea & Febiger, pp. 1680-1694.

Cisplatin

GENERAL USE: Advanced carcinoma of the prostate
RESPONSE RATE: 43%
SCHEDULE AND DOSE:

	Week*														
	1	2	3	4	5	6	7	8	9	10	11	12	13	14	15†
Cisplatin 1 mg/kg Slow IV infusion over 6 to 8 hours, mixed with 37.5 g mannitol, 40 mEq potassium chloride, and 2,000 ml D5W in ⅓ NS	X	X	X	X	X	X				X				X	

*X indicates week(s) to administer drug(s) indicated.
†Continue every 3 weeks until lesions progress or until toxicity requires that cisplatin be discontinued.

REFERENCE:

Merrin, C.: Treatment of advanced carcinoma of the prostate (stage D) with infusion of cis-diamminedichloroplatinum (II NSC 119875): a pilot study, J. Urol. **119:**522, 1978.

Cisplatin, cyclophosphamide, and doxorubicin (Adriamycin) (CISCA)

GENERAL USE: Metastatic bladder carcinoma

RESPONSE RATE: 83%

SCHEDULE AND DOSE: Repeat cycle every 21 days.

	Day*			
	1	2	→	21
Cyclophosphamide 650 mg/m² BSA† IV	X		No therapy, 3-week rest period	
Doxorubicin‡ 50 mg/m² BSA† IV	X			
Cisplatin§ 100 mg/m² BSA† IV infusion over 2 hours		X		

*X indicates day(s) to administer drug(s) indicated.

†BSA = body surface area.

‡Discontinue doxorubicin when it reaches a total cumulative dose of 450 mg/m², at which time increase cyclophosphamide dosage to 1,000 mg/m² IV.

§CAUTION: Prehydration and a sustained mannitol diuresis is necessary to prevent kidney damage with cisplatin infusions (see Section 6, Renal Dysfunction, and Table 6-18).

NOTE: There have been no phase III studies demonstrating that any combination of drugs is superior to any single drug.

REFERENCES:

Sternberg, J. J., et al.: Combination chemotherapy (CISCA) for advanced urinary tract carcinoma, J.A.M.A. **238**:2282-2287, 1977.

Cummings, K. B., et al.: Current concepts in the management of patients with deeply invasive bladder carcinoma, Semin. Oncol. **6**:220-228, 1979.

Cisplatin, doxorubicin (Adriamycin), and 5-fluorouracil

GENERAL USE: Metastatic bladder carcinoma

RESPONSE RATE: 62.5% (duration 5 to 37 weeks)

SCHEDULE AND DOSE: Continue to repeat cycle every 4 weeks.

	Week*					
	1 →	5 →	9 →	13 →	17 →	21
Cisplatin† 20 mg/m^2 BSA‡ IV *for 5 days* with continuous IV hydration	X	X	X			
Cisplatin† 50 to 75 mg/m^2 BSA‡ IV, single dose with continuous IV hydration				X	X	X
Doxorubicin§ 50 mg/m^2 BSA‡ IV, single dose	X	X	X	X	X	X
5-Fluorouracil 500 mg/m^2 BSA‡ IV, single dose	X	X	X	X	X	X

*X indicates week(s) to administer drug(s) indicated.

†CAUTION: Prehydration and a sustained mannitol diuresis is necessary to prevent kidney damage with cisplatin infusions (see Section 6, Renal Dysfunction, and Table 6-18). Cisplatin is given at a dosage of 20 mg/m^2 for 5 days for the first 3 cycles only, then 50-75 mg/m^2 as a single dose for the latter cycles.

‡BSA = body surface area.

§CAUTION: In adult patients with total cumulative doses of doxorubicin of 550 mg/m^2 (or 450 mg/m^2 in patients with previously irradiated heart tissue) there is a more common occurrence of cardiomyopathy or CHF or both.

NOTE: There have been no phase III studies clearly demonstrating that any combination of drugs is superior to any single drug.

REFERENCES:

Williams, S. D., et al.: Chemotherapy of bladder cancer with cis-diammine dichloroplatinum (DDP), Adriamycin (ADR), and 5-fluorouracil (5-FU), Proc. Am. Soc. Clin. Oncol. **19:**316, 1978.

Cummings, K. B., et al.: Current concepts in the management of patients with deeply invasive bladder carcinoma, Semin. Oncol. **6:**220-228, 1979.

Cisplatin

GENERAL USE: Metastatic bladder carcinoma
RESPONSE RATE: 57% (no prior therapy), 36% (prior therapy)
SCHEDULE AND DOSE:

	Day*			
	1	→	21 or 28	
Cisplatin† 70 mg/m² BSA‡ IV	X	No therapy, 3 to 4 weeks		

*X indicates day(s) to administer drug(s) indicated.
†CAUTION: Prehydration and a sustained mannitol diuresis is necessary to prevent kidney damage with cisplatin infusions (see Section 6, Renal Dysfunction, and Table 6-18).
‡BSA = body surface area.
NOTE: There have been no phase III studies clearly demonstrating that any combination of drugs is superior to any single drug. Cisplatin is considered the most active single agent.

REFERENCES:

Yagoda, A., et al.: Cis-dichlorodiammineplatinum (II) in advanced bladder cancer, Cancer Treat. Rep. **60:**917-923, 1976.

Yagoda, A., et al.: Cis-Platinum (DDP) regimens in bladder cancer, Proc. Am. Soc. Clin. Oncol. **20:**347, 1979.

Cummings, K. B., et al.: Current concepts in the management of patients with deeply invasive bladder carcinoma, Semin. Oncol. **6:**220-228, 1979.

Cyclophosphamide

GENERAL USE: Metastatic bladder carcinoma

RESPONSE RATE: 52%

SCHEDULE AND DOSES: Repeat cycle every 3 weeks.

	Day*			
	1	→	21	
Cyclophosphamide 1 g/m^2 BSA† IV	X	No therapy, 3 weeks		

*X indicates day(s) to administer drug(s) indicated.
†BSA = body surface area.
NOTE: There have been no phase III studies clearly demonstrating that any combination of drugs is superior to any single drug.

REFERENCES:

Merrin, C., et al.: Chemotherapy of bladder carcinoma with cyclophosphamide and Adriamycin, J. Urol. **114:**884-887, 1975.

Cummings, K. B., et al.: Current concepts in the management of patients with deeply invasive bladder carcinoma, Semin. Oncol. **6:**220-228, 1979.

Thiotepa (triethylene thiophosphoramide) (bladder instillation treatment program)

GENERAL USE: Well-differentiated papillary tumors
RESPONSE RATE: 71% (33% complete remission)
SCHEDULE AND DOSE:

	Weeks*												
	1	2	3	4	5	6	7	8	9	10	11	12	
Thiotepa 60 mg in 60 ml of sterile distilled water†	X	X	X	X					X	X	X	X	

*X indicates week(s) to administer drug(s) indicated.
†Instill once weekly. Retain in bladder 2 hours after instillation.

REFERENCES:

Carter, S. K., et al.: The chemotherapy of urologic cancer, Cancer **36:** 729-747, 1975.

Veenema, R. J.: The role of thiotepa instillations in bladder cancer, J.A.M.A. **204:**73-75, 1968.

Koontz, W. W.: Intravesical chemotherapy and chemoprevention of superficial, low grade, low stage bladder carcinoma, Semin. Oncol. **6**(2):217-219, 1979.

Actinomycin D and vincristine

GENERAL USE: Wilms' tumor (pediatric)

RESPONSE RATE: 81% disease free in 2 years, 86% alive

SCHEDULE AND DOSE: Alternate this 2-month schedule with the schedule for month 3 given on p. 155. The schedule below is given during months 1, 2; 4, 5; 7, 8; 10, 11; and 13, 14 only.

	Day*															
	1	2	3	4	5	→	8	→	15	→	22	→	29	→	36	→
Actinomycin D 15 μg/kg IV	X	X	X	X	X											
Vincristine 1.5 mg/m^2 BSA† IV (max. dose 2.0 mg)							X		X		X		X		X	

	Day*								
	43	44	45	46	47	→	50	→	57
Actinomycin D 15 μg/kg IV	X	X	X	X	X				
Vincristine 1.5 mg/m^2 BSA† IV (max. dose 2.0 mg)	X						X		X

*X indicates day(s) to administer drug(s) indicated.

†BSA = body surface area.

SCHEDULE AND DOSE: Start with month 3 and repeat for months 6, 9, 12, and 15.

	Day*				
	1	**2**	**3**	**4**	**5**
Actinomycin D† 15 μg/kg IV *for 5 days*	X	X	X	X	X
Vincristine† 1.5 mg/m² BSA‡ IV *on day 1 and day 5*	X				X

*X indicates day(s) to administer drug(s) indicated.

†NOTE: Beginning with month 3 of therapy, actinomycin D is given for 5 days at the start of months 3, 6, 9, 12, and 15, and vincristine is given on days 1 and 5 concurrently with actinomycin D.

‡BSA = body surface area.

REFERENCES:

D'Angio, G. J., et al.: The treatment of Wilms' tumor—results of the national Wilms' tumor study, Cancer **38:**633-646, 1976.

Al-Rashid, R. A.: Chemotherapy of Wilms' tumor. In Pediatric cancer chemotherapy, Flushing, N.Y., 1979, Medical Examination Publishing Co., p. 214.

SOFT TISSUE SARCOMAS
Doxorubicin (Adriamycin) and dacarbazine (DTIC)

GENERAL USE: Soft tissue sarcomas

RESPONSE RATE: 42% (adult)

SCHEDULE AND DOSE: Repeat cycle every 3 weeks.

	Day*						
	1	2	3	4	5	→	21
Doxorubicin† 60 mg/m² BSA‡ IV	X					No therapy, 2-week rest period	
Dacarbazine 250 mg/m² BSA‡ IV	X	X	X	X	X		

*X indicates day(s) to administer drug(s) indicated.

†NOTE: In adult patients with total cumulative doses of doxorubicin of 550 mg/m² (or 450 mg/m² in patients with previously irradiated heart tissue) there is a more common occurrence of cardiomyopathy or CHF or both.

‡BSA = body surface area.

REFERENCE:

Gottlieb, J. A., et al.: Adriamycin used alone and in combination for soft tissue and bony sarcomas, Cancer Chemother. Rep. **6**:271-282, 1975.

Cyclophosphamide, vincristine (Oncovin), doxorubicin (Adriamycin), and dacarbazine (DTIC, DIC) (CY-VA-DIC)

GENERAL USE: Soft tissue sarcomas (adult)

RESPONSE RATE: 37%

SCHEDULE AND DOSE: Repeat cycle every 21 days.

	Day* 1	2	3	4	5	→	21†
Cyclophosphamide 500 mg/m² BSA‡ IV	X					No therapy, 2 weeks	
Vincristine 1.4 mg/m² BSA‡ (max. dose 2.0 mg)	X				X		
Doxorubicin§ 50 mg/m² BSA‡ IV	X						
Dacarbazine 250 mg/m² BSA‡ IV	X	X	X	X	X		

*X indicates day(s) to administer drug(s) indicated.
†May be delayed 1 week if recovery of the granulocytes and platelets is not complete by day 21.
‡BSA = body surface area.
§CAUTION: In adult patients when cyclophosphamide and adriamycin are given concurrently, with total cumulative doses of 450 mg/m² of doxorubicin there is a more common occurrence of cardiomyopathy or CHF or both.

REFERENCES:

Gottlieb, J., et al.: An effective new four drug combination regimen (CY-VA-DIC) for metastatic sarcomas, Proc. Am. Soc. Clin. Oncol. **15:**162 (abstract 713), 1974.

Wilbur, J. R., et al.: Chemotherapy of sarcomas, Cancer **36:**765-769, 1975.

Pinedo, H. M., et al.: Re-evaluation of the CYVADIC regimen for metastatic soft tissue sarcoma, Proc. Am. Soc. Clin. Oncol. **20:**346, 1979.

Vincristine, actinomycin D, and cyclophosphamide (pulse VAC)

GENERAL USE: Rhabdomyosarcoma and other soft tissue sarcomas
RESPONSE RATE: 95% (pediatric)
SCHEDULE AND DOSE:

	Week*													
	1	2	3	4	5	6	7	8	9	10	11	12	13	→
Vincristine 2 mg/m² BSA† IV, single dose (max. dose 2.0 mg)	X	X	X	X	X	X	X	X	X	X	X	X		Discontinue
Actinomycin D 0.015 mg/kg/day IV *for 5 days* (max. dose 0.5 mg/day)	X												X	Continue 5-day therapy every 3 months for 5 or 6 courses
Cyclophosphamide 10 mg/kg/day IV or orally *for 7 days*	X						X						X	Continue 7-day therapy every 6 weeks for 2 years

*X indicates week(s) to administer drug(s) indicated.
†BSA = body surface area.

REFERENCES:

Wilbur, J. R., et al.: Chemotherapy of sarcomas, Cancer **36:**765-769, 1975.
Maurer, J. M.: Rhabdomyosarcoma, Pediatr. Ann. **8:**35-48, 1979.

Vincristine, actinomycin D, and cyclophosphamide (Standard VAC)

GENERAL USE: Rhabdomyosarcoma and undifferentiated sarcoma
RESPONSE RATE: 68% pediatric, less than or equal to 20% adult
SCHEDULE AND DOSE:

	Week*													
	1	2	3	4	5	6	7	8	9	10	11	12	13	→
Vincristine 2 mg/m² BSA† IV, single dose (max. dose 2.0 mg)	X	X	X	X	X	X	X	X	X	X	X	X		Discontinue
Actinomycin D 0.015 mg/kg/day IV *for 5 days* (max. dose 0.5 mg/day)	X												X	Continue 5-day therapy every 3 months for 5 or 6 courses
Cyclophosphamide 2.5 mg/kg/day Orally *for 7 days*	X	X	X	X	X	X	X	X	X	X	X	X	X	Continue daily for 2 years

*X indicates week(s) to administer drug(s) indicated.
†BSA = body surface area.

REFERENCES:

Wilbur, J. R., et al.: Chemotherapy of sarcomas, Cancer **36**:765, 1975.
Maurer, H. M.: Rhabdomyosarcoma, Pediatr. Ann. **8**:35-48, 1979.

Vincristine and actinomycin D

GENERAL USE: Rhabdomyosarcoma (pediatric)

RESPONSE RATE: 86%

SCHEDULE AND DOSE:

	Day*									
	1	→ 5	→ 21	→ 28	→ 35	→ 42	→ 49	→ 56	→	63†
Actinomycin D 0.015 mg/kg IV	X Daily →								1-week rest period	
Vincristine 0.075 mg/kg IV			X	X	X	X	X	X		

*X indicates day(s) to administer drug(s) indicated.

†Repeat every 63 days (9 weeks) for 1 year (six cycles) *or* until there is evidence of recurrence or metastasis.

REFERENCE:

Heyn, R., et al.: The role of combined chemotherapy in the treatment of rhabdomyosarcoma in children, Cancer **34:**2128-2142, 1974.

Actinomycin D, vincristine, cyclophosphamide, and doxorubicin (Adriamycin) (T-2 protocol) (Memorial Sloan-Kettering)

GENERAL USE: Nonmetastatic rhabdomyosarcoma (pediatric)

RESPONSE RATE: 84%

SCHEDULE AND DOSE: Repeat cycle every 90 days for 2 years (8 cycles).

	Day*																
	1	→	5	→	21	22	23	→	54	→	60	→	67	→	74	→	90
Dactinomycin 450 $\mu g/m^2$ BSA† IV	X	Daily	→														
Doxorubicin‡ 20 mg/m^2 BSA† IV					X	X	X Cycles 2-7									No therapy, 2 weeks	
Vincristine 1.5 to 2.0 mg/m^2 BSA† IV (max. dose 2.0 mg)									X		X		X		X		
Cyclophosphamide 1200 mg/m^2 BSA† IV									X				X				

*X indicates day(s) to administer drug(s) indicated.

†BSA = body surface area.

‡NOTE: Doxorubicin is given in cycles 2 to 7 only. CAUTION: In pediatric patients with a total cumulative dose of doxorubicin of 350 mg/m^2 when given concurrently with cyclophosphamide there is a more common occurrence of cardiomyopathy or CHF or both.

REFERENCES:

Exelby, P. R.: Management of embryonal rhabodmyosarcoma in children, Surg. Clin. North Am. **54:**849-857, 1974.

Al-Rashid, R. A.: Pediatric cancer chemotherapy, Flushing, N.Y., 1979, Medical Examination Publishing Co., p. 255.

CENTRAL NERVOUS SYSTEM CANCER
Carmustine (BCNU)

GENERAL USE: Brain gliomas (adult and pediatric)

RESPONSE RATE: 46%

SCHEDULE AND DOSE: Continue cycle every 6 weeks until tumor regression.

	Week*													
	1	2	3	4	5	6	7	8	9	10	11	12	13	→
Carmustine† 100 mg/m² BSA‡ IV *for 2 days*	X						X						X	

*X indicates week(s) to administer drug(s) indicated.

†CAUTION: The nadir of carmustine (BCNU) may be *delayed* 6 weeks after drug administration.

‡BSA = body surface area.

REFERENCE:

Goldsmith, M. A., et al.: Glioblastoma multiforme—a review of therapy, Cancer Treat. Rev. **1**:153-165, 1974.

Lomustine (CCNU)

GENERAL USE: Brain gliomas (adult and pediatric)

RESPONSE RATE: 41%

SCHEDULE AND DOSE: Continue cycle every 6 weeks until tumor regression.

	Week*													
	1	**2**	**3**	**4**	**5**	**6**	**7**	**8**	**9**	**10**	**11**	**12**	**13**	→
Lomustine† 130 mg/m² BSA‡ Orally, single dose	X						X						X	

*X indicates week(s) to administer drug(s) indicated.
†CAUTION: The nadir of lomustine (CCNU) may be *delayed* 6 weeks after drug administration.
‡BSA = body surface area.

REFERENCE:

Goldsmith, M. A., et al.: Glioblastoma multiforme—a review of therapy, Cancer Treat. Rev. **1**:153-165, 1974.

Procarbazine

GENERAL USE: Brain gliomas

RESPONSE RATE: 50%

SCHEDULE AND DOSE: Repeat cycle every 28 days until tumor regression.

	Day*														
	1	2	3	4	5	6	7	8	9	10	11	12	13	14	→ 28
Procarbazine 100 mg/m^2 BSA† Orally	X	X	X	X	X	X	X	X	X	X	X	X	X	X	No therapy, 2 weeks

*X indicates day(s) to administer drugs indicated.
†BSA = body surface area.

REFERENCE:

Gutin, P. H., et al.: Phase II study of procarbazine, CCNU, and vincristine combination chemotherapy in the treatment of malignant brain tumors, Cancer **35:**1398-1404, 1975.

Teniposide (VM-26)

GENERAL USE: Brain gliomas—secondary therapy (pilot study)
RESPONSE RATE: 48%
SCHEDULE AND DOSE: Continue once weekly until tumor regression.

	Week*								
	1	2	3	4	5	6	7	8	→
Teniposide 100 to 130 mg/m² BSA† IV infusion in D5W over 30 minutes, single dose	X	X	X	X	X	X	X	X	

*X indicates week(s) to administer drug(s) indicated.
†BSA = body surface area.

REFERENCE:

Kessinger, A., et al.: VM-26 as a second drug in the treatment of brain gliomas, Proc. Am. Soc. Clin. Oncol. **20**:295, 1979.

Dexamethasone

GENERAL USE: Brain tumors—reduction of cerebral edema (adult and pediatric)

SCHEDULE AND DOSE:

	Day*							
	1	2	3	4	5	6	7	→
Dexamethasone† 4 to 16 mg Orally, IM or IV in divided doses	X	X	X	X	X	X	X	Continue daily

*X indicates day(s) to administer drug(s) indicated.
†See Section 7, Intracerebral Metastases, and Table 7-5.

REFERENCE:

Carter, S. K., et al.: Chemotherapy of cancer, New York, 1977, Wiley Medical Co., 1977, p. 84.

Cyclophosphamide and vincristine

GENERAL USE: Neuroblastoma

RESPONSE RATE: 55%

SCHEDULE AND DOSE:

	Week*											
	1	2	3	4	5	6	7	8	9	10	11	12†
Cyclophosphamide 1,000 mg/m² BSA‡ IV single dose	X		X		X		X		X		X	
Vincristine 1.5 mg/m² BSA‡ IV single dose (max. dose 2.0 mg)		X		X		X		X		X		X

*X indicates week(s) to administer drug(s) indicated.

†Continue alternating cyclophosphamide with vincristine for 6 months or longer after complete tumor regression or until evidence of progressive disease.

‡BSA = body surface area.

REFERENCES:

Sawitsky, et al.: Vincristine and cyclophosphamide therapy in generalized neuroblastoma, Am. J. Dis. Child. **119:**308-313, 1970.

James, D. H., et al.: Combination chemotherapy for childhood neuroblastoma, J.A.M.A. **194:**123-126, 1965.

MISCELLANEOUS MALIGNANCIES

Vincristine, bleomycin, methotrexate, hydrocortisone, 5-fluorouracil, leucovorin, and doxorubicin (Adriamycin)

GENERAL USE: Cancer of the head and neck

RESPONSE RATE: 82%

SCHEDULE AND DOSE:

	Hour*							
	0 →	12 →	15 →	18 →	26 →	32 →	38 →	44
Vincristine 2 mg IV (max. dose 2.0 mg)	X							
Doxorubicin 50 mg IV	X							
Bleomycin 60 mg IV infusion over 6 hours		X						
Methotrexate 100 mg IV		X	X	X				
Hydrocortisone 500 mg IV		X		X				
5-Fluorouracil 500 mg IV				X				
Leucovorin 15 mg IM					X	X	X	X

*X indicates hour(s) to administer drug(s) indicated.

REFERENCE:

Price, L. A., et al.: Improved results in combination chemotherapy of head and neck cancer, Proc. Am. Soc. Clin. Oncol. **18:**271, 1977.

Methotrexate, bleomycin, and cisplatin (cis-diamminedichloroplatinum) (MBD)

GENERAL USE: Advanced cancer of the head and neck

RESPONSE RATE: 63%

SCHEDULE AND DOSE: Repeat cycle every 21 days.

	Day*							
	1	→	4	→	8	→	15	16 → 21
Methotrexate 40 mg/m^2 BSA† IM	X						X	No therapy, 1 week
Bleomycin 10 mg IM	X				X		X	
Cisplatin‡ 50 mg/m^2 BSA† IV with hydration			X					

*X indicates day(s) to administer drug(s) indicated.
†BSA = body surface area.
‡Given 30 minutes after starting a 2-hour infusion of 2 liters of 5% dextrose in 0.45% sodium chloride containing 10 mEq KCl/liter. Furosemide 40 mg IV is given at the start of the infusion and 12.5 g of mannitol is given IV prior to cisplatin. (See Section 6, Renal Dysfunction.)

REFERENCES:

Kaplan, B. H., et al.: Chemotherapy of advanced cancer of the head and neck (HNCa) with methotrexate (M), bleomycin (B) and cis-diamminedichloroplatinum (D) in combination—MBD, Proc. Am. Soc. Clin. Oncol. **20:**384, 1979.

Vogl, S. E., et al.: Chemotherapy of advanced head and neck cancer with methotrexate, bleomycin and cis-diamminedichloroplatinum II in an effective outpatient schedule, Cancer **44:**26-31, 1979.

Doxorubicin (Adriamycin)

GENERAL USE: Thyroid carcinoma

RESPONSE RATE: 36%

SCHEDULE AND DOSE: Repeat every 21 days.

	Day*		
	1	⟶ 21†	
Doxorubicin‡ 60 to 75 mg/m² BSA§ IV as a single dose (or divided into 3 consecutive daily doses)	X	No therapy, 3 weeks	

*X indicates day(s) to administer drug indicated.

†May be delayed 1 week if recovery of the granulocytes and platelets is not complete by day 21.

‡CAUTION: In adult patients with total cumulative doses of 550 mg/m² of doxorubicin (or 450 mg/m² in patients with previously irradiated heart tissue) there is a more common occurrence of cardiomyopathy or CHF or both.

§BSA = body surface area.

REFERENCES:

Gottlieb, J., et al.: Chemotherapy of thyroid cancer with Adriamycin, N. Engl. J. Med. **290:**193-197, 1974.

Gottlieb, J., et al.: Chemotherapy of thyroid cancer, Cancer **30:**848-853, 1972.

Section 4

HORMONAL THERAPY

The use of hormones in cancer therapy has been largely empirical, probably because some tumors have been closely associated with endocrine pathogenesis, such as breast cancer. However, other tumors such as renal cell cancer do not have an endocrine basis and yet exhibit a small but real response to progestin hormones. This section will discuss the results of hormonal therapy in those tumors listed in Table 4-1.

BREAST CANCER

Breast cancer is the most common malignancy in the United States, Canada, and Europe. Hormonal therapy produces the best quality and duration of response in a substantial percentage of patients. Two general types of hormonal therapy are presently in use in breast cancer: (1) *additive therapy,* which consists of estrogens, antiestrogens, androgens, progestins, and corticosteroids, and (2) *ablative therapy,* which consists of oophorectomy, hypophysectomy, surgical adrenalectomy, and medical adrenalectomy with aminoglutethimide.

Strategy in the treatment of breast cancer

The sequential treatment of breast carcinoma has been notably changed by the development of the estrogen receptor assay.[1] Prior to this assay the response rate of all patients to any hormone manipulation ranged from 20% to 40%.[2] The relationship of response rate to the presence (ER+) or absence (ER−) of estrogen receptor binding, however, has separated patients into high-response and low-response groups.[3,4] The objective responses in advanced disease and ER status are shown in Table 4-2.[5] These results now allow the oncologist the benefit of predicting those patients who could be spared hormone therapy or a surgical procedure.

Even with positive ER data, as many as 40% of these patients may still not respond to hormonal therapy. Other receptors or markers such as progesterone and glucocorticoid receptors may increase the response predictability to almost 90%.[6,7] However, the value of multiple receptors requires

Table 4-1. General response of hormonal therapy in hormone responsive tumors*

Disease	Therapy	Response rate (%)
Breast cancer	Oophorectomy	30-45
	Adrenalectomy	40
	Hypophysectomy	40
	Estrogens	36
	Androgens	20
	Antiestrogens	40
	Progestins	25
	Glucocorticoids	20
Renal cell cancer	Progestins	16
Endometrial cancer	Progestins	37
Prostatic carcinoma	Estrogens	80 (subjective improvement)
Lymphoma	Prednisone (part of MOPP)	5
Leukemia, acute lymphocytic	Prednisone	63 (complete)
Multiple myeloma	Prednisone	10-20

*Hormone receptor status is not considered.

Table 4-2. Estrogen receptor status and response to hormone therapy*

Hormone therapy	ER+	ER−	ER±
Ablative surgery			
Adrenalectomy	40/76	4/41	3/8
Oophorectomy	28/43	2/74	0/2
Hypophysectomy	9/14	0/12	—
	77/133 (58%)	6/127 (5%)	3/10 (30%)
Hormone therapy			
Androgen	10/28	2/22	0/1
Estrogen	38/60	2/49	0/2
Glucocorticoid	15/32	0/19	—
	63/120 (52%)	4/90 (4%)	0/3
Antiestrogens			
Nafoxidine	12/17	0/16	—
Tamoxifen	18/40	5/27	—
	30/57 (53%)	5/43 (11%)	

*Modified from Legha.[5]

further study before these will be accepted markers for predicting response to treatment.

A rational approach to the management of metastatic breast cancer is diagrammed in Fig. 5. This scheme will probably be altered slightly in the near future by the development of even newer tumor markers if correlated with the current hormone receptor assays.

Currently the preferred initial treatment of the premenopausal patients is oophorectomy, which produces a 40% remission rate.[3] Patients with ER positivity will respond with a mean duration of response of approximately 12 months.[8] In the postmenopausal patient with positive estrogen receptor, the preferred treatment is additive hormone therapy with estrogens or antiestrogens, which gives about a 60% response for about 10 to 12 months.[8] Only 8% of estrogen receptor negative patients respond to additive therapy.[8] Patients who relapse from either estrogen or antiestrogen are usually treated with the other agent, if indicated.

Following relapse from a previous hormonal therapy, such as castration or additive hormone, the patient may next receive surgical adrenalectomy or hypophysectomy. Both approaches give between a 40% and 50% response

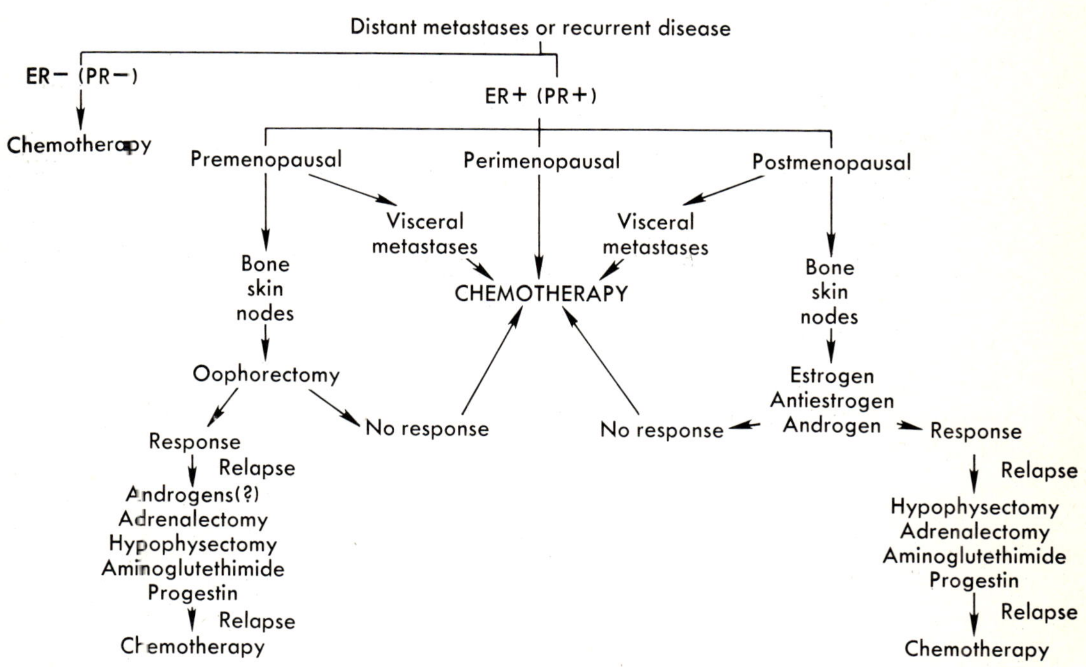

Fig. 5. General approach in treatment of breast cancer.

rate with median survival of about 2 years.[5,8] Some oncologists prefer the approach of using medical adrenalectomy prior to surgical adrenalectomy or hypophysectomy. Medical adrenalectomy is accomplished with the use of aminoglutethimide (Elipten), which is reported to give a 46% response rate in hormonally responsive cases.[9]

After relapse from surgical hormone maneuvers, progestins may be tried. They give a 20% response rate with minimal side effects.[10]

Chemotherapy is reserved for patients who develop visceral metastases or who have progressed rapidly or who are ER negative at the start of treatment.[11] The chemotherapy used for metastatic breast cancer is outlined in Section 3.

Hormones as additive therapy

Estrogens. Ethinyl estradiol and diethylstilbestrol (DES) are the most commonly used estrogens. Both drugs are given orally, although one estrogen preparation, Stilphostrol, is given intravenously if this route is necessary. Dose equivalents for Stilphostrol and DES have not been determined.[12] Oral estrogens initially cause nausea and vomiting, which usually diminish after the first 2 weeks of therapy.[13] If patient intolerance is observed, the dosage can be decreased by 50% and retitrated more slowly. Another potential problem from DES or ethinyl estradiol is salt and water retention, which can exacerbate congestive heart failure or hypertension. Mild diuretics, such as hydrochlorothiazide, may be added to manage fluid retention. Patients with a history of thromboembolic disease should probably not receive estrogens because of the increased risk of clotting. Such patients may receive adequate hormone therapy with antiestrogens while avoiding the risk of thromboembolism or stroke.[14]

Antiestrogens. Antiestrogens are primarily used in the treatment of metastatic breast cancer in postmenopausal women with positive estrogen receptors. As a class antiestrogens are nonsteroidal compounds, which are mainly derivatives of polycyclic phenols. The presumption that antiestrogens should be effective in premenopausal patients, an estrogen-rich milieu, rather than postmenopausal patients is countered by the favorable responses in the latter group.[5] It appears that although estrogen secretion is decreased considerably after menopause, the levels may fluctuate, and estrogen secretion may not stop completely.[15] The persistence of estrogens during the postmenopause period is probably due to the conversion of adrenal androgens to estrogens in the peripheral tissues.[15] Antiestrogens have been shown to block the uptake of the estrogen estradiol in human tumors.[16] Although the mechanism of action of antiestrogens is not completely understood, they bind to estrogen receptors in the cytosol of mammary tissue and eventually alter nuclear-directed protein synthesis.[17] The end result is a decrease in tumor replication. The antiestrogens that have been studied in breast cancer are clomiphene, nafoxidine, and tamoxifen.[5]

Tamoxifen is currently the only antiestrogen approved for clinical use in the United States. It is available as 10 mg oral tablets. In doses of 10 to 20 mg twice daily it produces a 50% to 60% objective regression in ER+ metastatic breast cancer.[5,18] Responses have been most frequent in postmenopausal patients with soft tissue metastases, while visceral and bone metastases respond less frequently.[19]

Tamoxifen is generally well tolerated with relatively uncommon side effects of hot flushes (14%) and nausea (10%).[5] Mild leukopenia and thrombocytopenia have been observed in 5% to 10% of cases; the myelosuppressive mechanism of tamoxifen is unknown.[20] About 10% of patients may elicit a tumor "flare" and hypercalcemia, as is seen occasionally in androgen or estrogen therapy. Vaginal bleeding is uncommon (5%) and skin rashes occasionally occur (20%). Treatment lasting longer than 1 year has led to decreased visual acuity because of corneal opacities and retinopathy.[21]

Androgens. Androgens are used in the treatment of perimenopausal and postmenopausal metastatic breast cancer. Responses are seen in 30% to 50% of patients with positive estrogen receptor protein and in less than 10% of patients with negative estrogen receptor.[22] The effectiveness of androgens is dependent on the site of the lesions and to some extent on the patient's age. The most beneficial responses are seen in patients with bone metastases.[21] Patients with soft-tissue or visceral metastases respond to a lower degree, 36% and 10% respectively. Generally response to androgen therapy is observed within 6 weeks.

Many androgen preparations are available (Table 4-3). Since no difference in response rate has been observed after either parenteral or oral therapy, the latter method seems preferable.[2,23] The most commonly used agents are fluoxymesterone, testosterone propionate, dromostanolone propionate, and testolactone. Testolactone differs from the other three agents in that it does not cause masculinization or fluid retention. However, it is the least effective of the androgens, 19% versus 30% for testosterone propionate, and responses are also surprisingly short (12 weeks).

Another androgen, calusterone, produces fewer virilizing side effects, but as with testolactone, responses occur in only 28% of patients and are extremely short (12 weeks).[24]

Androgen side effects include nausea and vomiting, virilization (hoarseness, acne, hirsutism), fluid retention, and increased libido. In addition, the 17-alkyl testosterone derivatives produce cholestatic jaundice, which is usually reversible upon discontinuation of therapy. In patients who may be

Table 4-3. Androgens commonly used in breast cancer

	Dose	Comment
Parenteral preparations		
Testosterone propionate (25, 50, 100 mg/ml in oil)	50-100 mg IM 3 times weekly	17-alkyl derivative
Testosterone enanthate (Delatestryl)	600-1,200 mg IM weekly	17-alkyl derivative
Testolactone (Teslac) 100 mg/ml	100 mg IM 3 times weekly	Nonhepatotoxic
Dromostanolone (Drolban) (25, 50 mg/ml)	100 mg IM 3 times weekly	Nonhepatotoxic
Nandrolone phenpropionate (Durabolin)	25-50 mg 3 times weekly	Nonhepatotoxic
Oral preparations		
Fluoxymesterone (Halotestin) 2, 5, 10 mg tablets	10-30 mg PO daily	17-alkyl derivative
Testolactone (Teslac) 50, 250 mg tablets	250 mg PO 4 times daily	Nonhepatotoxic

likely to respond to an androgen but should avoid hepatotoxicity, dromostanolone, nandrolone, or testolactone may be employed. As in estrogen therapy, hypercalcemia and tumor flare can occur, usually in the first week of treatment with androgens.[2,25]

Progestins. Progestins usually produce responses in 20% to 40% of unselected postmenopausal patients who have responded to previous hormonal manipulation.[2,26] In contrast to treatment with estrogens and androgens, soft-tissue metastases respond more frequently to progestins than do bone or visceral metastases.[26] Studies are in progress to define the role of progesterone receptors to predict response to exogenous progestins.[27] It is likely that the frequency of responses will increase in the presence of such protein-binding markers.

The following are preparations most commonly used (in order of popularity):

	Dose
1. Megestrol acetate (Megace) 20 and 40 mg tablets	40 mg 4 times daily orally
2. Medroxyprogesterone acetate (Depo-Provera) 50 mg/ml suspension	400-1000 mg/week IM
3. Hydroxyprogesterone caproate (Delalutin) 125 and 250 mg/ml suspension in oil	1 g twice weekly IM
4. Medroxyprogesterone acetate (Provera) 2.5 and 10 mg tablets	400-1000 mg/week orally

Side effects are uncommon and include nausea, sodium and fluid retention, and vaginal bleeding. In addition, tumor "flare" with associated hyper-

Table 4-4. Glucocorticoid side effects

Infections	Fungal, bacterial, viral
Mental reactions	Irritability, insomnia, depression
Cushingoid effects	Weight gain, trunkal obesity, moon facies, striae, acne, ecchymoses, poor wound healing
Gastrointestinal effects	Possible peptic ulcer disease, pancreatitis
Musculoskeletal effects	Muscle weakness, myopathy, osteoporosis, slowed linear growth in children
Metabolic disorder	Hyperglycemia, hyperlipidemia
Fluid and electrolyte imbalance	Edema, sodium retention, hypokalemia
Ophthalmologic effects	Glaucoma, cataracts

calcemia can occasionally occur. This reverses quickly within several days after discontinuation of therapy.

Glucocorticoids. Glucocorticoids play a small but important role in the treatment of metastatic breast cancer. Their use is usually reserved for the latter stages of disease or as a follow-up to other hormone therapy that has been effective initially. However, with the recent development of the glucocorticoid receptor and its potential predictive value, glucocorticoids may prove even more effective in selected patients than their usual 15% to 20% response rate.[17]

The most commonly used glucocorticoids are prednisone and dexamethasone. Both these agents produce less salt and water retention than hydrocortisone. Doses equivalent to 10 to 40 mg of prednisone produce responses in 15% to 20% of patients but for short periods of time, about 8 weeks.[2]

The adverse side effects ascribed to glucocorticoid therapy are listed in Table 4-4. They will *not* be discussed in detail in this manual.

Medical adrenalectomy with aminoglutethimide

Aminoglutethimide was originally developed as a sedative hypnotic and anticonvulsant in the early 1960s. Because it led to substantial adrenal insufficiency, it was withdrawn from clinical use until its recent resurgence in the treatment of advanced breast cancer. Although surgical adrenalectomy has been an established treatment for advanced breast cancer, many patients are poor candidates for this major surgical procedure. In addition, mortality is almost 10%. Thus "medical" adrenalectomy seems more attractive than surgery.

Aminoglutethimide inhibits steroidogenesis primarily by (1) blocking the conversion of cholesterol to pregnenolone in the adrenal gland and by (2) blocking Δ^4-androstenedione to estrone and estradiol in the peripheral tissues.[28,29] The end result of these actions is to decrease the extragonadal and adrenal production of estrogens and androgens and their effects on breast cancer. Aminoglutethimide does not affect gonadal hormone production and thus would fit into the scheme of breast cancer treatment in patients who are status-postoophorectomy or postmenopausal. Responses are seen in 26% to 55% of patients with positive estrogen-binding protein[30,31] and are best in patients with bone metastases. Doses of 250 mg four times daily can produce subjective responses (relief of bone pain) within 4 days. Objective tumor regression may last from 3 to 20 months and occurs predominantly in skin lesions but may also occur in bone and visceral lesions as well.[30]

Because aminoglutethimide decreases serum cortisol levels, reflex increases in ACTH occur, which can override the effect of the drug on the adrenal gland. Thus concurrent exogenous glucocorticoid must be administered along with aminoglutethimide.[32] Santen originally used replacement doses of dexamethasone because it did not interfere with the serum and urinary analysis of cortisol.[33] Unfortunately, aminoglutethimide was shown to enhance the hepatic metabolism (6-hydroxylation) of dexamethasone, and the dose of the latter had to be increased to between 2 and 3 mg per day. Since the interaction is variable among patients, adrenal suppression became difficult to control.

Recently Santen and co-workers demonstrated that hydrocortisone (40 mg daily) can be used as an effective replacement steroid, probably because 6-hydroxylation was not an important step in its metabolism,[34] whereas prednisone, prednisolone, and betamethasone would potentially interact with aminoglutethimide through 6-hydroxylation. The recommended dose of hydrocortisone is 20 mg at bedtime and 10 mg at 8 AM and 5 PM.

The usual side effects of aminoglutethimide are lethargy, ataxia, and nystagmus, which occur in about 40% of patients.[34] These can be controlled with dose reduction to 750 mg daily.[35] After long-term therapy, thyroid stimulating hormone (TSH) is suppressed and subsequent hypothyroidism may be evident, requiring thyroid hormone replacement.[36]

Adrenal suppression with the aminoglutethimide-hydrocortisone combination is reversible on discontinuation of therapy, but patients should be monitored for adequate recovery with dehydroepiandrosterone (DHEA).[37] The DHEA assay can be used to monitor effective adrenal suppression during aminoglutethimide-hydrocortisone therapy.[37]

PROSTATE CANCER

Estrogens are useful in the palliative management of metastatic prostatic carcinoma. Responses are seen in about 80% of patients with bone involvement and prostatic enlargement.[38] In most cases the treatment is palliative with responses lasting from 12 to 18 months.[38,39]

The mechanism of action of estrogen is not completely clear but is related to the inhibition of androgen synthesis, thus abolishing androgen stimulation of prostatic growth.[40]

The drug of choice is diethylstilbestrol (DES) in a dose of 1 to 3 mg three times daily. Higher doses (for example, 5 mg three times daily) are associated with increased mortality because of cardiovascular complications, such as pulmonary emboli and myocardial infarction.[41]

In patients who fail DES therapy, large doses of intravenous estrogen (Stilphostrol) may produce a response.[42] Initial doses of 500 to 1000 mg IV for 5 days are given followed by 250 to 1000 mg IV weekly. The drug should be administered over 30 to 60 minutes.[43]

The major complication from estrogen is cardiovascular, as discussed above. Acute side effects are nausea and vomiting, salt and water retention, and hypercalcemia. Other side effects include decreased libido and potency.

ENDOMETRIAL CARCINOMA

Progestins have almost a 40% response rate in endometrial cancer. A median duration of survival of 27 months occurs in responders and only 7 months in nonresponders.[44,45]

The mechanism of action of progestins is presumed to be a direct effect on endometrial tissue. Progesterone binding tumors may differentiate patients who are apt to respond.[46] Further study in this area is ongoing.

The progestins commonly used are the same as those listed in the section on breast cancer. Side effects are minimal as described previously.

RENAL CELL CARCINOMA (HYPERNEPHROMA)

Although no relation exists between the production of renal carcinomas and exogenous hormones, the progestin medroxyprogesterone acetate has been used in patients with metastatic disease. On the basis of progesterone-inhibited growth of transplantable renal adenocarcinomas in the hamster, a human study was done by Bloom and co-workers, who reported a 16% objective response rate as well as 55% subjective improvement.[47] Unfortunately, responders did not have an increased survival from progestin therapy, but the quality of life was enhanced by its palliation of bone pain and ureteral bleeding.

The dose of medroxyprogesterone is 500 to 1000 mg IM or orally weekly. Side effects are mild nausea or sterile abscesses in patients receiving injections.

LEUKEMIAS AND LYMPHOMAS

Glucocorticoids are well established as effective drugs in Hodgkin's disease, non-Hodgkin's lymphoma, and both acute and chronic leukemias.[47,48] In none of these diseases are they used alone. They offer a definite addition to the response rate, but their primary benefit is lack of myelosuppressive effect. Their long-term side effects are frequently avoided through the use of intermittent therapy. Good examples of combination regimens are MOPP, CVP, and VP (see Section 3).

Side effects of glucocorticoids are listed in the discussion on breast cancer (Table 4-4).

REFERENCES

1. Folca, P. J., et al.: Studies with tritium-labelled hexoestrol in advanced breast cancer, Lancet **2:**796-798, 1961.
2. Kennedy, B. J.: Hormonal therapies in breast cancer, Semin. Oncol. **1:**119-130, 1974.
3. McGuire, W. L., et al.: Hormone dependence in breast cancer, Metabolism **23:** 75-100, 1974.
4. Lippman, M.: Steroid hormone receptors in human malignancy, Life Sci. **18:** 143-152, 1976.
5. Legha, S. S., et al.: Hormonal therapy of breast cancer: new approaches and concepts, Ann. Intern. Med. **88:**69-77, 1978.
6. McGuire, W. L., et al.: Current status of estrogen and progesterone receptors in breast cancer, Cancer **39:**2934, 1977.
7. Allegra, J. C., et al.: Steroid hormone receptors in human breast cancer, Proc. Am. Assoc. Cancer Res. **19:**336, 1978.
8. McGuire, W. L., et al., editors: Estrogen receptors in human breast cancer, New York, 1975, Raven Press, pp. 1-7.
9. Harvey, A., et al.: A comparative trial of medical adrenalectomy vs. transphenoidal hypophysectomy in advanced breast cancer, Proc. Am. Assoc. Cancer Res. **17:**219 (abstract), 1976.
10. Ansfield, F. J., et al.: Further clinical studies with megestrol acetate in advanced breast cancer, Cancer **38:**53-55, 1976.
11. Carter, S. K., et al.: Chemotherapy of cancer, New York, 1977, John Wiley & Sons, pp. 138-148.
12. Dome Laboratories, West Haven, Conn., distributors of Stilphosterol, personal communication, May, 1980.
13. Carter, A. C., et al.: Diethylstilbestrol: recommended dosages for different categories of breast cancer patients, J.A.M.A. **237:**2079-2085, 1977.
14. Legha, S. S., et al.: Antiestrogens in the treatment of breast cancer, Cancer Treat. Rev. **3:**205-216, 1976.
15. Santen, R. J., et al.: Aminoglutethimide inhibits extraglandular estrogen production in postmenopausal women with breast carcinoma, J. Clin. Endocrinol. Metab. **47:**1257-1265, 1978.
16. Luman, C. B., et al.: Antioestrogens. A review, J. Clin. Endocrinol. Metab. **4:** 551-572, 1975.
17. Cash, R., et al.: Aminoglutethimide as an inhibitor of adrenal steroidgenesis: mechanism of action and therapeutic trial, J. Clin. Endocrinol. Metab. **27:**1239, 1967.
18. Kiang, D. T., et al.: Tamoxifen (antiestrogen) therapy in advanced breast cancer, Ann. Intern. Med. **88:**69, 1978.

19. Band, P., et al.: Treatment of advanced breast cancer with tamoxifen—10 mg BID. Preliminary report, Proc. Am. Assoc. Cancer Res. **17:**237, 1976.
20. Cole, M. P., et al.: Tamoxifen (ICI 46474) clinical experience in 129 patients with advanced breast cancer. In Namer, M., et al., editors: Hormones and breast cancer, Paris, 1976, INSERM, p. 245.
21. Kaiser-Kupfer, M. I., et al.: Tamoxifen retinopathy, Cancer Treat. Rep. **62:**315, 1978.
22. Henderson, I. C., and Canellos, G. P.: Cancer of the breast, N. Engl. J. Med. **302:** 78-90, 1980.
23. Kline, M. J., and Haskel, C. M.: Cancer chemotherapy, ed. 2, Philadelphia, 1975, W. B. Saunders Co.
24. Goldenberg, I. S., et al.: Androgenic therapy for advanced breast cancer in women, J.A.M.A. **223:**1267-1268, 1973.
25. Murad, F., and Gilman, A. G.: In Goodman, H., and Gilman, A. G., editors: Pharmacologic basis of therapeutics, ed. 5, New York, 1975, Macmillan Publishing Co., pp. 1451-1471.
26. Edelstyro, R. A.: Norethisterone in advanced breast cancer, Cancer **32:**1317, 1973.
27. Horowitz, K. B., et al.: In McGuire, W. L., Raymond, J. P., and Baulieu, F. E., editors: Progesterone receptor in normal and neoplastic tissues, New York, 1977, Raven Press.
28. Fishman, L. M., et al.: Effects of aminoglutethimide on adrenal function in man, J. Clin. Endocrinol. Metab. **27:**481, 1967.
29. Harvey, H. A., et al.: A comparative trial of transphenoidal hypophysectomy and estrogen suppression with aminoglutethimide in breast cancer, Cancer **43:**2207-2214, 1979.
30. Lipton, A., et al.: Medical adrenalectomy using aminoglutethimide and dexamethasone in advanced breast cancer, Cancer **33:**503-512, 1974.
31. Smith, I. E., et al.: Aminoglutethimide in treatment of metastatic breast carcinoma, Lancet **2:**646-649, 1978.
32. Santen, R. J., et al.: Kinetic, hormonal and clinical studies with aminoglutethimide in breast cancer, Cancer **39:**2948-2958, 1977.
33. Santen, R. J., et al.: Successful medical adrenalectomy with aminoglutethimide: role of altered drug metabolism, J.A.M.A. **230:**1661-1665, 1974.
34. Santen, R. J., et al.: Adrenal suppression with aminglutethimide. I. Differential effects of aminoglutethimide on glucocorticoid metabolism, J. Clin. Endocrinol. Metab. **45:**469-479, 1977.
35. Gale, K. E., et al.: Treatment of advanced breast cancer with aminoglutethimide, Clin. Res. **24:**376A, 1976.
36. Santen, R. J., et al.: Compensatory increase in TSH excretion without effect on prolactin secretion in patients treated with aminoglutethimide, J. Clin. Endocrinol. Metab. **45:**739-746, 1977.
37. Griffiths, C. T., et al.: Preliminary trial of aminoglutethimide in breast cancer, Cancer **32:**31-37, 1973.
38. Prout, G. R.: Prostate gland. In Holland, J. F., editor: Cancer medicine, Philadelphia, 1973, Lea & Febiger, pp. 1680-1694.
39. Chrisholm, G. D.: Conservative treatment of cancer of the prostate. In Castro, J. E., editor: The treatment of prostatic hypertrophy and neoplasia, Baltimore, 1974, University Park Press, pp. 121-146.

40. Pratt, W. B.: The steroid hormones. In Pratt, W. B., editor: The anticancer drugs, New York, 1979, Oxford University Press, pp. 195-197.
41. Bailar, J. C., et al.: Veterans Administration Cooperative Urological Research Group: estrogen treatment for cancer of the prostate—early results with 3 doses of diethylstilbestrol and placebo, Cancer **26:**257-261, 1970.
42. Carter, S. K.: Prostatic carcinoma. In Carter, S. K., et al., editors: Chemotherapy of cancer, New York, 1977, John Wiley & Sons, pp. 174-177.
43. Physicians' desk reference, vol. 34, Oradell, N.J., 1980, Medical Economics Co., pp. 841-842.
44. Reifenstein, E. C.: Hydroxyprogesterone caproate therapy in advanced endometrial cancer, Cancer **27:**485-502, 1971.
45. DeVita, V. T., et al.: Perspectives on research in gynecologic oncology. Treatment protocols, Cancer **38:**161-177, 1976.
46. Friedman, M. A., et al.: The clinical value of hormone receptor assays in malignant disease, Cancer Treat. Rev. **5:**185-194, 1978.
47. Bloom, H. J., et al.: Medroxyprogesterone acetate in the treatment of metastatic renal cancer, Br. J. Cancer **25:**250, 1971.
48. DeVita, V. T., et al.: Combination versus single-agent chemotherapy: a review of the basis for selection of drug treatment of cancer, Cancer **35:**98, 1975.
49. Talley, R. W.: Corticosteroids. In Holland, J. F., editor: Cancer medicine, Philadelphia, 1973, Lea & Febiger, pp. 933-945.

Section 5

DRUG PREPARATION AND ADMINISTRATION

This section is designed to aid clinicians in drug acquisition, drug name recognition, prescription writing, and drug preparation and administration. References to sources for this information are given at the end of the chapter. They should be referred to if further information is needed. The drugs have been alphabetized in two sections—Established Anticancer Drugs and Drugs in Early Investigation. Information on stability and on physical and chemical compatibility is included in the monographs. Biologic incompatibilities and drug toxicity are not included in this section; the reader is referred to Sections 6 and 9 for this information. Dosages cited in this section should not be used in place of those given in specific drug regimens outlined in Section 3.

ESTABLISHED ANTICANCER DRUGS

There are over thirty drugs that demonstrate activity against a variety of tumors. The selection of a single agent or combination of drugs is based primarily on experience derived from clinical trials. The standard as well as new regimens were outlined in Section 3. This discussion outlines the important physical and chemical factors that affect the preparation and administration of the established antineoplastic agents. The following drug monographs were collated from information in the literature as well as from information received from the major cancer centers throughout the United States.

L-Asparaginase

SYNONYMS: Elspar, L-ASP, crasnitin, asparaginase, NSC-109229, amidohydrolase, coalspase[3,9]

MANUFACTURER: Merck Sharp & Dohme

DOSAGE FORMS AND STRENGTHS: 10,000 IU vial with 80 mg of mannitol[1]

STORAGE: Refrigerate (2° to 8° C).[1,2]

SOLUTION PREPARATION: Reconstitute with 5 ml of unpreserved normal saline solution or sterile water for injection to produce a 2,000 unit/ml concentration for IV administration. Reconstitute with 2 ml of sodium chloride 0.9% for IM administration. Gently rotate the vial to assure complete dissolution. Vigorous shaking may result in the loss of some potency. *Cloudy solutions should be discarded.*[1,2,4]

STABILITY:

Prior to mixing: Intact vials are stable for 2 years at refrigeration temperature (2° to 8° C) and at least 6 weeks at room temperature (22° to 25° C).[4]

At different concentrations: Reconstituted solution is stable for 20 days at room temperature and at refrigerated temperatures. When it is further diluted with normal saline solution or 5% dextrose injection to 35 IU/ml, stability becomes 4 days at room temperature and at refrigerated temperatures. The manufacturer recommends that the reconstituted solution should be used within 8 hours after preparation as long as it is clear. Discard turbid solutions.[1,4]

DOSAGE: As single agent: Adult: 5,000 to 10,000 units/m^2 daily for 7 days every 3 weeks or 10,000 to 40,000 units/m^2 as a single dose every 2 to 3 weeks. Pediatrics: 500 to 6,000 units/m^2 daily for 14 days as induction or consolidation; 10,000 units/m^2 twice weekly during remission induction; 60,000 units/m^2 every second day for 12 doses in non-Hodgkin's lymphoma. When L-asparaginase is used as the sole induction agent for adults or children, the recommended dosage regimen is 200 IU/kg daily IV for 28 days.[2,6]

ROUTES OF ADMINISTRATION: IV push, IV infusion, or IM. With IM the volume should be limited to 2 ml at a single injection site. IM route is less likely to result in anaphylaxis. If the volume is greater than 2 ml, two injection sites should be used. IV infusion should be given over a period of 30 minutes or more through the side arm of a running IV infusion of sodium chloride or 5% dextrose injection.[1,6]

SPECIAL PRECAUTIONS: Anaphylactic reactions may occur. Intradermal skin testing should be done prior to the initial administration of the drug and between doses if the drug interval is a week or more. Intradermal skin testing does not preclude the possibility of developing an allergic reaction. Withdraw 0.1 ml of the reconstituted solution as described above in Solution Preparation for IV solutions and inject 0.1 ml into a vial containing 9.9 ml of diluent, resulting in a skin test solution of 20 IU/ml. Use 0.1 ml of this solution (about 2 IU) for the intradermal skin test. The test site should be observed for at least 1 hour for the appearance of a wheal or erythema, either of which indicates a positive reaction.[1,6]

COMPATIBILITY: 5% dextrose injection, USP, sodium chloride injection, USP, and sterile water for injection, USP.[1,6]

Bleomycin sulfate

SYNONYMS: Blenoxane, Bleo, BLM-2, NSC-125066[3,5,9]

MANUFACTURER: Bristol[5]

DOSAGE FORMS AND STRENGTHS: For injection: 15 units (15 mg) of bleomycin sulfate powder per ampule. It is a cream-colored, hygroscopic powder.[5]

STORAGE: Room temperature.[1,5]

SOLUTION PREPARATION:

For IM or SC: Reconstitute ampule with 1 to 5 ml of sterile water for injection, USP, *or* sodium chloride for injection, USP, *or* 5% dextrose injection, USP, *or* bacteriostatic water for injection, USP, to yield a solution containing 3 to 15 units (3 to 15 mg)/ml.[1,5,6]

For IV or intra-arterial injection: Reconstitute ampule with a minimum of 5 ml of sodium chloride for injection, USP, *or* 5% dextrose injection, USP, to yield a solution of 3 units (3 mg)/ml.[1,5,6]

STABILITY:

Prior to mixing: Unopened ampules are stable for 18 months.[5]

At different concentrations: Reconstituted solutions are stable for 2 weeks at room temperature and 4 weeks when stored at 2° to 8° C (use bacteriostatic diluent). But because of the possibility of contamination it has been recommended that solutions be used immediately and leftover portions be discarded or transferred aseptically into a sterile, sealed container. For IV infusions further dilute with 50 to 100 ml of 5% dextrose injection, USP, or sodium chloride 0.9%.[1,8,28]

pH: Varies from 4.5 to 6.0 depending on the diluent.[8]

DOSAGE: Usual SC, IM, or IV dose: 0.25 to 0.50 units/kg (10 to 20 units/m^2) once or twice weekly. Continuous IV infusion: up to 15 to 20 units/m^2 over 24 hours for 5 to 14 days. Intra-arterial: usual dose, 10 to 20 units/m^2 over 12 to 24 hours for 5 to 14 days. Intracavitary: 15 to 240 units in 100 ml normal saline once per course. Usual dose, 60 to 120 units. See Special Precautions given below before administration in lymphoma patients and the elderly.[1,5,8]

ROUTES OF ADMINISTRATION: SC, IM, IV, intra-arterial, and intracavitary injections. Rate of Infusion: IV push and intra-arterial injections should be given slowly over a 10-minute period. IV infusions can be given over 15 to 30 minutes or slowly over 24 hours.[1,5,8]

SPECIAL PRECAUTIONS:

1. Pulmonary fibrosis is the most severe toxicity of bleomycin; even though it is found mostly in elderly patients and those receiving

greater than 400 units total cumulative dose, it is unpredictable. It presents itself initially as pneumonitis and can progress to death.

2. In 1% of lymphoma patients a severe idiosyncratic reaction consisting of hypotension, mental confusion, fever, chills, and wheezing has occurred. A test dose of 1 to 5 units 24 hours apart for two doses should be given to lymphoma patients before therapeutic doses are given.
3. Patients who experience fever and chills, which are common side effects with bleomycin injections, can be given Benadryl 50 mg orally 30 minutes prior to bleomycin administration to minimize these symptoms. Safe use in pregnancy has not been established.[5,8]

COMPATIBILITY: Sterile water for injection, USP, dextrose 5% in water for injection, USP, and sodium chloride 0.9% for injection, USP, have been recommended as diluents for bleomycin sulfate. Bleomycin has been found to be compatible with heparin sulfate, 100 to 1,000 units/ml in 5% dextrose.[1,5,8]

INCOMPATIBILITY: Bleomycin sulfate is inactivated in vitro by agents containing sulfhydryl groups, hydrogen peroxide, and ascorbic acid.[8]

Busulfan

SYNONYMS: Myleran, BUS, BSF, busulphan, BAN, NSC-750[7,9]

MANUFACTURER: Burroughs Wellcome[5]

DOSAGE FORMS AND STRENGTHS: 2 mg white scored tablets[5]

STORAGE: Room temperature.[2,5]

STABILITY: Tablets are stable for 1 year.[2]

DOSAGE: As a single agent: Usual adult dosage is 4 to 8 mg daily, taken by mouth, but doses ranging from 1 to 12 mg daily have been used. Alternatively, some clinicians have recommended dosages of 0.065 to 0.1 mg/kg daily. There is little agreement on whether busulfan should be administered continually or intermittently. With both dosage schedules, WBCs and platelets must be monitored at least every week. Therapy is discontinued when the leukocyte count falls below 10,000/mm^3. If continual therapy (maintenance) is used, 1 to 3 mg daily is recommended by the manufacturer if the remission is less than 3 months, while others suggest a maintenance dosage range from 2 mg weekly to 4 mg daily to prevent rapid relapses. Blood counts are monitored monthly, and therapy is discontinued when the leukocyte count falls below 50,000/mm^3. Pediatric dosage range: 0.06 to 0.120 mg/kg daily. Alternatively, 1.8 to 4.6 mg/m^2 daily has been recommended.[5,8]

ROUTES OF ADMINISTRATION: Oral route only[5]

SPECIAL PRECAUTIONS: Weekly blood counts (monthly counts during maintenance schedule) are essential while patient is on busulfan to prevent unanticipated severe myelosuppression. Drug is known to have delayed refractory pancytopenia. Busulfan is potentially teratogenic.[5,8]

Carmustine

SYNONYMS: BiCNU, BCNU, bischloroethyl nitrosourea, NSC-409962[5,9]
MANUFACTURER: Bristol[5]
DOSAGE FORMS AND STRENGTHS: 100 mg vial for injection with a separate 3 ml vial of absolute alcohol as the sterile diluent[5]
STORAGE: Refrigerate and protect from light.[1,5]
SOLUTION PREPARATION: Add the accompanying 3 ml vial of absolute alcohol to the carmustine powder. Add 27 ml of sterile water for injection, USP, or sodium chloride for injection, USP, to yield a 3.3 mg/ml solution (or add the 3 ml of absolute alcohol and then 17 ml of sterile water for injection, USP, to yield a 5 mg/ml solution). A clear, colorless solution should result. These concentrations should be further diluted with at least 100 to 200 ml of sodium chloride for injection, USP, or 5% dextrose for injection, USP, for drug administration. Carmustine should be protected from light.[1,4,5]
STABILITY:

Prior to mixing: Unopened vials are stable for 4 years under refrigeration and protected from light. When carmustine is kept at room temperature and protected from light, approximately 3% degradation per 36 days occurs. Exposure to temperatures of 27° C (80.6° F) or greater will result in liquefication of the drug. An oily film will appear on the vial.[1,4,5] *If this occurs, the drug should be discarded.*

At different concentrations[1,4,5]:

Concentration	Temperature	Time	Decomposition
3.3 mg/ml	2°-8° C	24 hr	4%
	20° C	3 hr	6%
	20° C	6 hr	8%
Further dilution in 500 ml of sodium chloride for injection, USP, or 5% dextrose injection, USP	2°-8° C	48 hr	Stable
	20° C	2 hr	4%

pH: 5.6 to 6.0 at 3.3 mg/ml concentration[1,5]
DOSAGE: As single agent: In previously untreated patients 200 mg/m² is given every 6 weeks as a single dose or divided into daily injections such as 100 mg/m² on 2 successive days.[5] A dosage of 200 to 300 mg/m² IV given every 6 to 8 weeks has also been reported.[2] With other neoplastic agents, doses of 30 to 60 mg/m² every 6 weeks are frequently used.
ROUTES OF ADMINISTRATION: Should be administered by IV drip over a 1- to 2-hour period. Short infusions over 15 to 45 minutes can be used. Local

burning pain at the site of injection or along the course of the vein and venospasms occur commonly and can be minimized by slowing the rate of the infusion and further dilution of the drug. Rapid IV infusion may produce intensive flushing of the skin and suffusion of the conjunctiva. These effects occur within 2 hours and may persist for 4 hours after carmustine administration.[5]

SPECIAL PRECAUTIONS: Carmustine has delayed and cumulative bone marrow toxicity and should not be given any more frequently than every 6 weeks by an experienced individual. It should not be given until platelets and leukocytes have returned to acceptable levels (platelets > 100,000/mm^3 and leukocytes > 4,000/mm^3). Hypotension may occur.[5,2] Avoid contact with skin because brown staining results.[2]

COMPATIBILITY: Carmustine is slightly soluble in water, freely soluble in alcohol, and highly soluble in lipids. Carmustine is also compatible with sodium chloride for injection, USP, and 5% dextrose for injection, USP.[1,5]

SPECIAL APPLICATIONS: In the treatment of mycosis fungoides, carmustine in concentrations of 0.1% to 0.4% in 95% alcohol has been applied topically 1 to 2 times daily for 2 weeks. Total dosage should not exceed 200 mg per week for 6 weeks. After the dosage limit has been met, a rest interval of 4 weeks should follow.[65]

Chlorambucil

SYNONYMS: Leukeran, CHL, CB-1348, NSC-3088[3,5,9]

MANUFACTURER: Burroughs Wellcome[5]

DOSAGE FORMS AND STRENGTHS: 2 mg sugar-coated tablets[5]

STORAGE: Room temperature.[2]

STABILITY: Tablets are chemically stable for 1 year at room temperature.[2]

DOSAGE: As a single agent: Usual oral dose is 0.1 to 0.2 mg/kg daily for 3 to 6 weeks as required (4 to 10 mg daily for the average patient). The entire daily dose may be given at one time. These dosages are for initiation of therapy or for short courses of treatment. When lymphocytic infiltration of the bone marrow is present or bone marrow is hypoplastic, do not exceed 0.1 mg/kg daily (about 6 mg for the average patient). Short courses of treatment are safer than continuous maintenance therapy, although both methods have been effective. If maintenance dosage is used, it should not exceed 0.1 mg/kg daily and may be as low as 0.03 mg/kg daily (usually 2 to 4 mg daily or less).[5,8]

ROUTES OF ADMINISTRATION: Oral route only[5]

SPECIAL PRECAUTIONS: Blood counts should be taken weekly to avoid possible severe hematologic toxicity from occurring.[5,8]

Chlorotrianisene

SYNONYMS: Tace, NSC-10108[5,9]
MANUFACTURER: Merrell-National[5]
DOSAGE FORMS AND STRENGTHS: 12, 25, and 72 mg capsules.[5]
STORAGE: Store capsules in well-closed containers, protected from excessive heat and cold, in an area with no more than 50% humidity.[8]
DOSAGE: Prostatic carcinoma: 12 to 25 mg/day orally[5]
ROUTES OF ADMINISTRATION: Oral route only[5]

Cisplatin

SYNONYMS: Platinol; platinum, diamminedichloro-; CPDD; PDD; CPD; DDP; CACP; NSC-119875; cis-diamminedichloroplatinum (II); cis-DDP; cis-platinum[1,3,4,9]
MANUFACTURER: Bristol; Division of Cancer Treatment, National Cancer Institute[1,4]
DOSAGE FORMS AND STRENGTHS: 10 mg vial; 10 and 25 mg vials (investigational)[1,4]
STORAGE: Refrigerate.[1,4]
SOLUTION PREPARATION: Add 10 ml of sterile water for injection, USP, to both the commercial and investigational 10 mg vials and 24.5 ml to the investigational 25 mg vial to result in a concentration of 1 mg/ml (do not refrigerate the reconstituted solutions). Further dilute the reconstituted solutions in 50 to 250 ml of 5% dextrose in sodium chloride 0.9% injection, USP, or 5% dextrose in sodium chloride 0.45% injection, USP, or 5% mannitol with sodium chloride 0.45% or 0.9% or in sodium chloride 0.45%. *Do not use* intravenous solutions that *do not* contain chloride ions for administration of cisplatin. It is not recommended to add bicarbonate to cisplatin to adjust the pH of the solution, because of a precipitation that forms in 48 hours.[1,4]
STABILITY: Intact vials are stable for 12 months at room temperature and for 2 years when refrigerated. The commercial 10 mg vial is stable for 20 hours at room temperature after reconstitution. The investigational 10 mg and 25 mg vials are stable for 24 hours at room temperature after reconstitution. It is questionable whether light has any significant effect on cisplatin. The manufacturer recommends protecting it from direct sunlight.[1,4,28]
pH: 3.5 to 5.5 reconstituted solution[1,4]
DOSAGE: (a) 50 to 75 mg/m^2 once every 3 weeks; (b) 15 to 20 mg/m^2 daily for 5 days every 3 to 4 weeks; (c) up to 125 mg/m^2 every 4 to 6 weeks as a single dose or divided over 2 to 5 days.[1,2]

ROUTES OF ADMINISTRATION: IV push or by IV infusion. The IV infusion should be given over 30 to 60 minutes. It is essential that patients are well hydrated and have adequate renal function before receiving the drug and after drug administration. The drug is commonly given with mannitol or Lasix or both. (See Section 6, Renal Dysfunction.)[1,28]

COMPATIBILITY: 5% dextrose in sodium chloride 0.9%, 5% dextrose in sodium chloride 0.45%, 5% mannitol with sodium chloride 0.9% or 0.45%, sodium chloride 0.45%, and sodium chloride 0.9%[1,4]

INCOMPATIBILITY: 5% dextrose injection, USP,[34] sodium bicarbonate, any solution with *low* or *no* chloride ion content, and metal aluminum (see Special Precautions).[1,4]

SPECIAL PRECAUTIONS: Cisplatin should be administered with needles, syringes, catheters, and sets that are free of the metal aluminum. Cisplatin interacts with aluminum forming a black precipitate. Stainless steel and plated brass do not observably react with cisplatin in 24 hours.[1]

Cyclophosphamide

SYNONYMS: Cytoxan, CYC, Endoxan, CTX, CYT, CPM, NSC-26271[5,9]

MANUFACTURER: Mead Johnson[5]

DOSAGE FORMS AND STRENGTHS: For injection: 100, 200, and 500 mg vials. Tablets: 25 and 50 mg white and blue speckled.[5]

STORAGE: All products should be stored at room temperature (36° to 90° F).[2]

SOLUTION PREPARATION: Reconstitute the vials with sterile water for injection, USP, or bacteriostatic water for injection, USP (paraben-preserved only), in the following amounts: to the 100 mg vial add 5 ml of diluent; to the 200 mg vial add 10 ml of diluent; to the 500 mg vial add 25 ml of diluent. Shake the vials vigorously to dissolve the powder. The resultant solutions have a concentration of 20 mg/ml.[1,5,8]

Extemporaneous oral liquid preparations containing 1 mg/ml or 5 mg/ml may be prepared by dissolving the powder for injection in aromatic elixir, USP. Store under refrigeration and use within 14 days.[5,8]

STABILITY: At different concentrations reconstituted solutions are stable for 24 hours when stored at room temperature and for 6 days under refrigeration. If reconstituted to a concentration of 21 mg/ml with sterile water for injection, USP, or bacteriostatic water for injection, USP (paraben-preserved), less than 1.5% of cyclophosphamide decomposition will occur within 8 hours at 24° to 27° C and within 6 days at 5° C.[31] Solutions of 21 mg/ml may be heated to 50° C or 60° C for 15 minutes and have negligible loss of potency. Heating the solutions to 70° C or 80° C for 15 minutes, however, results in decomposition equal to or greater than 10%. The use of heat to speed dissolution is therefore not recommended.[1,30]

PH: Reconstituted solution, 3.9 to 6.7[1]

DOSAGE: As a single agent: 500 to 1500 mg/m² IV every 2 to 4 weeks or 10 to 20 mg/kg IV daily for 2 to 5 days every 3 weeks. If induction therapy is administered orally, the usual dose is 1 to 5 mg/kg daily. Patients with compromised bone marrow function may require a reduction in the initial loading dose by 33% to 50%. Adult maintenance dosage has various schedules. Doses consist of 10 to 15 mg/kg IV every 7 to 10 days, 3 to 5 mg/kg IV twice weekly, or 1 to 5 mg/kg orally per day. Children: Initial dose is 2 to 3 mg/kg/24 hours (60 to 90 mg/m²/24 hours) orally or IV for 6 or more days. Resistant neoplasms: 4 to 8 mg/kg/24 hours (125 to 250 mg/m²/24 hours) orally or IV for 6 days. Maintenance: 2 to 5 mg/kg/week (50 to 150 mg/m² twice weekly orally).[2,5,8,66]

ROUTES OF ADMINISTRATION: Primarily orally, direct IV, or IV infusion; less frequently IM, intrapleural, and intraperitoneal. Some clinicians believe the drug should not be administered via routes that bypass activation in the liver.[8]

SPECIAL PRECAUTIONS: Administer only a clear solution. May cause dizziness if given too rapidly intravenously. The patient should be well hydrated before and 72 hours after administration to reduce the possibility of hemorrhagic cystitis developing. Cyclophosphamide is potentially teratogenic and is excreted in breast milk.[5,8]

COMPATIBILITY: Dextrose 5% in water, sodium chloride 0.9%, and dextrose 5% in sodium chloride 0.9% have been recommended as diluents for IV infusions. Amino acids 4.25%, dextrose 25%.[1,5]

Cytarabine

SYNONYMS: Cytosar-U, cytosine arabinoside, Ara-C, C.A., arabinosyl cytosine, NSC-63878[5,7,9]

MANUFACTURER: Upjohn[1,5]

DOSAGE FORMS AND STRENGTHS: For injection: 100 and 500 mg multidose vials[5]

STORAGE: Refrigerate. However, studies have shown that cytarabine can be stored at room temperature not exceeding 25° C for 36 months.[1,5]

SOLUTION PREPARATION: The 100 mg vial is reconstituted with 5 ml of bacteriostatic water for injection, USP, containing benzyl alcohol 0.9% to yield a 20 mg/ml solution, and the 500 mg vial is reconstituted with 10 ml of bacteriostatic water for injection, USP, to yield a 50 mg/ml solution. Minimum dilution volumes of 1 to 2 ml can be used. Other diluents acceptable are normal saline solution, 5% dextrose for injection, USP, Elliott's B solution, and Ringer's injection, lactated. Hazy solutions should be discarded.[1,5]

STABILITY:

Prior to mixing: Unreconstituted vials have an expiration date of 2 years.[1,8] At room temperature not exceeding 25° C no potency loss occurs for at least 36 months or more.[1,12]

At different concentrations: The reconstituted solution is stable for 48 hours at room temperature.[5] However, studies have shown the stability at this concentration to be good for several weeks and months. One study revealed a 90% potency of cytarabine for 6.5 months at a pH of 6.9 at 25° C.[13] Cytarabine decomposes about 10 times faster in alkaline solutions than in acid solutions.[13] At a concentration of 500 mg/liter, cytarabine is stable for 7 days at room temperature in dextrose 5% in water, sodium chloride 0.9%, and sterile water for injection, USP.[1]

pH: Reconstituted solution, pH 5; 2.5 mg/ml in Elliott's B solution, pH 7; 2.5 mg/ml in Ringer's injection, lactated, pH 5.6; 2.5 mg/ml in sodium chloride 0.9%, pH 5.3[1]

DOSAGE: Most commonly used in doses of 100 mg/m^2 to 200 mg/m^2 per day given for 5 to 10 days either by continuous IV infusion or by IV push in divided doses every 6 to 8 hours for acute leukemia *inductions* every 2 to 3 weeks. Higher doses of 4 mg/kg IV have been reported. For *maintenance therapy,* weekly or semiweekly SC injections of 1 mg/kg are used, which may be increased to 2 mg/kg daily.[2,5] For *IT injections for CNS metastasis* in leukemia and lymphoma, doses range from 4.5 mg/m^2 to 73 mg/m^2 given at 3- to 7-day intervals. At doses above 27 mg/m^2 side effects are more likely to appear. Doses of 5 to 10 mg/m^2 are most commonly employed.[67,68]

ROUTES OF ADMINISTRATION: Doses are administered by direct IV, IV infusion, SC, or IT injection. A patient receiving rapid IV injections can tolerate higher total doses as compared to patients receiving IV infusions but will experience a higher frequency of nausea and vomiting. Even though bone marrow depression appears to occur more frequently in patients receiving IV infusions rather than rapid IV injections, pharmacologically IV infusions maximize the therapeutic effect of cytarabine in patients. Children appear to tolerate higher doses than adults do; where dose ranges are quoted, children should receive the higher dose and adults the lower.[5,67]

The minimum dilution volumes (1 to 2 ml) are used for IM and SC routes. IT solutions should be prepared with preservative-free solutions such as Elliott's B solution or Ringer's lactate, USP. Volumes of 5 to 10 ml are most commonly employed.[1,67]

SPECIAL PRECAUTIONS: Cloudy or hazy solutions should be discarded. Cytarabine is potentially teratogenic.[5]

COMPATIBILITY: Dextrose 5% in water; sodium chloride 0.9%; water for injection, USP; amino acids 4.25%; dextrose 25%; dextrose 5% in Ringer's injection, lactated; dextrose 5% in sodium chloride 0.9%; Ringer's injection, lactated; *1 g cephalothin* in 1,000 ml 5% dextrose in water; *200 mg methotrexate* in 1,000 ml 5% dextrose in water; *250 mg methylprednisolone sodium succinate* in 1,000 ml of 5% dextrose in normal saline, 10% dextrose in normal saline, or normal saline; *200 mg prednisolone sodium phosphate* in 1,000 ml of 5% dextrose in water; 4 mg *vincristine sulfate* in 1,000 ml of 5% dextrose in water[1]

INCOMPATIBILITY: 250 mg 5-fluorouracil in 1 liter of 5% dextrose in water; 250 mg methylprednisolone in 1,000 ml of Ringer's injection or sodium lactate 1/6M.

Dacarbazine

SYNONYMS: DTIC-Dome, DIC, NSC-45388, imidazole carboxamide[5,9]

MANUFACTURER: Dome Division of Miles Laboratories[5]

DOSAGE FORMS AND STRENGTHS: Injection: 100 and 200 mg vials[5]

STORAGE: Refrigerate and protect from light.[8,38] Stable at room temperature 6 to 8 months.[2]

SOLUTION PREPARATION: Add 9.9 ml sterile water for injection, USP, to the 100 mg vial and 19.7 ml to the 200 mg vial to produce a 10 mg/ml solution. If necessary, either strength may be reconstituted with a minimum of 2 ml. The reconstituted solution may be further diluted with 5% dextrose in water, USP, or sodium chloride 0.9% to result in a 50 to 250 ml volume for IV infusion.[1,5,38]

STABILITY:

Prior to mixing: Dacarbazine is stable 4 years when refrigerated (2° to 8° C) and protected from light. At room temperature it is stable for 4 to 6 months in the intact vials.[1,2]

At different concentrations: The manufacturer states reconstituted solutions are stable for 8 hours at room temperature and 72 hours refrigerated.[5] Other studies have revealed that the reconstituted solutions are stable at least 24 hours at room temperature (1% decomposition) and at least 96 hours under refrigeration (less than 1% decomposition) protected from light. With further dilution with 5% dextrose in water or normal saline solution to 50 to 250 ml volumes the solution is stable 24 hours protected from light, at room temperature or in refrigeration. Without light protection there is a 5% decomposition over a 24-hour period at room temperature. Extensive decomposition can be noted by a color change from pale yellow to pink in the solution.[1,8]

pH: 3-4.0, reconstituted solutions with sterile water for injection, USP[5]

DOSAGE: 2 to 4.5 mg/kg IV per day for 10 days every 4 weeks *or* 250 mg/m^2 IV for 5 days every 3 weeks *or* 850 to 1,000 mg/m^2 IV one time only (in combination with other agents, i.e., ABVD regimen, to minimize toxicity) every 3 weeks. Use lower doses in patients with impaired marrow or renal function. (See Section 6, Dose Modification in Renal or Hepatic Disease.)[5,38]

ROUTES OF ADMINISTRATION: IV only. Dacarbazine can be given by IV push over 1 to 2 minutes or by IV infusion of 50 to 250 ml over 15 to 30 minutes. Infusions are generally less painful than rapid IV pushes.[1,5]

SPECIAL PRECAUTIONS: Protect from light. Avoid extravasation. Severe necrosis may result.[1,5]

COMPATIBILITY: 5% dextrose in water and normal saline solution as diluents[1]

INCOMPATIBILITY: Forms an immediate precipitate with hydrocortisone sodium succinate (Solu-Cortef).[69]

Dactinomycin

SYNONYMS: Cosmegen, actinomycin D, ACT-D, ACT, DACT, ACD, NSC-3053[5,9]

MANUFACTURER: Merck Sharp & Dohme[5]

DOSAGE FORMS AND STRENGTHS: 0.5 mg vials[1]

STORAGE: Room temperature. Protect from light.[1,8]

SOLUTION PREPARATION: Reconstitute with 1.1 ml of sterile water for injection, USP (preservative free), to yield a solution with a concentration of 0.5 mg/ml.[1,8] *Only sterile water for injection without preservative should be used as the solvent because other solvents may cause precipitation.*[14]

STABILITY:

Prior to mixing: Dactinomycin is stable for more than 1 year at room temperature when protected from light.[1,8]

At different concentrations: The reconstituted solution is also stable for 1 year at room temperature; however, it contains no preservative, so it has been suggested that unused portions be discarded within 8 hours.[1,8,10]

pH: 5.5 to 7.0 in a 1:2,000 solution[1]

DOSAGE: As a single agent: Usual adult dose is 0.5 mg IV daily for up to 5 days. It is also given as a single weekly dose of 2 mg for 3 to 4 weeks. In children the usual dose is 0.015 mg/kg (maximum dose 0.5 mg) given daily for 5 days over 3 to 5 weeks or a total dose of 2.4 mg/m^2 given in divided doses over 1 week. A repeated course (in adults and children) may be given after 2 weeks if toxicity does not develop. For an isolation perfusion technique, doses of 0.05 mg/kg for the lower extremities and pelvis and 0.035 mg/kg for the upper extremities should be given.[1,6,8]

ROUTES OF ADMINISTRATION: Direct IV, IV infusion, and by the isolation perfusion technique. IV infusions should take place over 10 to 15 minutes. Preferably dactinomycin should be administered by slow IV push directly into the vein using the double syringe technique (see Section 7, Ancillary Therapy—Extravasation) with the administration of 5 to 10 ml of normal saline solution before and after drug administration, or into the tubing of a running IV solution of normal saline solution or 5% dextrose in water.[1,6,8]

SPECIAL PRECAUTIONS: Avoid extravasation. Severe tissue necrosis may result. Avoid administration at time of chickenpox infection as severe generalized disease may result.[1,6,8]

COMPATIBILITY: Dextrose 5% in water and sodium chloride 0.9% are recommended diluents for the reconstituted solution.[1]

INCOMPATIBILITY: Solvents such as sodium chloride 0.9% and bacteriostatic water for injection may cause precipitation when used to reconstitute dactinomycin; therefore, they should be avoided.[1,14] Cellulose ester filters bind about 95% to 99% of dactinomycin in the first 10 ml. After 12 hours 13% of the total amount of the drug is bound. No significant reduction of potency is lost using stainless steel filters (IVEX-2 Filter Set, Argyle Filter Connector, and In-Sure Filter Set).[1]

Daunorubicin hydrochloride

SYNONYMS: Cerubidine, daunomycin, rubidomycin, DNR, NSC-82151[4,9]

MANUFACTURER: Ives Laboratories; Division of Cancer Treatment, National Cancer Institute[1,4]

DOSAGE FORMS AND STRENGTHS: 20 mg/10 ml vial with mannitol 100 mg[4,32]

STORAGE: Room temperature.[4,32]

SOLUTION PREPARATION: Reconstitute with 10 ml of sterile water for injection USP or normal saline to yield a 2 mg/ml solution, or 4 ml to yield a 5 mg/ml solution. Further dilution with 100 to 1,000 ml of normal saline solution or 5% dextrose in water for IV infusion can be prepared. Isotonic diluents should be used for IV push solutions.[1,4,32]

STABILITY:

Prior to mixing: Intact vials are stable for at least 2 years at room temperature (22° to 25° C).[1]

At different concentrations: Reconstituted solutions are stable for 7 days at room temperature. Since no preservatives are present, it is recommended for use within 8 hours, with discard of unused portions. Further dilution of reconstituted solutions with 5% dextrose in sodium chloride injection, USP, results in a solution that is stable for 24 hours.

At pH greater than 8.0, daunorubicin decomposes, resulting in a color change from red to blue-purple.[1,4,32]

PH: Reconstituted solution, pH 5.0 to 6.0[4,32]

DOSAGE: 30 to 60 mg/m^2 IV once weekly; 60 mg/m^2 per day for 3 days or 60 to 150 mg/m^2 single dose and repeat every 2 to 3 weeks. 1 mg/kg/day IV for 5 days every 3 to 4 weeks. Dosage adjustments are necessary with hepatic and renal impairment (see Section 6, Dose Modification in Renal and Hepatic Disease.)[2,3,7]

ROUTES OF ADMINISTRATION: Preferred route is IV push to be administered in not less than 2 to 3 minutes in 5 to 15 ml of isotonic diluent, either directly into the vein by double syringe technique with 5 to 10 ml of normal saline given before and after drug administration or into the tubing of a running IV. Short IV infusions in 50 to 200 ml of diluent over 10 to 45 minutes have also been used, but this method has a greater risk of serious extravasation. If stinging or burning occurs, the infusion should be stopped and restarted in another vein.[1,3,32]

SPECIAL PRECAUTIONS: Avoid extravasation. Severe necrosis of tissues may result. The total cumulative dose should be checked before administration, and it should not exceed a total dose of 550 mg/m^2 in adults or 450 mg/m^2 in children.[1,2,32] Patients should be informed that their urine will be red for 1 to 2 days after administration.

COMPATIBILITY: Sterile water for injection, USP, sodium chloride injection, USP, 5% dextrose in sodium chloride injection, USP, and 5% dextrose in water. Contrary to doxorubicin, daunorubicin has been found to be compatible when 20 mg is mixed with 40 mg of hydrocortisone sodium succinate (Solu-Cortef) in 100 ml of 5% dextrose in water.[3]

INCOMPATIBILITY: Daunorubicin forms an immediate precipitate with heparin sodium and with dexamethasone sodium phosphate.[3]

Diethylstilbestrol

SYNONYMS: Diethylstilbestrol, Stilphostrol, DES[5,9]

MANUFACTURER: Lilly, Dome Division of Miles Laboratories[5]

DOSAGE FORMS AND STRENGTHS: Diethylstilbestrol Enseals (enteric coated tablets): 0.1, 0.25, 0.5, 1, and 5 mg. Tablets: 0.1, 0.25, 0.5, 1, and 5 mg. Stilphostrol (diphosphate salt), tablets: 50 mg mottled gray-white. Injection: 0.25 g/5 ml ampule. One milligram of diethylstilbestrol is approximately equivalent to 1.6 mg of diethylstilbestrol diphosphate.[5,6,8]

STORAGE: Room temperature. Store solutions away from heat and light.[5,8]

SOLUTION PREPARATION: Dissolve a single daily dose in 300 ml of normal saline or 5% dextrose in water to be given by IV infusion.[5]

DOSAGE:

Prostatic carcinoma. Oral (diethylstilbestrol): Initial therapy, 1 to 3 mg daily. This dosage may be increased in advanced cases. Maintenance therapy, 1 mg daily. Oral (diethylstilbestrol diphosphate): Initial therapy, 50 mg orally three times daily. This dosage may be increased to 200 mg orally three times daily. IM: Initial therapy, 5 mg twice weekly. Maintenance therapy, 2 to 4 mg twice weekly.[5,8] IV infusion: Initial therapy, 500 mg on day 1 followed by 1 g daily for 5 days. Maintenance therapy: 250 to 500 mg once or twice weekly.[8]

Breast carcinoma. Oral (diethylstilbestrol): 10 to 20 mg daily. Usual dose is 15 mg daily in divided doses for a minimum of 3 months.[5,8]

ROUTES OF ADMINISTRATION: Orally, IM, and IV infusion. IV infusions should be given slowly 1 to 2 ml per minute for the first 10 to 15 minutes and then the rate should be adjusted so that the entire amount is given within 1 hour.[5,8]

SPECIAL PRECAUTIONS: Do not use darkened solutions. Use with caution in cardiac, liver, or renal disease.[5,8]

COMPATIBILITY: Normal saline solution and 5% dextrose in water[5,8]

Doxorubicin

SYNONYMS: Doxorubicin hydrochloride, Adriamycin, ADR, Adriablastina, hydroxydaunorubicin, hydroxyldaunomycin, NSC-123127[5,9]

MANUFACTURER: Farmitalia S.p.A., Italy, distributed by Adria Laboratories[5,9]

DOSAGE FORMS AND STRENGTHS: 10 and 50 mg vials[5]

STORAGE: Room temperature in a dry place protected from sunlight.[1,8]

SOLUTION PREPARATION: Reconstitute with 0.9% sodium chloride, sterile water for injection, USP, or 5% dextrose in water. Add 5 ml to the 10 mg vial and 25 ml to the 50 mg vial to yield a 2 mg/ml concentration. For IV push administration, use 10 to 20 ml of an isotonic solution (normal saline or 5% dextrose in water). Shake the vial vigorously after reconstitution to allow the drug to dissolve.[1]

STABILITY:

Prior to mixing: Intact vials are stable 2 years.[1,8]

At different concentrations: Reconstituted solutions protected from sunlight are stable for 24 hours at room temperature and for 48 hours with refrigeration (4° to 10° C). Doxorubicin is unstable at pH values less than 3 and those greater than 7.[8]

pH: 3.8 to 6.5, reconstituted with sodium chloride 0.9%[8]

DOSAGE: Usual dose is 60 to 75 mg/m^2 given every 3 to 4 weeks; alternatively, 25 to 30 mg/m^2 for 3 successive days every 3 to 4 weeks.[5,8]

Dosage adjustments with hepatic impairment[5]:

Serum bilirubin levels	BSP retention	Recommended dose
1.2 to 3.0 mg/dl	9%-15%	½ normal dose
>3 mg/dl	>15%	¼ normal dose

ROUTES OF ADMINISTRATION: Adriamycin should be administered by IV push or into the tubing of a running IV infusion of 5% dextrose in water or 0.9% sodium chloride. The rate of administration is dependent on the size of the vein and the dosage. However, the dose should be administered in *not less* than 3 to 5 minutes. Local erythematous streaking along the vein as well as facial flushing may indicate too rapid administration. If stinging or burning occurs, the infusion should be stopped and restarted in another vein. The double syringe technique should be employed with 5 to 10 cc of normal saline flush before and after administration. Patients should be informed that their urine will be red for 1 to 2 days after administration.[1,5]

SPECIAL PRECAUTIONS: Avoid extravasation. Severe necrosis of tissues may result. The total cumulative dose should be checked before administration. It should not exceed 550 mg/m² in adults or 450 mg/m² in children.[5,8]

COMPATIBILITY: Dextrose 5% in water and sodium chloride 0.9%[1,8]

INCOMPATIBILITY: Heparin sodium (a precipitate may form). Also, a color change to deep purple is reported when doxorubicin is mixed with fluorouracil in 5% dextrose in water. Dexamethasone sodium phosphate, hydrocortisone sodium phosphate and sodium succinate (Solu-Cortef), aminophylline, and cephalothin sodium (Keflin) have also been reported to be incompatible.[1,3,8]

Fluorouracil

SYNONYMS: Adrucil, Efudex (topical), 5-fluorouracil, Fluoroplex (topical), 5-FU, NSC-19893, Ro2-9757[5,9]

MANUFACTURER: Hoffmann-LaRoche; Adria Laboratories[5]

DOSAGE FORMS AND STRENGTHS: Injection: 500 mg/10 ml ampule.[5] Topical: Efudex—2% and 5% solutions and 5% 25 g cream, Fluoroplex—1% solution and 1% 30 g cream[5]

STORAGE: Room temperature (15° to 27° C) and protected from light.[1,5]

SOLUTION PREPARATION: Inspect the ampules of fluorouracil for discoloration and precipitate. If present, it does not mean decomposition has occurred. Discard only if the solution is dark yellow. Resolubilize the precipitate by heating to 60° C with vigorous shaking and allow to cool to body temperature before using. No dilution is required for drug administration. Filter the solution before use.[5]

STABILITY:

Prior to mixing: Intact ampules are stable for 2 years from the date of manufacture.[8]

At different concentrations: Solutions of further dilutions with 5% dextrose in water or normal saline are stable for 24 hours.[2]

pH: 8.6 to 9.0[1,5]

DOSAGE: Initial dose: 400 to 500 mg/m²/day (12 mg/kg/day; maximum dose 800 mg/day) for 4 to 5 days repeated every 4 weeks. Maintenance: (a) 200 to 500 mg/m² (6 mg/kg) every second day for 4 days repeated every 4 weeks; (b) 500 to 600 mg/m² (10 to 15 mg/kg) IV or orally every week (maximum dose 1 g per week). Topical (actinic keratoses): Apply cream or solutions twice daily in an amount sufficient to cover lesions. Onset of inflammatory response begins in 2 to 3 days. Continue application for 2 to 4 weeks until inflammatory response reaches the erosion, necrosis, and ulceration stage; then discontinue. Healing will be evident in 1 to 2 months after cessation of topical 5-fluorouracil.[2,5]

ROUTES OF ADMINISTRATION: IV push, IV infusion, oral, and topical application. For IV infusion the infusion rate and volume of 5% dextrose in water or normal saline is not crucial. Oral administration of the IV solution has been used infrequently. It has been found that response rates are not as high as the IV route or the remission durations as long. Doses of 15 mg/kg are commonly put in 120 ml of water, juice, or carbonated drinks. Fruit juices have a pH around 4, and 5-FU has a pH of 9. When 5-FU and fruit juices are mixed together, 5-FU precipitates out. A buffered bicarbonated solution or water is better than the commonly recommended vehicles for administration.[3,5]

SPECIAL PRECAUTIONS: Observe ampule for clarity and filter before use.[5]

COMPATIBILITY: 5% dextrose injection and sodium chloride 0.9% as infusion vehicles. Amino acids 4.25%, dextrose 25%, dextrose 5% in Ringer's injection, lactated, 1 g cephalothin sodium in 1,000 ml 5% dextrose in water, 200 mg prednisolone sodium phosphate in 1,000 ml of 5% dextrose in water, and 4 mg vincristine sulfate in 1,000 ml of 5% dextrose in water.[1]

INCOMPATIBILITY: The mixture of doxorubicin HCl 10 mg with 250 mg of 5-fluorouracil in 1 liter of dextrose 5% in water causes a color change in the solution to deep purple. Fluorouracil has also been reported to alter the ultraviolet spectrum with cytarabine 400 mg in 1,000 ml D_5W and methotrexate 200 mg in 1,000 ml D_5W within 1 hour at room temperature. *The-*

oretical incompatibilities: mixing the alkaline solution of 5-fluorouracil with acidic drugs such as tetracycline, insulin, multivitamins, amino acid solutions, and so on.[1]

Fluoxymesterone

SYNONYMS: Halotestin, Ora-Testryl, Ultandren, NSC-12165[5,9]

MANUFACTURER: Upjohn; Squibb; Ciba-Geigy[5,9]

DOSAGE FORMS AND STRENGTHS: Halotestin 2, 5, and 10 mg tablets,[5] Ora-Testryl 5 mg tablets[6]

STORAGE: Room temperature.[5]

DOSAGE: As a single agent: 15 to 30 mg orally in 2 to 3 divided doses daily. Divided doses ensure more stable blood levels. Continue a minimum of 1 month for a subjective response and 2 to 3 months for an objective response.[5]

ROUTES OF ADMINISTRATION: Oral only.[5]

Hydroxyurea

SYNONYMS: Hydrea, HYD, HU, HUR, NSC-32065[3,5,9]

MANUFACTURER: Squibb[5]

DOSAGE FORMS AND STRENGTHS: 500 mg capsule[5]

STORAGE: Room temperature.[5]

DOSAGE: As single agent: Intermittent therapy: 80 mg/kg as a single dose every 3 days. Continuous therapy: 20 to 30 mg/kg as a single dose daily. Adequate trial period for determining the antineoplastic effectiveness is 6 weeks of therapy.[5]

ROUTES OF ADMINISTRATION: Oral[5]

SPECIAL PRECAUTIONS: Therapy should be interrupted if the WBC count drops below 2500/mm^3 or the platelet count below 100,000/mm^3. Safety in pregnancy has not been established.[5]

Leucovorin calcium

SYNONYMS: Leucovorin calcium injection, folinic acid, citrovorum factor, SF, CF, 5-formyl FH_4, NSC-3590, formyltetrahydrofolate[3-5,9]

MANUFACTURER: Lederle; Division of Cancer Treatment, National Cancer Institute (to obtain 50 mg injection)[4,5]

DOSAGE FORMS AND STRENGTHS: 3 mg/ml ampules for IM injection (preservatives: propylparaben 0.02% and methylparaben 0.08%); 50 mg vial (powder) (preservatives: propylparaben 0.02% and methylparaben 0.08%); 50 mg vial (powder) (investigational) (preservatives: propylparaben 0.2 mg/ml, methylparaben 0.8 mg/ml, and sodium chloride 9 mg/ml)[4,5]; 5 mg tablets (investigational)

STORAGE: Room temperature.[4,5]

SOLUTION PREPARATION: None for the 1 ml ampule. To both of the 50 mg vials add 5 ml of sterile water for injection, USP, which results in a concentration of 10 mg/ml.[4,5]

STABILITY:

Prior to mixing: The ampule and both vials are stable at least 2 years.[3,4]

At different concentrations: Reconstituted solution of the 50 mg vial (Lederle) should be used as soon as possible since it may precipitate with prolonged standing. Reconstituted solution of the 50 mg vial (investigational) is stable at least 7 days at room temperature.[4,5]

pH: Ampules are approximately 7.8. Reconstituted solution of 50 mg vial (Lederle) is also approximately 7.8. Reconstituted solution (investigational) has a pH of 6.0 to 8.0.[4,5]

DOSAGE: For high dose methotrexate with leucovorin rescue or methotrexate overdosage, many leucovorin schedules have been used to reverse methotrexate toxicity. Leucovorin is also sometimes used to counter the systemic toxic effects of intrathecal methotrexate or for normal intravenous or oral doses of methotrexate. The following are common schedules and principles in the administration of leucovorin.

For high dose methotrexate: Leucovorin is initiated anywhere from 0 to 72 hours after methotrexate and continued for 36 to 96 hours depending on the dose of methotrexate, methotrexate serum levels, and creatinine clearance of the patient (see Section 7, Ancillary Therapy—Leucovorin Rescue).

Common schedules[1]:

a. 40 mg/m² 24 hours after methotrexate followed by 25 mg/m² every 6 hours for 72 hours
b. 6 to 15 mg/m² every 6 hours for 72 hours begun 2 hours after methotrexate
c. 9 mg orally every 6 hours for 12 doses begun 6 hours after methotrexate

For methotrexate overdosage: In general, leucovorin doses to counter toxicity from methotrexate overdosage should be equal to or greater than the dose of methotrexate given to the patient. Leucovorin should be administered immediately. It is optimal to be able to administer it within the first hour after methotrexate was administered. Leucovorin is less effective if administered after the first hour. Leucovorin should be administered until methotrexate toxic serum levels fall to normal.[5] A 75 mg IV infusion should be administered within 12 hours, followed by 12 mg IM every 6 hours for 4 doses or more if needed.

For average or intrathecal methotrexate doses: In general the leucovorin dose is equal to the methotrexate dose given. It may be initiated every 6 hours for a total of 4 to 12 doses from 0 to 72 hours after methotrexate administration. An example of a common schedule often given is a 6 to 12 mg dose IM or orally every 6 hours for 4 doses begun 24 hours after intrathecal methotrexate administration.

ROUTES OF ADMINISTRATION: IM, IV push, IV infusion, or orally. IV infusion should be given over 1 to 3 minutes. The injectable products can be taken orally.[70] (See Section 6, Renal Dysfunction, Table 6-15, and Section 7, Leucovorin Rescue).

COMPATIBILITY: 50 mg of leucovorin is compatible in 1,000 ml of dextrose 10% in sodium chloride 0.9%, dextrose 10% in water, Ringer's injection, and Ringer's injection, lactated.

Lomustine

SYNONYMS: CCNU, CeeNU, NSC-79037[4,5]

MANUFACTURER: Bristol[5]

DOSAGE FORMS AND STRENGTHS: CeeNU comes in a 6-capsule dose pack: two 100 mg capsules (green/green), two 40 mg capsules (green/purple), and two 10 mg capsules (purple/purple). The drug occurs as a yellow powder.[5]

STORAGE: Room temperature or below in well-closed containers. Avoid excessive heat (over 40° C).[5]

DRUG PREPARATION: The dose pack provides enough medication for a single dose. The total dose prescribed can be obtained (to within 10 mg) by determining the proper combination of the capsule strengths in the dose pack. The appropriate number of capsules of each size should be placed in a single vial to which is attached the patient information label (provided with the pack) explaining the differences in the appearance of the capsules. The remaining capsules (if any) should be discarded and not given to the patient. Patients should be cautioned not to expose CeeNU to temperatures greater than 40° C or to moisture.[5]

STABILITY: Capsules are stable for at least 4 years when stored at room temperature in well-closed containers.[4]

DOSAGE: As single agent: Usual dosage for adults and children is 130 mg/m^2 orally as a single dose given every 6 weeks. If there is prior radiation or chemotherapy, dosage should be reduced to 100 mg/m^2 every 6 weeks.[5]

ROUTES OF ADMINISTRATION: *Oral route only.* Nausea, vomiting, and anorexia are common with CeeNU; their frequency and duration can be minimized by administering the drug to a patient who has been premedicated with antiemetics or a patient in a fasting state. CeeNU absorption is rapid; therefore, vomiting after 30 to 60 minutes does not decrease efficacy.[3,5]

SPECIAL PRECAUTIONS: Lomustine has delayed and cumulative bone marrow toxicity and should not be given any more frequently than every 6 weeks by an experienced individual. It should not be given until platelets and leukocytes have returned to acceptable levels (platelets ≥ 100,000/mm^3 and leukocytes ≥ 4,000/mm^3). More than one dose of lomustine should not be dispensed at any one time because of its severe hematologic toxicities. Safe usage in pregnancy has not been established.[5]

Mechlorethamine hydrochloride

SYNONYMS: Mustargen, nitrogen mustard, HN2, mustine, NSC-762[5,9]

MANUFACTURER: Merck Sharp & Dohme[5]

DOSAGE FORMS AND STRENGTHS: 10 mg vial also containing 100 mg of sodium chloride (dry powder)[6]

STORAGE: Room temperature.[2]

SOLUTION PREPARATION: Reconstitute with 10 ml of sterile water for injection, USP, or normal saline solution, which produces a 1 mg/ml solution. Because solution is unstable, prepare immediately before use. Discard unused portions. Further dilution is discouraged except for intracavitary instillation.[1,6]

STABILITY: A 1 mg/ml solution is stable for 1 hour at room temperature (22° to 25° C).[2]

pH: 3.0 to 5.0 in a 1:50 solution.[1,8]

DOSAGE: Usual dose is 0.4 mg/kg as a single dose IV every 4 to 6 weeks. The single dose may be given in two divided daily doses. Intracavitary dose: 0.2 to 0.4 mg/kg IV.[1,5,8]

ROUTES OF ADMINISTRATION: IV or intracavitary.[1,5] When given by IV push, give into a vein or into the tubing of a running infusion solution over 3 to 5 minutes. It is given intracavitary to control pleural, peritoneal, and pericardial malignant effusions. Mechlorethamine has been instilled in a 1 mg/1 ml concentration and also in further dilutions of 50 to 100 ml in normal saline solution.[1,5,8]

SPECIAL PRECAUTIONS: Do not use solution if discolored. Avoid extravasation. Severe tissue necrosis may result. (See Section 7, Ancillary Therapy—Extravasation.)[5]

COMPATIBILITY: Sodium chloride 0.9% up to 50 to 100 ml.[1]

INCOMPATIBILITY: More unstable in neutral and alkaline solutions than in acid solutions. Specifically incompatible with methohexital sodium. It is recommended that one avoid giving mechlorethamine HCL by infusion because of rapid decomposition.[1,8]

Melphalan

SYNONYMS: Alkeran, L-PAM, L-phenylalanine mustard, L-Sarcolysin, CB-3025, NSC-8806, MPL[4,5,9]

MANUFACTURER: Burroughs Wellcome (oral)[5]; Burroughs Wellcome (London, England) for the Division of Cancer Treatment, National Cancer Institute (injection)[4,5]

DOSAGE FORMS AND STRENGTHS: 2 mg tablet; 100 mg vial (investigational) with a 1 ml ampule of acid-alcohol solvent and a 9 ml ampule of phosphate buffer[4,5]

STORAGE: Room temperature.[2,4]

SOLUTION PREPARATION: Add to 100 mg vial, 1 ml of acid-alcohol solvent and then further dilute with 9 ml of phosphate buffer resulting in a 10 mg/ml concentration. May dilute further with 5% dextrose injection, USP, or normal saline solution. Discard if precipitation occurs.[1,4]

STABILITY:

Prior to mixing: Intact injectable vials are stable up to 4 years at room temperature[4]

At different concentrations: Reconstituted solution is stable for 24 hours at room temperature (8.5% hydrolysis in 24 hours). Further dilution with 5% dextrose injection, USP, is stable also for 24 hours at room temperature. Melphalan injectable solution does not contain a preservative. Solutions should be discarded after use or within 8 hours.[4]

pH: Reconstituted solution pH of about 7[4]

DOSAGE:

Oral: Initial therapy: (a) 6 mg daily for 2 to 3 weeks followed by a rest period of 4 weeks; (b) 10 mg daily orally for 7 to 10 days every 4 to 6 weeks; (c) 0.1 to 0.15 mg/kg orally for 7 days every 2 to 6 weeks; (d) 0.25 mg/kg orally for 4 days every 4 to 6 weeks; (e) 20 to 30 mg/m^2 every 4 to 6 weeks (IV or orally). Maintenance therapy: 0.05 mg/kg or less orally daily adjusted according to the blood count.[2,5,7]

IV: Doses appear to be similar in effect to equivalent oral doses. However, due to less bioavailability when given orally and less hepatic clearance when given IV, caution should be used equating the two routes.[3]

ROUTES OF ADMINISTRATION: Oral, IV infusion, and regional perfusion. IV infusion should be given in 100 to 150 ml of 5% dextrose in water or normal saline solution over 15 to 30 minutes.[1,5]

SPECIAL PRECAUTIONS: If the leukocyte count falls below 3,000/mm^3 or the platelet count below 100,000/mm^3, the drug should be discontinued until bone marrow recovery. Safe use in pregnancy has not been established.[5]

COMPATIBILITY: 5% dextrose in water and normal saline solution[1,4]

6-Mercaptopurine

SYNONYMS: Purinethol, 6-MP, mercaptopurine, NSC-755, purine-6-thiol monohydrate[4,5]

MANUFACTURER: Burroughs Wellcome (oral); Burroughs Wellcome for the Division of Cancer Treatment, National Cancer Institute (injection)[4,5]

DOSAGE FORMS AND STRENGTHS: 50 mg tablet, 500 mg vial (investigational)[4,5]

STORAGE: Room temperature.[2,4]

SOLUTION PREPARATION: Reconstitute with 49.8 ml of sterile water for injection, USP, resulting in 10 mg/ml concentration. Further dilute for administration to a concentration of 1 to 2 mg/ml with 250 to 500 ml of 5% dextrose injection, USP, or sodium chloride injection, USP.[4]

STABILITY:

Prior to mixing: Intact injectable vials are stable for at least 4 years.[4]

At different concentrations: Reconstituted solution is stable 21 days at room temperature or refrigeration temperature. Further dilution of solution as stated above results in a solution stable for 3 days at room temperature or refrigeration temperature. Since no antibacterial preservative is present, it is recommended that solutions be discarded in 8 hours.[4]

pH: Reconstituted solution 10.0 to 11.0[4]

DOSAGE:

Oral: (a) 2.5 mg/kg orally daily (100 to 200 mg in the average adult and 50 mg in the average 5-year-old child); if there is no improvement in 4 weeks, increase the dose to 5 mg/kg orally daily if blood counts permit. (b) 750 to 1000 mg/m² per day for 5 days every 3 weeks.

IV: 500 to 1500 mg/m² per day for 5 days; repeat as counts permit. Dosage of 6-mercaptopurine should be reduced to ⅓ or ¼ the usual dose if allopurinol (Zyloprim), 300 to 600 mg daily, is given concurrently in order to reduce or prevent hyperuricemia or to retard the metabolism of mercaptopurine.[2,5]

ROUTES OF ADMINISTRATION: Oral, IV infusion. IV infusion should be given *slowly* at 1 to 2 mg/ml concentration to reduce the incidence of vein irritation.[4,5]

SPECIAL PRECAUTIONS: Avoid extravasation. Severe tissue necrosis may result. Significant liver and renal impairment requires lower doses.[4,5] (See Section 6, Dose Modification in Renal or Hepatic Disease.)

COMPATIBILITY: Physically compatible with methotrexate sodium in 5% dextrose in water.[1]

INCOMPATIBILITY: Physically incompatible with allopurinol sodium and prednisolone sodium succinate in 5% dextrose in water.[1]

Methotrexate

SYNONYMS: Methotrexate, amethopterin, MTX, NSC-740, sodium methotrexate[3,7,9]

MANUFACTURER: Lederle; Bristol; Division of Cancer Treatment, National Cancer Institute (for investigational forms)[4,5]

DOSAGE FORMS AND STRENGTHS:

Oral: Lederle: 2.5 mg tablet, 50 mg tablet (investigational).

Injectable: Lederle: 5 mg and 50 mg vials with 0.9% weight volume benzyl alcohol, 20 mg vial lyophilized and preservative free; Bristol: 20, 50, and 100 mg vials lyophilized and preservative free; Investigational: 50 mg and 1 g vials lyophilized and preservative free.[1,4,5]

STORAGE: Room temperature.[4,5] Bristol recommends protection from light.[1]

SOLUTION PREPARATION:

Lederle: 5 and 50 mg vials with preservatives require no reconstitution. Reconstitute 20 mg vial with 20 ml of sodium chloride injection USP for a 1 mg/ml concentration.[5]

Bristol: reconstitute the 20, 50, and 100 mg vials with 2 to 10 ml depending on route of administration with a sterile preservative-free diluent such as sodium chloride 0.9%.[1]

Investigational: reconstitute the 50 mg vial with 5.0 ml of sodium chloride injection, USP, 5% dextrose in water, or Elliott's B solution for a 10 mg/ml concentration. Reconstitute the 1.0 g vial with 19.4 ml of sterile water for injection, USP, sodium chloride injection, USP, 5% dextrose injection, USP, 5% dextrose in sodium chloride injection, USP, or Elliott's B solution (simulated CSF) for a 50 mg/ml concentration.[4]

STABILITY:

Prior to mixing: Tablets are stable 5 years at room temperature.[8] Intact vials are stable at least 2 years at room temperature.[1,4,8]

At different concentrations: Reconstituted solutions are stable at room temperature for 1 week. Further dilution does not alter the stability. Since the reconstituted methotrexate preparations do not contain a preservative, it is recommended to discard them 8 hours after initial entry or immediately after use. Intrathecal preparations should be prepared prior to administration and used immediately to avoid risk of bacterial contamination.[1,4]

pH: Commercial injectable products, approximately 8.5. The reconstituted solutions of the 1.0 g vial have a pH of 7.8 to 8.8; the 50 mg vial, 7.0 to 8.8.[1,4,8]

DOSAGE:

a. 2.5 to 5.0 mg orally daily.

b. 0.4 mg/kg (maximum dose 25 mg) IV daily for 4 to 5 days.
c. 0.4 mg/kg IV twice weekly.[7]
d. 15 to 30 mg IM daily for 5 days every 1 or 2 or more weeks for 3 to 5 courses.[5,8]
e. Maintenance therapy of acute lymphocytic leukemia: 20 to 30 mg/m^2 orally or IM twice weekly or 2.5 mg/kg IV for 14 days.[8]
f. High dose requiring leucovorin rescue and urine alkalinization:
   (1) 100 to 750 mg/kg IV over 4 hours.
   (2) 300 mg/kg IV over 4 hours.
   (3) 1500 mg/m^2 IV over 6 hours.
   (4) 2 to 7 g/m^2 IV over 6 hours.
   (5) 1 to 15 g/m^2 IV over 20 hours.[1]
g. Intrathecal administration:
   (1) 6.25 to 12.5 mg/m^2 IT at 2- to 5-day intervals until cerebrospinal fluid cell counts return to normal; then give one additional dose
   (2) 12 mg/m^2 IT once weekly for 2 weeks, then once monthly[8]
   (3) 5 to 15 mg/m^2 IT every 3 to 7 days. Repeat every 6 to 8 weeks for CNS remission maintenance.[2] (See Section 7, Therapy of CNS Metastases.)

ROUTES OF ADMINISTRATION: IV push, IV infusion, IM, oral, IA (intraarterial—investigational), or IT. Most frequently high dose methotrexate is given in 1 to 2 liters of normal saline solution or 5% dextrose in water over 24 hours. *Only the nonpreserved preparations should be used.* Before administration the patient should be well hydrated and his urine made alkaline to pH 7 with 2 to 3 g of sodium bicarbonate given every 3 to 6 hours and continued during therapy to protect the kidneys.[71] Methotrexate serum levels should be taken at 24, 48, and 72 hours to monitor toxicity.[72] (See Section 6, Renal Dysfunction, Table 6-15 and Section 7, Leucovorin Rescue.)

For intrathecal administration, Elliott's B solution is often recommended as a diluent, but normal saline solution, lactated Ringer's, dextrose 5% lactated Ringer's, and the patient's own CSF are often used. Volume administered should be equal to the spinal fluid removed. Volumes used range from 2 to 20 ml. Usual range is 4 to 12 ml. Preservative-free preparations should be used.[1,5] (See Section 7, Therapy of CNS Metastasis.)

SPECIAL PRECAUTIONS: High dose methotrexate should be administered *by experienced persons in a hospital setting where methotrexate blood levels can be obtained.* Patients have died from lack of knowledge and vigilance of health professionals administering the drug. Death usually occurs 5 to 10 days after drug administration.

Pharmacist should dispense no more than a 7-day supply of methotrexate at one time. Refills of prescriptions should be by direct order of the physician only.[5]

COMPATIBILITY: Dextrose 5% in water, sodium chloride 0.9%, or dextrose 5% in sodium chloride 0.9% as diluents. Cephalothin sodium, cytarabine, 6-mercaptopurine, and vincristine have all been found to be physically compatible with methotrexate in the same solution.[1]

INCOMPATIBILITY: 5-Fluorouracil and prednisolone sodium phosphate have been found to alter the ultraviolet spectra within 1 hour, noting a chemical change when methotrexate is mixed with them. This possibly might be clinically significant.[1]

Mithramycin

SYNONYMS: Mithracin, NSC-24559[5,9]

MANUFACTURER: Pfizer Laboratories for Dome Division of Miles Laboratories[5]

DOSAGES FORMS AND STRENGTHS: 2.5 mg vial with 100 mg mannitol and disodium phosphate[5]

STORAGE: Refrigerate.[5]

SOLUTION PREPARATION: Add 4.9 ml of sterile water for injection, USP, or normal saline to produce a 0.5 mg/ml concentration. Further dilute in 50 to 1,000 ml of 5% dextrose injection, USP, or sodium chloride injection, USP, for IV administration.[1,5]

STABILITY:

Prior to mixing: Intact vials are stable for 2 years when refrigerated and 3 months at room temperatures not exceeding 25° C.[1,8]

At different concentrations: Reconstituted solution is stable for 24 hours at room temperature and 48 hours when refrigerated.[1] Further diluted solutions to 1,000 ml with 5% dextrose in water are stable at room temperature for 4 to 6 hours.[15] Since no preservatives are present, it is recommended that solution be discarded immediately after use.[1,5]

pH: Reconstituted solution has a pH of 7.[5]

DOSAGE: *Tumors of testes:* 25 to 30 μg/kg IV for 8 to 10 days (maximum 30 μg/kg IV); 1 to 2 mg/m^2/day every 2 days for 5 doses repeated every 3 weeks. *Hypercalcemia and hypercalciuria:* 25 μg/kg/day IV for 3 to 4 days (maximum 30 μg/kg IV) repeated in 1 week, or as 2 to 3 doses per week[2,5]

ROUTES OF ADMINISTRATION: IV infusion only. Rapid IV push should be avoided as it is associated with a higher incidence and greater severity of gastrointestinal side effects. IV infusion is given slowly over a period of 4 to 6 hours in 1,000 ml of dextrose 5% in water.[1,5,8]

SPECIAL PRECAUTIONS: Mithramycin should only be administered to hospitalized patients or by experienced physicians because of the severe toxicities that have resulted in death. Avoid extravasation. Severe tissue necrosis may result.[5]

COMPATIBILITY: 5% dextrose in water as infusion solution.[1,5]

INCOMPATIBILITY: In acidic solutions below pH 5 mithramycin is hydrolyzed. Iron may be chelated by mithramycin. In general, mithramycin has a strong capacity for chelating metals.[1,8]

Mitomycin C

SYNONYMS: Mutamycin, Mitomycin, MTC, Ametycine, NSC-26980, Mitocin-C[5,9]

MANUFACTURER: Bristol[5]

DOSAGE FORMS AND STRENGTHS: Injection: 5 and 20 mg vials[5]

STORAGE: Room temperature. Avoid excessive heat (over 40° C).[5]

SOLUTION PREPARATION: Add 10 ml of sterile water for injection to the 5 mg vial and 40 ml to the 20 mg vial resulting in a final concentration of 0.5 mg/ml. If product does not dissolve immediately, allow to stand at room temperature until solution is obtained. Place 20 mg in 20 ml of sterile water for bladder instillation.[5,73]

STABILITY:

Prior to mixing: Stable for 2 years at room temperature.[5]

At different concentrations: Reconstituted solution is stable for 14 days refrigerated or 7 days at room temperature.[5]

With further dilution in various IV fluids at room temperature:[5]

IV fluid	Stability
5% Dextrose injection	3 hours
0.9% Sodium chloride injection	12 hours
Sodium lactate injection	24 hours

In combination (5 to 15 mg of mitomycin C) with heparin 1,000 units to 10,000 units in 30 ml of 0.9% sodium chloride injection, stability is 48 hours at room temperature.[5]

pH: Reconstituted solution has a pH of 6 to 8.[8]

DOSAGE:

a. 20 mg/m² IV as a single dose every 6 to 8 weeks.
b. 2 mg/m² daily IV for 5 days, 2 days no drug, then 2 mg/m² daily IV for another 5 days (total, 10 days of therapy). Repeat every 6 to 8 weeks.[5]
c. 20 mg in 20 ml sterile water instilled in bladder and retained 3 hours. Repeat 3 times a week up to 20 times per course.[73]

ROUTES OF ADMINISTRATION: IV. Give by slow IV push or in small volume (50 ml or less) short infusions.[5,8]

SPECIAL PRECAUTIONS: Avoid extravasation. Severe tissue necrosis may result. Mitomycin C has cumulative bone marrow toxicity.[5]

COMPATIBILITY: 5% dextrose injection, 0.9% sodium chloride injection, and sodium lactate injection have been recommended as diluents for IV infusions.[5]

Procarbazine hydrochloride

SYNONYMS: Matulane, NSC-77213, Natulan, MIH, Ibenzmethyzin, Methylhydrazine, Ro 4-6467[3,5,9]

MANUFACTURER: Hoffmann-La Roche[5]

DOSAGE FORMS AND STRENGTHS: 50 mg capsule[5]

STORAGE: Room temperature. Keep away from moisture.[2,8]

STABILITY: Capsules are stable for 4 years at room temperature.[8]

DOSAGE: As single agent.

Adult:

a. 150 mg/m^2/day for 14 to 21 days.[2]
b. Initial therapy: 2 to 4 mg/kg/day for 7 days. Maintenance: 4 to 6 mg/kg per day. Continue until maximum response or bone marrow toxicity. Resume treatment at 1 to 2 mg/kg per day.[5]
c. Initial therapy: 100 mg/m^2 orally daily, increasing over 1 week to 150 to 200 mg/m^2; maintain for 3 weeks, then reduce to 100 mg/m^2 orally daily until toxicity.[7]

Children: Initial: 50 mg daily for 7 days. Maintenance: 100 mg/m^2 daily until maximum response or bone marrow toxicity. Resume treatment at 50 mg daily (calculated dose to the nearest 50 mg).[5]

ROUTES OF ADMINISTRATION: Oral only. Dosage may be given in divided doses or in one single dose.[5]

SPECIAL PRECAUTIONS: Blood counts should be monitored closely.[5]

Thioguanine

SYNONYMS: Thioguanine, 6-TG, Lanvis, 6-thioguanine, NSC-752[4,5,7]

MANUFACTURER: Burroughs Wellcome; Division of Cancer Treatment, National Cancer Institute (to obtain injectable form)[4,5]

DOSAGE FORMS AND STRENGTHS: 40 mg tablet; 75 mg vial (investigational)[4,5]

STORAGE: Room temperature (oral tablets). Intact vials should be stored at refrigeration temperatures (2° to 8° C).[2,4]

SOLUTION PREPARATION: Add 5 ml of sodium chloride injection, USP, to 75 mg vial to produce a 15 mg/ml concentration. May further dilute with 5% dextrose in sodium chloride injection, USP.[4]

STABILITY:

Prior to mixing: Intact injectable vials are stable for 4 years at refrigerator temperatures and 2 years at room temperature.

At different concentrations: The reconstituted solution is stable for 24 hours under refrigeration. At room temperature precipitate may form upon standing. Further dilution in 500 ml of 5% dextrose in sodium chloride injection, USP, results in a solution stable for 24 hours at room temperature or refrigeration temperatures. Since no preservative is present, it is recommended that the solutions be discarded after 8 hours.[4]

pH: Reconstituted solution has a pH of 10.0-12.0[4]

DOSAGE: Initial therapy: 2 mg/kg daily for 4 weeks. If no improvement and no bone marrow depression, increase dosage to 3 mg/kg daily. Maintenance therapy: 2 mg/kg daily.[5]

ROUTES OF ADMINISTRATION: Oral, IV. May give by IV push or by IV infusion in 50 to 150 ml of 5% dextrose in water or normal saline solution over 15 to 45 minutes.[1,5]

COMPATIBILITY: Sodium chloride injection, USP, and 5% dextrose in sodium chloride injection, USP.[4]

Triethylene thiophosphoramide

SYNONYMS: Thiotepa, THIO, TESPA, TSPA, NSC-6396

MANUFACTURER: Lederle[5]

DOSAGE FORMS AND STRENGTHS: 15 mg vial[5]

STORAGE: Store at refrigeration temperatures (2° to 8° C).[8]

SOLUTION PREPARATION: Reconstitute with 1.5 ml of sterile water for injection, USP, to produce a 10 mg/ml concentration. Solution should be clear to slightly opaque but *not* grossly opaque or precipitated. The addition of sterile water for injection results in an isotonic solution. The addition of other diluents for reconstitution results in a hypertonic solution, which may cause mild to moderate discomfort at the injection site.[5]

Further dilution may be done to large volumes with sodium chloride injection, USP, dextrose injection, USP, dextrose and sodium chloride injection, USP, Ringer's injection, USP, or lactated Ringer's injection, USP. Do not use any other acidic diluent than those mentioned.[5]

For bladder instillation: put 30 to 60 mg of Thiotepa in 30 to 60 ml of sterile water. For intracavitary instillation: further dilute reconstituted solution with normal saline solution to 10 to 20 ml volumes for intrapleural and pericardial instillations.[3,5]

STABILITY: The reconstituted solution is stable for 5 days; however, since it does not contain a preservative, it is recommended that it be used immediately and that unused portions be discarded.[8]

DOSAGE: Initial therapy: 200 μg/kg IV, IM, IA daily for 5 days. Maintenance therapy: Depends on drug's slow onset of action, cumulative effects, and patient's clinical and hematologic response. Maximum dose is 200 μg/kg/week. Drug should not be administered more often than 1 to 3 weeks. *Chronic leukemia:* Initial therapy, 10 to 60 mg IV for 5 days. Maintenance therapy: 10 mg IV every 1 to 3 weeks. *Intracarotid injections for cerebral lesions:* 40 to 50 mg every 6 to 9 weeks. *Local intratumor injections:* 10 to 60 mg in one or multiple sites. *Intracavitary injections* (pleural, pericardial, or peritoneal): 10 to 50 mg injected into cavity following paracentesis.[8] *Topical application:* Initially 60 mg except in presence of surgical shock, chronic renal or cardiovascular disease, marked debility, or asthenia; then 45 mg is initiated. Doses are usually repeated weekly for 4 weeks. *Bladder doses:* Instill 60 mg into the bladder by catheter. Solution is retained for 2 hours. Instill once a week for 4 weeks (one course). The course may be repeated if necessary, but the second and third courses should be given with caution due to bone marrow toxicity.[5]

ROUTES OF ADMINISTRATION: IV push, IV infusion, IM, IA, intracavitary, topical application, intralesionally, intracarotid.[5,8]

SPECIAL PRECAUTIONS: Thiotepa has a slow onset of action; as a result, overdosage in a patient can happen easily. The maximum effect of the initial dosage should be observed before administering a second.[5,8]

COMPATIBILITY: Sodium chloride injection, USP, dextrose injection, USP, dextrose and sodium chloride injection, USP, Ringer's injection, USP, or lactated Ringer's injection, USP; procaine HCl 2% or epinephrine HCl 1:1,000 or both.[5]

INCOMPATIBILITY: Acidic diluents for initial reconstitution.[5]

Vinblastine sulfate

SYNONYMS: Velban, NSC-49842, VBL, Vincaleukoblastine sulfate, Velbe[5,9]

MANUFACTURER: Lilly[5]

DOSAGE FORMS AND STRENGTHS: Injection, 10 mg vial[5]

STORAGE: Store in refrigeration temperatures (2° to 8° C). Protect from light.[5,8]

SOLUTION PREPARATION: Add 10 ml of sodium chloride 0.9% (preserved with phenol or benzyl alcohol) to produce a concentration of 1 mg/ml. Other diluents are not recommended. Vinblastine should not be further diluted in large volumes of diluent (i.e., 100 to 250 ml). This increases the chance of extravasation.[5]

STABILITY: The reconstituted solution is stable 30 days at refrigeration temperatures.[8]

pH: Reconstituted solution has a pH of 3.5 to 5.0.[8]

DOSAGE: A *single dose should not be given any more frequently than once every 7 days.* Initial dose is 0.1 mg/kg (3.7 mg/m^2), then increased in increments of 0.05 mg/kg (1.8 mg/m^2) each week until a WBC count of 3,000/mm^3 is achieved. (Usual dose range is 0.15 to 0.2 mg/kg [5.5 to 7.4 mg/m^2]). For maintenance dose administer one increment lower than necessary to achieve a WBC count of 3,000/mm^3 and give weekly. Do not exceed 18.5 mg/m^2 for adults and 12.5 mg/m^2 for children.[5,8]

ROUTES OF ADMINISTRATION: IV push, rapid IV infusion in *small* volumes. IV push using the double syringe technique of administering 5 to 10 ml of normal saline before and after drug administration is preferred. Vinblastine should be administered over a 1-minute period by IV push and over 15 minutes or less by IV infusion.[8]

SPECIAL PRECAUTIONS: Avoid extravasation. Severe tissue necrosis can result.[5]

COMPATIBILITY: 5% dextrose in water or normal saline solution as small volume diluents for infusions.[5]

Vincristine sulfate

SYNONYMS: Oncovin, VCR, LCR, NSC-67574, leurocristine sulfate[5,9]

MANUFACTURER: Lilly[5]

DOSAGE FORMS AND STRENGTHS: 1 and 5 mg vials each with a 10 ml vial of bacteriostatic sodium chloride injection as a diluent for reconstitution[5]

STORAGE: Refrigeration temperatures of 2° to 8° C. Protect from light.[5]

SOLUTION PREPARATION: Add the 10 ml diluent to the 1 and 5 mg vials to obtain 0.1 and 0.5 mg/ml concentrations respectively. Sodium chloride 0.9% or sterile water for injection may also be used as diluents for reconstitution of vincristine. Further dilution in 50 ml of dextrose 5% in water or sodium chloride 0.9% can be done for rapid IV infusions.[1,5]

STABILITY:

Prior to mixing: Although refrigeration is recommended, vincristine has been found to be stable for at least 6 months at room temperature not exceeding 25° C.[8]

At different concentrations: Reconstituted solution is stable for 14 days under refrigeration without significant loss of potency.[5]

pH: Solution of 0.1% in water is 3.5 to 4.5.[1]

DOSAGE: 1.4 to 2 mg/m^2 in a single dose given weekly with a maximum dose of 2.0 mg[5]

ROUTES OF ADMINISTRATION: IV push and rapid IV infusion. IV push should be over 1 minute, rapid IV infusion over 15 minutes or less.[1,5,8]

SPECIAL PRECAUTIONS: Avoid extravasation. Severe tissue necrosis may result.[1,5,8]

COMPATIBILITY: Vincristine is compatible with 5% dextrose in water and normal saline solution for further dilution and with cytarabine 16 mg/liter in D_5W, fluorouracil 10 mg/liter in D_5W, and methotrexate 100 and 8 mg/liter in D_5W.[1]

DRUGS IN EARLY INVESTIGATION

The development of new, effective antineoplastic drugs has been slow and costly. The National Cancer Institute (NCI) performs most of the preclinical testing of these agents. Whether the drug is passed through preclinical toxicology studies depends on the priority listing by the NCI. When these drugs are available for clinical study, they are classified according to the following scheme:

Group A drugs: These are drugs in phase I and II clinical trials, and distribution is limited to intramural investigators and cooperative groups designated to carry out phase I and II studies.

Group B drugs: These are drugs in phase II studies and are available through protocol acceptance and distribution, which includes cooperative groups, NCI contractors, and cancer center directors.

Group C drugs: These drugs have demonstrated efficacy in several studies. They are distributed to oncologists for use in specific diseases.

Table 5-1 lists the current classification of these drugs as of 1981. The data sheets for group A, B, and C drugs are provided by the Pharmaceutical Resources Branch of the NCI.

Table 5-1. Investigational drug classification

Group A_1 (Phase I)		**Group A_2 (Phase II)**	
L-Alanosine	(NSC-153352)	Anguidine	(NSC-141537)
Amino-thiadiazole	(NSC-4728)	Bruceantin	(NSC-165563)
Cycloleucine	(NSC-1026)	Chlorozotocin	(NSC-178248)
Dichloroallyl lawsone	(NSC-126771)	3-Deazauridine	(NSC-126849)
DON	(NSC-7365)	Gallium nitrate	(NSC-15200)
Heroin	(NSC-302357)	Indicine N-oxide	(NSC-132319)
ICRF-187	(NSC-169780)	Maytansine	(NSC-153858)
Misonidazole (IV)	(NSC-261037)	Methyl-GAG	(NSC-32946)
PCNU	(NSC-95466)	Misonidazole (oral)	(NSC-261037)
Pentamethylmelamine	(NSC-118742)	PALA disodium	(NSC-224131)
α-TGdR	(NSC-71851)	Thymidine	(NSC-21548)
		Zinostatin (neocarzinostatin)	(NSC-157365)

Table 5-1. Investigational drug classification—cont'd

Drug	NSC number
Group B_1—drugs for the New Drug Studies Mechanism, Division of Cancer Treatment (DCT) contractors and cooperative groups	
Cyclocytidine	(NSC-145688)
Dianhydrogalactitol	(NSC-132313)
Dibromodulcitol	(NSC-104800)
Diglycoaldehyde	(NSC-118994)
Elliott's B solution	(NSC-V-7)
ICRF-159	(NSC-129943)
Melphalan (IV)	(NSC-8806)
TMCA	(NSC-36354)
Teniposide	(NSC-122819)
Group B_2—drugs available only to Division of Cancer Treatment contractors and cooperative groups	
AMSA	(NSC-249992)
BCG-Connaught	(NSC-B116341)
BCG-MER	(NSC-143769)
BCG-Pasteur (to be discontinued)	(NSC-B116328)
BCG-Tice	(NSC-B116327)
Calcium leucovorin	(NSC-3950)
C. parvum	(NSC-220537)
DES	(NSC-3070)
Tegafur	(NSC-148958)
Ifosfamide	(NSC-109724)
Methotrexate (high dose)	(NSC-740)
Phenestrin	(NSC-104469)
Prednisolone	(NSC-9151)
Prednisone	(NSC-10023)
Pyrazofurin	(NSC-143059)
THC	(NSC-134454)
Group B_3—drugs available only for existing studies	
Dichloromethotrexate	(NSC-29630)
Zorubicin	(NSC-164001)
Baker's antifol	(NSC-139105)
Levamisole	(NSC-177023)
Yoshi-864	(NSC-102627)
6-Mercaptopurine (IV)	(NSC-755)
Piperazinedione	(NSC-135758)
8-Azaquanine	(NSC-749)
DMSO	(NSC-763)
Dibromomannitol	(NSC-94100)
6-Thioguanine	(NSC-752)
Azapicyl	(NSC-68626)
Streptonigrin	(NSC-45383)
Nafoxidine	(NSC-70735)
Thalicarpine	(NSC-68075)
Procarbazine	(NSC-77213)
TIC-HN_2	(NSC-82196)
Group B_4—existing INDs will be closed	
Azaserine	
F_3TDR	
Group C drugs	
Azacitidine (NSC-102816) approved efficacy—refractory AML	
Erwinia Asparaginase (NSC-106977) approved efficacy—ALL in patients sensitive to *E. coli* L-asparaginase	
Hexamethylmelamine (NSC-13875) approved efficacy—ovarian carcinoma	
Semustine (NSC-95441) approved efficacy—carcinoma of the colon and stomach, melanoma	
Stretozocin (NSC-85998) approved efficacy—islet cell carcinoma of the pancreas, carcinoid	
Etoposide (NSC-141540) approved efficacy—small cell carcinoma of the lung	

Acridinyl anisidide

SYNONYMS: AMSA, NSC-249992, M-AMSA[1,4]

MANUFACTURER: Division of Cancer Treatment, National Cancer Institute[4]

DOSAGE FORMS AND STRENGTHS: 20 and 75 mg vials. Accompanying each is an additional vial containing 19.0 and 13.5 ml, respectively, of 0.008M of L-lactic acid diluent.[4]

STORAGE: Refrigerate.[4,19]

SOLUTION PREPARATION: The 20 mg vial is reconstituted with the 19.0 ml of 0.008M of L-lactic acid diluent provided, resulting in a final concentration of 1 mg/ml. The 75 mg vial is reconstituted with the 13.5 ml of 0.008M of L-lactic acid diluent provided, resulting in a final concentration of 5 mg/ml. Both reconstituted solutions may be further diluted with 5% dextrose injection, USP.[4,19]

STABILITY: Intact vials and diluents are stable at least 4 years when stored at room or refrigeration temperatures.[1] Both reconstituted and further diluted solutions in 500 ml of 5% dextrose injection, USP, are stable at least 48 hours at room temperature.[1,4] Since these solutions contain no preservatives, it is recommended that they be discarded after 8 hours.[4,19]

ROUTES OF ADMINISTRATION: IV. Give by IV infusion in 5% dextrose in water over 30 to 60 minutes.[1]

COMPATIBILITY: L-lactic acid, 5% dextrose injection, USP.[4]

INCOMPATIBILITY: Avoid solutions containing chloride. They may result in precipitation. Sodium chloride injection, USP.[1,4]

L-Alanosine

SYNONYMS: L-Alanosine, monosodium salt, NSC-153353[4,17]

MANUFACTURER: Division of Cancer Treatment, National Cancer Institute[4]

DOSAGE FORMS AND STRENGTHS: 100 mg vial[4,17]

STORAGE: Room temperature.[4,17]

SOLUTION PREPARATION: Reconstitute with 5 ml of sodium chloride injection, USP, to obtain a concentration of 20 mg/ml. This may be further diluted with 5% dextrose in sodium chloride injection, USP, to obtain a concentration of 1 mg/ml.[4,17]

STABILITY: Shelf life studies are in process. The reconstituted and further diluted solutions are stable at least 6 days at room temperature and under refrigeration. Since no preservative is present, it is recommended that the solution be discarded after 8 hours.[4,17]

pH: Reconstituted solution, 6.5 to 8.0[4,17]

ROUTES OF ADMINISTRATION: IV. Give by IV infusion over 30 minutes to 1 hour.[1]

COMPATIBILITY: Sodium chloride injection, USP, or 5% dextrose in sodium chloride injection, USP.[4,17]

Amino-thiadiazole

SYNONYMS: 2-amino-1,3,4-thiadiazole, NSC-4728[4,18]

MANUFACTURER: Division of Cancer Treatment, National Cancer Institute[4]

DOSAGE FORMS AND STRENGTHS: 200 mg vial[4,18]

STORAGE: Room temperature[4,18]

SOLUTION PREPARATION: Reconstitute with 20 ml of sterile water for injection, USP, sodium chloride injection, USP, or 5% dextrose injection, USP, to obtain a 10 mg/ml concentration.[4,18]

STABILITY: Intact vials are stable for at least *4 years* at room temperature. The reconstituted solution is stable for 72 hours at room temperature. Further dilution of the reconstituted solution does not alter solution stability. Since no preservative is present, the solution should be discarded after 8 to 24 hours.[4]

pH: Reconstituted solution, 5.5 to 7.0[4,18]

ROUTES OF ADMINISTRATION: IV[4,18]

COMPATIBILITY: Sterile water for injection, USP, sodium chloride injection, USP, 5% dextrose injection, USP, and 5% dextrose in sodium chloride injection, USP.[4]

Anguidine

SYNONYMS: NSC-141537, diacetoxyscirpenol[4,20]

MANUFACTURER: Division of Cancer Treatment, National Cancer Institute[4]

DOSAGE FORMS AND STRENGTHS: 5 mg vial[4]

STORAGE: Room temperature.[4,20]

SOLUTION PREPARATION: Reconstitute with 9.8 ml of sterile water for injection, USP, or sodium chloride injection, USP, to obtain a concentration of 0.5 mg/ml. This solution may be further diluted with 5% dextrose in sodium chloride injection, USP.[1,4]

STABILITY: Intact vials are stable for at least 2 years when stored at room temperature.[20] Reconstituted solutions are stable for 7 days at room temperature. When they are further diluted in 5% dextrose in sodium chloride, the solutions are stable for 24 hours at room temperature. Since there is no preservative present, the solution should be discarded 8 hours after preparation.[4]

pH: Reconstituted solution, 6.0 to 8.0[4,20]

ROUTES OF ADMINISTRATION: IV. If anguidine is given IV push, immediate side effects of vomiting, fever, chills, mental dysfunction, hypotension, and transient renal impairment may occur. When it is given by IV infusion, less vomiting, fever, and chills occur, but more myelosuppression occurs than with IV push. It can be given by an IV infusion in 50 ml of 5% dextrose in water, 5% dextrose in sodium chloride, or normal saline solution over 20 to 30 minutes or by a 4-hour infusion.[1,20]

SPECIAL PRECAUTIONS: Avoid skin contact due to irritation.[4,20]

COMPATIBILITY: 5% dextrose in sodium chloride injection, USP, 5% dextrose in water, sterile water for injection, USP, or sodium chloride injection, USP[1,4]

Erwinia asparaginase

SYNONYMS: NSC-106977, Porton asparaginase[4,21]

MANUFACTURER: Division of Cancer Treatment, National Cancer Institute[4]

DOSAGE FORMS AND STRENGTHS: 10,000 IU vial[4,21]

STORAGE: Refrigerate.[4,21]

SOLUTION PREPARATION: Reconstitute with 2 ml of sterile water for injection, USP, or sodium chloride injection, USP, to obtain a solution of 5,000 IU/ml. Further dilution may be done with 5% dextrose injection, USP, or sodium chloride injection, USP, to obtain a concentration of 35 IU/ml. Cloudy solutions should be discarded.[4,21]

STABILITY: Intact vials are stable 6 weeks at room temperature and 2 years when refrigerated. Reconstituted solution is stable up to 20 days at room temperature or when refrigerated. A further diluted solution with a concentration of 35 IU/ml is stable for 4 days at room temperature and at refrigeration temperatures. Turbid solutions should be discarded regardless of stability times.[4,21]

DOSAGE: (see page 184)

ROUTES OF ADMINISTRATION: IV push, IV infusion, or IM (see page 184)

SPECIAL PRECAUTIONS: Reconstituted solutions should be withdrawn within 15 minutes after preparation to minimize protein denaturation. Allergic reactions are the most common side effect encountered. *Erwinia* asparaginase appears to produce fewer allergic reactions and less nausea, vomiting, tremors, and drowsiness than *E. coli* asparaginase (see p. 184 for test doses).[4,21]

COMPATIBILITY: Sodium chloride injection, USP, 5% dextrose injection, USP, or sterile water for injection, USP[4,21]

5-Azacitidine

SYNONYMS: Aza-CR, 5-AZC, NSC-102816, ladakamycin, 5-azacytidine[3,9]

MANUFACTURER: Division of Cancer Treatment, National Cancer Institute[4]

DOSAGE FORMS AND STRENGTHS: For injection: 100 mg vial with 100 mg mannitol[1,2,4]

STORAGE: Store at refrigeration temperature (2° to 8° C).[1,2,4]

SOLUTION PREPARATION: Add 19.9 ml of sterile water for injection, USP, to the 100 mg vial, resulting in a 5 mg/ml concentration. The reconstituted solution can be further diluted in lactated Ringer's injection, USP, or normal saline solution. Lactated Ringer's injection, USP, provides optimal pH for solution stability of 5-azacitidine. Do *not* use 5% dextrose in water.[1,4]

STABILITY:

Prior to mixing: Stable for 2 years at room temperature (22° to 25° C) and 4 years at refrigeration temperatures (2° to 8° C). Because of degradation at elevated temperatures, refrigeration storage is recommended.[1,4]

At different concentrations: Reconstituted solutions are stable for 30 minutes at room temperature and should be used immediately for maximum potency. Decomposition is slowed by refrigeration. Infusion solutions of lactated Ringer's injection at room temperature should be used in 2 to 3 hours, during which 10% to 15% degradation can occur. Normal saline solutions are stable for less than 30 minutes.[1,4]

pH: Reconstituted solution, 6.0 to 7.5. 5-Azacitidine 100 mg/500 ml in lactated Ringer's injection, USP, has a pH of 6.4. The pH for optimal inhibition of degradation is about 6.5.[1,4]

DOSAGE: (a) 50 to 400 mg/m^2 per day for 5 days every 2 to 3 weeks (usual dosage range); (b) 150 to 200 mg/m^2 IV twice weekly for 2 to 8 weeks; (c) 200 to 633 mg/m^2 per week IV; (d) also 10-day IV and SC schedules.[2,62,64]

ROUTES OF ADMINISTRATION: SC, IV push, and IV infusion (preferred pharmacologically). (a) Normal saline solution can be used for infusions over a 15- to 30-minute period; (b) Lactated Ringer's injection, USP, should be used for continuous infusions longer than 30 minutes.[1,2,4,63]

SPECIAL PRECAUTIONS: Observe for possible hypotension and also observe the injection site for skin necrosis.[1,2,62]

COMPATIBILITY: Normal saline solution, sterile water for injection, USP, and lactated Ringer's injection, USP.[1,4]

INCOMPATIBILITY: 5% dextrose for injection, USP.[1,4]

Bacillus Calmette-Guérin vaccine

SYNONYMS: BCG, NSC-116327 (Tice), NSC-116328 (Pasteur), NSC-116341 (Connaught)[4]

MANUFACTURER: Division of Cancer Treatment, National Cancer Institute[4]

DOSAGE FORMS AND STRENGTHS:

1. Tice strain of BCG: 5 ± 3 × 10^8 colony forming units (cfu) per ampule

with 5 ml ampule of sterile diluent of buffering salts (produced by Institute for Tuberculosis Research at the University of Illinois).[4]

2. Pasteur strain of BCG: $3.75 - 15 \times 10^7$ cfu per ampule (low potency formulation) and $6 \pm 4 \times 10^8$ cfu per ampule (high potency formulation) with an ampule of sterile, isotonic sodium chloride solution as a diluent for reconstitution (produced by Institute Pasteur Production, Paris, France—U.S. distributor, Philips Roxane Laboratories, Columbus, Ohio). Note: this preparation is being phased out.[4]
3. Connaught strain of BCG: $8 \pm 4 \times 10^8$ cfu per vial with a sterile diluent of phosphate buffered saline vial for reconstitution (produced by Connaught Laboratories, Ontario, Canada).[4]
4. Glaxo strain of BCG: approximately 5×10^8 cfu with sterile diluent (produced by Glaxo Laboratories, Greenford, England, and Eli Lilly Co., Indianapolis, Ind.).[3]

STORAGE: Refrigerate at 5° C or lower and protect from direct or indirect sunlight or fluorescent light.[4]

SOLUTION PREPARATION: Reconstitute vaccines with 0.5 to 1.0 ml of the provided diluent. Complete preparation by aspirating the diluent and vaccine together until a uniform suspension is achieved. Vials with clumping or marked opacity should not be used. For intradermal administration a 10- to 12-fold dilution with the buffered solution is required. Sterile water for injection, USP, may be used but *not* bacteriostatic water for injection, USP, due to preservatives.[4] Autoclave all used syringes and needles in an aseptic manner prior to disposal.

STABILITY:

Prior to mixing: Expiration is 1 year from the manufacture date. Tice strain expiration is 6 months.[3,4]

At different concentrations: The suspension should be used immediately after reconstitution.[4]

DOSAGE: Doses are commonly listed as vials or ampules per administration. Scarification: usual dose is 5×10^8 cfu given weekly for 3 months, then every other week for 2 years. Monthly and bimonthly schedules are used. This is the preferred route since it has demonstrated greater responses. Intralesional, subcutaneous, and intracavitary: $10^6 - 10^7$ cfu. Oral: 1 to 4 vials of 10^8 cfu diluted in 50 to 100 ml of fluid (preferably isotonic) given weekly.[3,4]

ROUTES OF ADMINISTRATION: (1) dermal scarification, (2) intradermal or SC injection, (3) intrapleural, (4) intraperitoneal, (5) oral, (6) aerosol, (7) epilesional, (8) intralesional. *Scarification is preferred.*[3,4]

SPECIAL PRECAUTIONS: Care should be taken in handling BCG vaccine. Contracting BCG is remote; however, immunodeficient or suppressed persons might be affected. Contact with BCG may cause conversion to tuberculin reactivity with possible confusion as to the cause of the induced TB sensitivity.[4]

COMPATIBILITY: Sterile water for injection, USP, and normal saline solution.[4]

INCOMPATIBILITY: Bacteriostatic water for injection, USP, or any other solutions that contain an antibacterial preservative.[3,4]

BCG Scarification procedure*

Supplies

1. No. 18 gauge needle
2. 3 cc syringe
3. 1-inch paper tape
4. Sterile 4 × 4 inch gauze
5. Cover (petri dish or Frisbee)
6. Soap and water or acetone
7. Dryer with *cool cycle* (optional)
8. BCG (check expiration date) and diluent

Step 1: Resuspension of freeze-dried BCG vaccine

See Preparation.

Step 2: Placement

A. Upper arm and thigh (top and side).
B. Rotate sites: example—right arm, left arm, left leg, right leg, then repeat.
C. May be placed over previous scarification only if that site is very well healed (cannot feel scar).

Step 3: Preparation of site

A. Shave area if necessary. (You may wish to shave a large enough area to include tape.)
B. Cleanse a large area well with either soap and water or acetone. Allow to dry thoroughly.
C. *Do not* use alcohol as this agent will destroy the BCG.

Step 4: Scarification

A. The scarification should be approximately 5 cm square and when complete should have ten scratches down and ten across.
B. Holding the skin taut, make scratches with the cutting edge of the needle. Avoid using the point of the needle. Do this by bringing the whole hand across the surface, similar to drawing a line with a pen.
C. Exert enough pressure to produce capillary oozing (slight bleeding) from each scratch.
   1. You do not want free bleeding.
   2. If scratch is not deep enough to produce oozing, repeat the scratch in the same place.
   3. Proper bleeding can be checked by waiting after the first line has been made and judging the pressure.
D. The square should be made first in order to approximate the area—then

*Dorr, R. T., and Fritz, W. L.: *Cancer chemotherapy manual,* New York, 1977, American Elsevier Publishing Co., pp. 81-83. (Modification of M. D. Anderson BCG scarification procedure).

filled in with the eight scratches across and eight scratches down. (Continue to hold the skin taut while scratching.)

E. If excess bleeding should occur, hold slight pressure on the area with a sterile 4 × 4 inch gauze.

Step 5: Application of BCG

A. Push a few drops of the BCG through the needle with the plunger of the syringe onto the scarification.

B. Massage the BCG into the area (covering all scratches) with the flat of the needle. Repeatedly pull the skin taut to allow penetration of the vaccine. Continue adding vaccine a few drops at a time, massaging until all vaccine is on scarification.

C. You may direct a cool flow of air to area. (Use the dryer on cool as heat destroys the BCG.) This will shorten the drying time.

D. If medicine should roll off scarified area, push back with the needle or air flow.

E. Dry scarified area well. A glaze will form, and the site will not be sticky.

Step 6: Cover

A. If desired for comfort, place a folded 4 × 4 inch gauze at the top and bottom edges of the scarification, but not touching the area.

B. Place a petri dish over the area with its edges resting on the 4 × 4 inch gauze. If using a Frisbee, the 4 × 4 inch gauze is not necessary.

C. Tape securely but not tightly with paper tape. Do not eliminate all ventilation.

After care

1. Leave shield in place for 48 hours if possible.
2. Do not wash or get the area wet for 48 hours.
3. At the end of 48 hours, wash area well with soap and water.
4. Wash twice daily until healed.
5. Do not scratch site.
6. If area becomes dry or itchy, rub area with small amount of lotion (non–highly perfumed lotion such as Vaseline Intensive Care). Do not use alcohol.

Possible and common reactions

1. Itching
2. Redness
3. Swelling
4. Warmth at the site
5. Scaling or thickened scab
6. Discomfort at site
7. Scarring
8. Flu-like symptoms
   a. Fever to 101° for 24 to 48 hours
   b. Chills
   c. Headache
   d. Aching
9. Previous scarification sites may flare up with repeated treatments.
10. May have swelling or tenderness in lymph nodes in the groin or under the arm.

NOTE: *Dispose of equipment in an aseptic manner.*

Grading of BCG scarification response

The local response to BCG scarification can vary considerably, and a means of standardized reporting is necessary. One such scheme involves the use of a local response scale. This grading system should not be confused with BCG toxicity evaluation.

Grade 0: Normal healing at the scarification. No overt signs of skin inflammation.
Grade 1: Patchy erythema and induration at the scarification site.
Grade 2: Confluent erythema and induration.
Grade 3: Extension of inflammatory skin involvement to greater than 10 mm beyond the edges of the scarification site.
Grade 4: Local tissue ulceration or involvement of regional lymph nodes.

BCG toxicity grading

Because of the potential for varied and significant adverse reactions to BCG, various toxicity grading scales have been developed. Generally a numerical scale with increasing severity is utilized, such as:

Grade 0: Well-tolerated local inflammatory reaction. Mild to moderate fever, malaise, or transient liver enzyme elevations.
Grade 1: Local inflammatory reaction with lymph node involvement or systemic symptoms (fever, malaise) necessitating a delayed or reduced dosage scheme.
Grade 2: Local inflammatory response with the formation of abscesses (cutaneous drainage).
Grade 3: Above (grade 2) plus regional lymph node involvement.
Grade 4: Systemic BCG infection, noted by marked temperature elevation, elevated liver enzymes, severe flulike syndrome, local and distant abscesses, cough with pulmonary infiltrates—also, anaphylaxis or recurrent erythema nodosum.

Baker's antifol

SYNONYMS: Triazinate, NSC-139105, TZT, soluble Baker's antifol, BAF, ethanesulfonic acid compound[4,22]

MANUFACTURER: Division of Cancer Treatment, National Cancer Institute[4]

DOSAGE FORMS AND STRENGTHS: 100 and 250 mg vials[4,22]

STORAGE: Room temperature.[4,22]

SOLUTION PREPARATION: Reconstitute the 100 mg vial with 5 ml of sterile water for injection, USP, to obtain a concentration of 20 mg/ml. Reconstitute the 250 mg vial with 10 ml of sterile water for injection, USP, to obtain a concentration of 25 mg/ml. These may be further diluted with 5% dextrose in sodium chloride injection, USP.[4,22]

STABILITY: Intact vials are stable for at least 4 years at room temperature. Reconstituted and further diluted solutions of 500 ml are stable for at least 4 days at room temperature. Since the solutions contain no preservatives, it is recommended to discard them after 8 hours.[4]

pH: Reconstituted solutions, 5.0 to 7.0[4]

ROUTES OF ADMINISTRATION: IV infusion. May give by IV infusion in 50 to 100 ml of 5% dextrose in water or normal saline solution over 30 to 60 minutes.[1,22]

COMPATIBILITY: Sterile water for injection, USP, 5% dextrose in sodium chloride injection, USP, and 5% dextrose in water, USP[4,22]

Bruceantin

SYNONYMS: NSC-165563[4,24]

MANUFACTURER: Division of Cancer Treatment, National Cancer Institute[4]

DOSAGE FORMS AND STRENGTHS: 3 mg vial accompanied by an ampule of 1.5 ml of absolute ethanol as a diluent[4,24]

STORAGE: Deep freeze (−10° to −20° C).[4,24]

SOLUTION PREPARATION: Dissolve the contents of the 3 mg vial in 1.5 ml of absolute ethanol and further dilute with 13.5 ml of sodium chloride injection, USP, resulting in a concentration of 0.2 mg/ml. This may be further diluted with 5% dextrose in sodium chloride injection, USP.[4,24]

STABILITY: Intact vials are stable for at least 12 months at −20° C. Reconstituted and diluted (to 500 ml) solutions are stable for at least 4 days at room temperature. Since no preservative is present, it is recommended that the solution be discarded after 8 hours.[4,24]

pH: Reconstituted solution, 5.2 to 6.2[4,24]

ROUTES OF ADMINISTRATION: IV[24]

COMPATIBILITY: 5% dextrose in sodium chloride injection, USP, and sodium chloride injection, USP[4,24]

Chlorozotocin

SYNONYMS: DCNU, NSC-178248, the 2-chloroethyl analog of streptozotocin[4,26]

MANUFACTURER: Division of Cancer Treatment, National Cancer Institute[4]

DOSAGE FORMS AND STRENGTHS: 50 and 200 mg vials[1]

STORAGE: Refrigerate.[4,26]

SOLUTION PREPARATION: Reconstitute the 50 mg vial with 5 ml of sterile water for injection, USP, or sodium chloride injection, USP, to obtain a concentration of 10 mg/ml. Reconstitute the 200 mg vial with 9.8 ml of sterile water for injection, USP, to obtain a concentration of 20 mg/ml. These may be further diluted to a concentration of 0.1 mg/ml with 5% dextrose injection, USP, or 5% dextrose in sodium chloride injection, USP.[1,4]

STABILITY: Intact vials are stable for 2 years when refrigerated. Reconstituted and diluted solutions are stable for 3 hours at room temperature and 24 hours when refrigerated.[1,4]

pH: Reconstituted solutions, 3.8 to 4.2[4,26]

ROUTES OF ADMINISTRATION: IV. Give IV infusion rapidly every 6 weeks.[1]

COMPATIBILITY: Sterile water for injection, USP, sodium chloride injection, USP, 5% dextrose injection, USP, and 5% dextrose in sodium chloride injection, USP[4,26]

Corynebacterium parvum

SYNONYMS: *C. parvum* Wellcome, Wellcome CN6134, NSC-220537.[4]

MANUFACTURER: Burroughs Wellcome for the Division of Cancer Treatment, National Cancer Institute[4]

DOSAGE FORMS AND STRENGTHS: Suspension, 7 mg/ml, 1.2 ml per ampule with 0.01% thimerosal[4]

STORAGE: Refrigerate, storing upright. Protect from sunlight and ultraviolet radiation.[4]

SOLUTION PREPARATION: Ampules should be shaken vigorously before use to resuspend the suspension.[4]

STABILITY: Manufacturer recommends not using after two years of storage. Light (sunlight and ultraviolet) degrades the preservative (0.01% thimerosal), discoloring the suspension.[4]

ROUTES OF ADMINISTRATION: SC and IV.[4] Febrile responses to IV administration are common. Aggregates of bacteria often form; therefore IV administration requires an in-line blood filtration unit that filters particles >50 μm. Plastic bags or self-vented infusion bottles are recommended. Vacuum-containing intravenous solution bottles are not recommended for administration. ULTIPOR Blood Transfusion Filter manufactured by Pall Biomedical Products Corporation has been tested for *C. parvum* administration and found suitable.[4] Give by IV infusion in 150 to 250 ml of 5% dextrose in water over 60 minutes.[1]

SPECIAL PRECAUTIONS: *C. parvum* is a suspension of bacteria bodies and should be administered cautiously with aseptic technique and disposal precautions.[4]

COMPATIBILITY: 5% dextrose in water[1]

Cyclocytidine

SYNONYMS: Cyclo-C, NSC-145668, cyclocytidine hydrochloride[4,29]

MANUFACTURER: Division of Cancer Treatment, National Cancer Institute[4]

DOSAGE FORMS AND STRENGTHS: 200 and 500 mg vials, prepared as a lyophilized powder[4]

STORAGE: Room temperature.[4,29]

SOLUTION PREPARATION: Reconstitute the 200 mg vial with 5.0 ml of sterile water for injection, USP, sodium chloride injection, USP, or 5% dextrose injection, USP, to obtain a concentration of 40 mg/ml. Reconstitute the 500 mg vial with 10 ml of any of the three diluents above to obtain a concentration of 50 mg/ml.[4,29] Either vial may be further diluted with 5% dextrose in sodium chloride injection, USP.[4] For subcutaneous administration: the 200 and 500 mg vials should be reconstituted with 1.2 and 3 ml of normal saline respectively to yield a concentration of 167 mg/ml.[29]

STABILITY: Intact vials are stable for 4 years at room temperature. The reconstituted and further diluted solutions of 500 ml are stable for 24 hours at room temperature. Since no preservative is present, it is recommended that the solution be discarded after 8 hours.[4,29]

pH: Reconstituted solutions, 4.0 to 6.0[4,29]

ROUTES OF ADMINISTRATION: IV or SC. Can give by IV infusion in 50 to 150 ml 5% dextrose in water over 15 to 30 minutes.[1,4,29]

COMPATIBILITY: Sterile water for injection, USP, sodium chloride injection, USP, 5% dextrose injection, USP, and 5% dextrose in sodium chloride injection, USP[4,29]

Cycloleucine

SYNONYMS: NSC-1026, 1-aminocyclopentanecarboxylic acid[4]

MANUFACTURER: Division of Cancer Treatment, National Cancer Institute[4]

DOSAGE FORMS AND STRENGTHS: 20 g/500 ml infusion bottle (40 mg/ml)[4]

STORAGE: Room temperature.[4]

SOLUTION PREPARATION: None[4]

STABILITY: Infusion solution is stable for 4 years at room temperature.[4]

pH: 5.5 to 7.5[4]

ROUTES OF ADMINISTRATION: IV infusion. Self-venting administration sets are required for administration of drug (for example, Venoset, Saftiset)[1]

INCOMPATIBILITY: The chemical and physical compatibilities have not been evaluated; therefore other medication and combinations with cycloleucine should be avoided.[1]

3-Deazauridine

SYNONYMS: NSC-126849, 3-DAUR, deazaUR, deazaUMP, 3-deazauridine 5′-monophosphate, 3-deazauridine 5′-diphosphate, deazaUDP, deazaUTP, 3-deazauridine 5′-triphosphate.[33]

MANUFACTURER: Division of Cancer Treatment, National Cancer Institute[4]

DOSAGE FORMS AND STRENGTHS: 500 mg vial and a 2.0 g vial[4,33]

STORAGE: Refrigerate.[4,33]

SOLUTION PREPARATION: Reconstitute the 500 mg vial with 9.8 ml of sodium chloride injection, USP, or sterile water for injection, USP, to obtain a concentration of 50 mg/ml. If reconstituted with 4.7 ml or 2.2 ml, solutions containing concentrations of 100 mg/ml and 200 mg/ml respectively will result. Reconstitute the 2.0 g vial with 18.8 ml of sterile water for injection, USP, or sodium chloride injection, USP, to obtain a concentration of 100 mg/ml. Both vials may be further diluted with 5% dextrose in sodium chloride injection, USP.[4,33]

STABILITY: Intact vials when refrigerated are stable at least 2 years pending ongoing studies. At room temperature they are stable 6 months. Reconstituted solutions are stable 7 days at room temperature. Further diluted solutions up to 500 ml are stable for at least 4 days at room temperature. Since no preservative is present, it is recommended that the solutions be discarded after 8 hours.[4]

pH: 6.0 to 8.0[4]

ROUTES OF ADMINISTRATION: IV. Give by 24-hour continuous IV infusion.[33]

COMPATIBILITY: Sodium chloride injection, USP, sterile water for injection, USP, and 5% dextrose in sodium chloride injection, USP[4,33]

Dianhydrogalactitol

SYNONYMS: NSC-132313, DAG[4]

MANUFACTURER: Division of Cancer Treatment, National Cancer Institution[4]

DOSAGE FORMS AND STRENGTHS: 50 mg vial[4]

STORAGE: Refrigerate.[4]

SOLUTION PREPARATION: Reconstitute with 5 ml of sterile water for injection, USP, or sodium chloride injection, USP, to obtain a concentration of 10 mg/ml. Further dilution may be achieved with 5% dextrose in sodium chloride injection, USP.[4]

STABILITY: Intact vials are stable for at least 2 years when refrigerated and 3 months at room temperature. Reconstituted solutions are stable for 24 hours. Solutions further diluted up to 500 ml with 5% dextrose in sodium chloride injection, USP, are stable 8 hours. Since the solutions contain no preservative, it is recommended that they be discarded after 8 hours.[4]

pH: Reconstituted solution 5.0 to 7.0[4]

ROUTES OF ADMINISTRATION: IV[4]

COMPATIBILITY: Sterile water for injection, USP, sodium chloride injection, USP, and 5% dextrose in sodium chloride injection, USP[4]

Dibromodulcitol

SYNONYMS: NSC-104800; mitolactol; D-galactitol; 1,6-dibromo-1,6-dideoxy-; DBD[9,34]

MANUFACTURER: Division of Cancer Treatment, National Cancer Institute[34]

DOSAGE FORMS AND STRENGTHS: 50 and 100 mg tablets[34]

STORAGE: Room temperature.[34]

STABILITY: Tablets are stable for at least *2 years* when stored at room temperature. Partial bottles are also stable for extended periods if caution is observed to avoid exposure to heat and moisture.[34]

ROUTES OF ADMINISTRATION: Oral[34]

Dichloroallyl lawsone

SYNONYMS: DCL, NSC-126771[4,35]

MANUFACTURER: Division of Cancer Treatment, National Cancer Institute[4]

DOSAGE FORMS AND STRENGTHS: 250 mg vial[4,35]

STORAGE: Room temperature.[35]

SOLUTION PREPARATION: Reconstitute with 10 ml of sterile water for injection, USP, to obtain a concentration of 25 mg/ml. Further dilute with 5% dextrose injection, USP, for a final concentration of 1 mg/ml before drug administration.[4]

STABILITY: Intact vials are stable at least 2 years at room temperature. The reconstituted and diluted (1 mg/ml) solutions are stable 4 days at room temperature. Since no preservative is present, it is recommended that the solution be discarded after 8 hours.[4]

pH: Undiluted solution, 11.0 to 11.7.[4] Solutions of 0.1 to 10 mg/ml in 5% dextrose injection, USP, 7.5 to 9.5. Solutions in the pH range 7.5 to 9.5 are necessary to prevent reversion to the less soluble free acid (evidenced by a yellow precipitate).[35]

ROUTES OF ADMINISTRATION: IV. Give by slow IV infusion over 1 hour.[35]

SPECIAL PRECAUTIONS: Orange-yellow precipitate indicates reversion to the less soluble free acid due to a shift outside the optimum pH range of 7.5 to 9.5. *Only administer clear solutions.*[35]

COMPATIBILITY: Sterile water for injection, USP, and 5% dextrose injection, USP[35]

INCOMPATIBILITY: A precipitation has been observed after dilution with 5% dextrose in sodium chloride injection, USP. Therefore it is not recommended to use solutions with a chloride ion present for reconstitution or dilution.[4]

Dichloromethotrexate

SYNONYMS: NSC-29630[36]

MANUFACTURER: Division of Cancer Treatment, National Cancer Institute[4]

DOSAGE FORMS AND STRENGTHS: 250 mg vial[36]

STORAGE: Room temperature.[36]

SOLUTION PREPARATION: Reconstitute with 10 ml of sterile water for injection, USP, or 5% dextrose injection, USP, to obtain a 25 mg/ml concentration.[4,36]

STABILITY: Intact vials are stable at room temperature for at least 4 years. Reconstituted solution is stable for at least 7 days at room temperature. Since no preservative is present, solutions should be discarded 8 hours after preparation.[4]

pH: Reconstituted solution, 7.0 to 8.0[4,36]

ROUTES OF ADMINISTRATION: Parenteral. Can be given by rapid IV infusion over 5 to 10 minutes.[1]

COMPATIBILITY: Sterile water for injection, USP, and 5% dextrose injection, USP[36]

Diglycoaldehyde

SYNONYMS: Inosine dialdehyde, NSC-118994, INOX, Wyeth WY-5321[4]

MANUFACTURER: Division of Cancer Treatment, National Cancer Institute[4]

DOSAGE FORMS AND STRENGTHS: 1.0 g vial[4]

STORAGE: Room temperature.[49]

SOLUTION PREPARATION: Reconstitute with 9.0 ml of sterile water for injection, USP, to obtain a concentration of 100 mg/ml. The reconstituted solution is further diluted with 500 ml of a buffered solution of pH 7.0 to 8.0 of 5% dextrose injection, USP, or sodium chloride injection, USP, to minimize local irritation upon IV administration. Five hundred milligrams of sodium bicarbonate per 1.0 g of diglycoaldehyde results in a pH of 7.5 to 8.0. *Sodium bicarbonate solutions should not be used for reconstitution.*[4]

STABILITY: Intact vials are stable for at least 4 years at room temperature.[4] Reconstituted and diluted solutions as recommended are stable for at least 48 hours at either room or refrigeration temperatures.[37] Since no preservative is present, it is recommended that the solution be discarded after 8 hours.[4]

pH: Reconstituted solution, 3.0 to 4.0; diluted buffered solution, 7.0 to 8.0.[4]

ROUTES OF ADMINISTRATION: IV. Give the buffered solution by a 6-hour infusion because of local tissue reaction.[37]

COMPATIBILITY: Sterile water for injection, USP, 5% dextrose in sodium chloride injection, USP, sodium chloride injection, USP, and 5% dextrose injection, USP[4]

DON

SYNONYMS: NSC-7365, 6-Diazo-5-oxo-L-norleucine[4]

MANUFACTURER: Division of Cancer Treatment, National Cancer Institute[4]

DOSAGE FORMS AND STRENGTHS: 100 mg vial[4]

STORAGE: Deep freeze temperatures (−20° to −10° C).[4]

SOLUTION PREPARATION: Reconstitute with 5 ml of sodium chloride injection,

USP, to obtain a concentration of 20 mg/ml. This may be further diluted with 5% dextrose in sodium chloride injection, USP.[4]

STABILITY: Intact vial shelf-life studies are still in progress. Both the reconstituted and diluted solutions (concentration 0.2 to 1 mg/ml) are stable for at least 24 hours at refrigeration temperatures.[1,4]

pH: Reconstituted solution, 5.4 to 5.8[4]

ROUTES OF ADMINISTRATION: Parenteral. Can be given by rapid IV infusion.[1]

COMPATIBILITY: Sodium chloride injection, USP, and 5% dextrose in sodium chloride injection, USP[4]

Etoposide

SYNONYMS: VP 16-213, NSC-14150, Ethylidene-Lignan P, EPEG[4,59]

MANUFACTURER: Sandoz, Basle, Switzerland, distributed by Bristol in the U.S., provided by the Division of Cancer Treatment, National Cancer Institute.[4,59]

DOSAGE FORMS AND STRENGTHS: 100 mg ampule[4]

STORAGE: Room temperature.[4,59]

SOLUTION PREPARATION: Dilute with at least a 1:20 dilution of sodium chloride injection, USP, before administration. Discard solutions that have a precipitate.[4,59]

STABILITY: The intact ampules are chemically stable at room temperature for approximately 5 years from the date of manufacture.[1] Dilution in sodium chloride injection, USP, results in the following solution stability before precipitation occurs:

1:20 —30 minutes
1:50 — 3 hours
1:100— 6 hours

VP16-213 is less stable in 5% dextrose injection, USP, than sodium chloride injection, USP. Discard solutions with a precipitate.[4]

DOSAGE: 75 to 200 mg/m^2 per day for 3 days every 3 to 5 weeks[2]

ROUTES OF ADMINISTRATION: IV. Give by slow IV infusion over 30 minutes.[1]

SPECIAL PRECAUTIONS: Observe the prepared solution for clarity before use. Hypotension is possible; therefore patient should be recumbent. Anaphylaxis is possible.[2]

COMPATIBILITY: Sodium chloride injection, USP

INCOMPATIBILITY: In 5% dextrose solutions, etoposide is less stable than in normal saline solution. Contact with buffered aqueous solutions with a pH above 8 should be avoided.[4,59]

Gallium nitrate

SYNONYMS: NSC-15200[4,40]

MANUFACTURER: Division of Cancer Treatment, National Cancer Institute[4]

DOSAGE FORMS AND STRENGTHS: 100 mg ampules (10 mg/ml) and 500 mg ampules (25 mg/ml)[4,40]

STORAGE: Room temperature.[4,40]

SOLUTION PREPARATION: None. Can be further diluted with 5% dextrose in sodium chloride injection, USP.[4]

STABILITY: Ampules are stable for 3 years at room temperature. If further diluted up to 500 ml, the solution is stable for 24 hours at room temperature.[4]

pH: 6.0 to 7.0[4,40]

ROUTES OF ADMINISTRATION: IV infusion. Give slowly at a rate of 1 ml per minute.[4]

SPECIAL PRECAUTIONS: Give only clear solution.[4,40]

COMPATIBILITY: 5% dextrose in sodium chloride injection, USP[4]

Hexamethylmelamine

SYNONYMS: HXM, HMM, NSC-13875[4,41]

MANUFACTURER: Division of Cancer Treatment, National Cancer Institute[4]

DOSAGE FORMS AND STRENGTHS: 50 and 100 mg capsules[4,41]

STORAGE: Room temperature.[4,41]

STABILITY: Intact bottles of capsules are stable for at least 4 years when stored at room temperature.[4]

DOSAGE: 160 to 320 mg/m^2 per day continuously; 240 to 320 mg/m^2 per day for 21 days, repeated every 6 weeks.[2]

ROUTES OF ADMINISTRATION: Oral[4,41]

ICRF-187

SYNONYMS: NSC-169780; ICRF-187 is the (+) enantiomer of the racemic ICRF-159[4,43]

MANUFACTURER: Division of Cancer Treatment, National Cancer Institute[4]

DOSAGE FORMS AND STRENGTHS: 250 mg vial[4,43]

STORAGE: Room temperature.[4,43]

SOLUTION PREPARATION: Reconstitute with 25 ml of sodium chloride injection, USP, to obtain a concentration of 10 mg/ml.[4,43]

STABILITY: Shelf-life studies of the intact vials are in process. Reconstituted solutions are stable for at least 8 hours at room temperature. It is recommended that they be discarded after 8 hours since no preservative is present.[4]

pH: Reconstituted solution, 5.0 to 6.5[4,43]

ROUTES OF ADMINISTRATION: IV push and slow IV infusion over 30 minutes[1]

COMPATIBILITY: Sodium chloride injection, USP, and 5% dextrose injection, USP[4,43]

Ifosfamide

SYNONYMS: NSC-109724, Z4942, isophosphamide, M5F9325 (Mead Johnson)[4,45]

MANUFACTURER: Division of Cancer Treatment, National Cancer Institute[4]

DOSAGE FORMS AND STRENGTHS: 1.0 and 3.0 g vials

STORAGE: Room temperature. Heat (temperatures above 35° C) will liquefy or degrade the material or do both.[4,45]

SOLUTION PREPARATION: 1.0 g/vial: reconstitute with 20 ml of sterile water for injection, USP, to produce a concentration of 50 mg/ml. These may be further diluted with 5% dextrose in Ringer's injection, USP, 5% dextrose in sodium chloride injection, USP, 5% dextrose in water, USP, lactated Ringer's injection, USP, half normal saline solution, normal saline solution, or sodium lactate.[1,4] 3.0 g/vial: reconstitute with 30 ml of sterile water for injection, USP, to produce a concentration of 100 mg/ml.[4]

STABILITY: Intact vials are stable for at least 5 years at room temperature. When reconstituted as recommended, the solution is stable for 7 days at room temperature. Further dilution of the reconstituted solution to a concentration of 16 mg/ml or 0.6 mg/ml results in a solution stable at room temperature for 7 days and for 6 weeks under refrigeration.[1] No preservative is present; so it is recommended that the solution be discarded 8 hours after preparation.[4]

pH: Reconstituted solutions, 5.5 to 6.5[4,45]

DOSAGE: 1,000 to 1,500 mg/m^2/day for 5 days as continuous or intermittent IV infusion; repeated every 2 to 3 weeks[2,45]

ROUTES OF ADMINISTRATION: IV.[45] May be given by IV infusion, varying from 30 minutes to 5 hours.[1]

COMPATIBILITY: Sterile water for injection, USP, lactated Ringer's injection, USP, 5% dextrose injection, USP, sodium chloride injection, USP, 0.45% sodium chloride injection, USP, 5% dextrose in Ringer's injection, USP, and 5% dextrose in sodium chloride injection, USP[1]

Indicine N-oxide

SYNONYMS: NSC-132319[4,44]

MANUFACTURER: Division of Cancer Treatment, National Cancer Institute[4]

DOSAGE FORMS AND STRENGTHS: 1.0 g vial[4,44]

STORAGE: Refrigerate.[4,44]

SOLUTION PREPARATION: Reconstitute with 9.2 ml of sterile water for injection, USP, to result in a concentration of 100 mg/ml. This may be further diluted with 5% dextrose in sodium chloride injection, USP, or sodium chloride injection, USP.[4,44]

STABILITY: Intact vials are stable at least 6 months when refrigerated. Reconstituted and diluted solutions are stable at least 48 hours at room temperature. Since no preservative is present, it is recommended that the solution be discarded after 8 hours.[4]

pH: Reconstituted solution, 6.0 to 8.0[4,44]

ROUTES OF ADMINISTRATION: IV push and rapid IV infusion[1]

COMPATIBILITY: Sterile water for injection, USP, sodium chloride injection, USP, 5% dextrose in sodium chloride injection, USP[4]

Levamisole hydrochloride

SYNONYMS: NSC-177023, R 12,564 (Janssen Pharmaceutica, Belgium), Tramisol (American Cyanamid)[4,9,63]

MANUFACTURER: Supplied by Janssen Pharmaceutica, New Brunswick, N.J., for the Division of Cancer Treatment, National Cancer Institute[4]

DOSAGE FORMS AND STRENGTHS: 50 mg film-coated tablets[4,46]

STORAGE: Room temperature. Protect from light.[4]

STABILITY: Stable for at least 3 years at room temperature, protected from light.[4]

DOSAGE: Usually 150 mg daily

ROUTES OF ADMINISTRATION: Oral. At daily doses in excess of 2.5 mg/kg the incidence of gastrointestinal side effects is increased. To reduce these side effects the drug is divided over 2 to 3 doses. It is generally given intermittently on 2, 3, or 4 consecutive days every week, every fortnight, or at each disease episode.[46]

Maytansine

SYNONYMS: NSC-153858[4,48]

MANUFACTURER: Bristol for the Division of Cancer Treatment, National Cancer Institute[4]

DOSAGE FORMS AND STRENGTHS: 0.25 mg vial[4,48]

STORAGE: Refrigerate.[4,48]

SOLUTION PREPARATION: Reconstitute with 5 ml of sterile water for injection, USP, or sodium chloride injection, USP, to obtain a concentration of 0.05 mg/ml. This solution may be further diluted to a concentration of 10 μg/ml with 5% dextrose in sodium chloride injection, USP.[4]

STABILITY: Intact vials are stable for at least 2 years under refrigeration. Reconstituted and diluted solutions are stable at least 4 days at room temperature or refrigeration temperatures. Since no preservative is present, it is recommended that the solution be discarded after 8 hours.[4]

pH: Reconstituted solution, 5.0 to 7.0[4]

ROUTES OF ADMINISTRATION: IV. Give by a single IV bolus or continuous IV infusion.[48]

SPECIAL PRECAUTIONS: Avoid extravasation.[48]

COMPATIBILITY: Sterile water for injection, USP, sodium chloride injection, USP, and 5% dextrose in sodium chloride injection, USP[4]

Methyl-GAG

SYNONYMS: NSC-32946, Mitoguazone[1,49]

MANUFACTURER: Division of Cancer Treatment, National Cancer Institute[1]

DOSAGE FORMS AND STRENGTHS: 1.0 g vial[1,49]

STORAGE: Room temperature.[49]

SOLUTION PREPARATION: Reconstitute the 1.0 g vial with 9.1 ml of sodium chloride injection, USP, to obtain a concentration of 100 mg/ml. May be further diluted with 5% dextrose in sodium chloride injection, USP.[1]

STABILITY: Intact vials are stable for at least 2 years at room temperature. Once reconstituted, solutions are stable for 48 hours at room or refrigerated temperatures. Further diluted solutions at a concentration of 2 mg/ml are stable 7 days at room and refrigeration temperatures.[1]

pH: Reconstituted solution, 3.5 to 5.5[1]

ROUTES OF ADMINISTRATION: IV. Can give by IV infusion over 30 to 45 minutes.[1,49]

COMPATIBILITY: Sodium chloride injection, USP, and 5% dextrose in sodium chloride injection, USP[1]

Misonidazole

SYNONYMS: NSC-261037, formerly RO-7-0582[1,4,50]

MANUFACTURER: Hoffmann-LaRoche for the Division of Cancer Treatment, National Cancer Institute[4]

DOSAGE FORMS AND STRENGTHS: 100 and 500 mg capsules[4]; 500 mg vial[1]

STORAGE: Room temperature (22° to 25° C).[4,50]

SOLUTION PREPARATION: Reconstitute with 19.7 ml sodium chloride injection, USP, or sterile water for injections, USP, to obtain a concentration of 25 mg/ml. May be further diluted with 5% dextrose in water.[1]

STABILITY: Shelf-life studies are in process. Injectable drug is stable 14 days after reconstitution and with further dilution to a concentration of 1 g/liter in 5% dextrose in water.[1]

pH: Reconstituted solution, 4.0 to 7.0[1]

ROUTES OF ADMINISTRATION: Oral,[50] IV[1]

Nafoxidine hydrochloride

SYNONYMS: Upjohn U-11100A, NSC-70735[4,47]

MANUFACTURER: Upjohn for the Division of Cancer Treatment, National Cancer Institute[4]

DOSAGE FORMS AND STRENGTHS: 60 mg tablets[4,47]

STORAGE: Room temperature.[4,47]

STABILITY: The tablets are stable at least 4 years at room temperature.[4]

ROUTES OF ADMINISTRATION: Oral[4,47]

PALA disodium

SYNONYMS: NSC-224131, N-phosphonoacetyl-L-aspartate disodium[4,52]

MANUFACTURER: Division of Cancer Treatment, National Cancer Institute[4]

DOSAGE FORMS AND STRENGTHS: 1 g ampule[4,52]

STORAGE: Refrigerate.[4,52]

SOLUTION PREPARATION: May be further diluted to a concentration of 1 mg/ml in 5% dextrose injection, USP, or sodium chloride injection, USP.[4]

STABILITY: Shelf-life stability studies are in process. Diluted solutions to 1 mg/ml concentration are stable for 2 weeks at room temperature.[4]

pH: Reconstituted solution, 6.5 to 7.5[4,52]

ROUTES OF ADMINISTRATION: IV. May give by rapid or continuous IV infusions over 15 minutes daily for 5 days.[1]

COMPATIBILITY: Sterile water for injection, USP, 5% dextrose injection, USP, and sodium chloride injection, USP[4,52]

PCNU

SYNONYMS: NSC-95466[4]

MANUFACTURER: Division of Cancer Treatment, National Cancer Institute[4]

DOSAGE FORMS AND STRENGTHS: 50 mg vial. An ampule containing 1 ml of sterile anhydrous N,N-dimethyl-acetamide (DMA) and another ampule containing 3 ml of sterile propylene glycol accompany the 50 mg vial to be used as diluents.[53]

STORAGE: Refrigerate.[53]

SOLUTION PREPARATION: Reconstitute with 0.25 ml of sterile N,N-dimethyl-acetamide (DMA) and 2.25 ml of sterile propylene glycol to obtain a 20 mg/ml concentration of PCNU. Further dilute with 5% dextrose injection, USP, so that the final concentration is not more than 0.5 mg/ml.[4,53]

STABILITY: Shelf-life stability studies are ongoing. The reconstituted solution further diluted in 5% dextrose injection, USP, is stable for at least 4 hours at room temperature (approximately 4% to 6% decomposition).[4]

ROUTES OF ADMINISTRATION: IV. Give by slow IV infusion.[4]

COMPATIBILITY: 5% dextrose injection, USP[4]

Pentamethylmelamine hydrochloride

SYNONYMS: PMM, NSC-118742, pentamethylmelamine hydrochloride[54]

MANUFACTURER: Division of Cancer Treatment, National Cancer Institute[4]

DOSAGE FORMS AND STRENGTHS: 500 mg vial, with mannitol 300 mg[54]

STORAGE: Room temperature.[54]

SOLUTION PREPARATION: Reconstitute with 9.5 ml of sterile water for injection, USP, to obtain a concentration of 50 mg/ml. The reconstituted solution may be further diluted with 5% dextrose injection in sodium chloride injection, USP. Since no preservative is present, the solution should be discarded after 8 hours after preparation.[4,54]

STABILITY: Shelf-life studies are ongoing. The reconstituted solution is stable for at least 7 days at room temperature or refrigeration temperature. Further dilution does not alter solution stability.[54]

pH: Reconstituted solution, 4.5 to 5.5[4,54]

ROUTES OF ADMINISTRATION: IV. May give by slow IV infusions over 1 to 2 hours.[1]

COMPATIBILITY: Sterile water for injection, USP, and 5% dextrose in sodium chloride injection, USP[54]

Piperazinedione

SYNONYMS: NSC-135758, crystalline antibiotic, *Actinomycete* Fermentation Product, Merck Compound 593A[55]

MANUFACTURER: Division of Cancer Treatment, National Cancer Institute[4]

DOSAGE FORMS AND STRENGTHS: 5 mg vial[55]

STORAGE: Room temperature.[4]

SOLUTION PREPARATION: Reconstitute with 5 ml of sterile water for injection, USP, to obtain a concentration of 6 mg/ml. If necessary, the drug may be dissolved in a minimum of 2 ml of sterile water for injection, USP. The solution may be further diluted in 5% dextrose in sodium chloride injection, USP. Since no preservative is present, it is recommended that the solution be discarded after 8 hours.[4,55]

STABILITY: Intact vials are stable for at least 24 months when stored at room temperature.[4]

pH: Reconstituted solution, 3.0 to 4.5[4]

ROUTES OF ADMINISTRATION: IV[55]

COMPATIBILITY: Sterile water for injection, USP, and 5% dextrose in sodium chloride injection, USP[55]

Pyrazofurin

SYNONYMS: NSC-143095, Lilly XW 8791-AMX[4]

MANUFACTURER: Lilly for the Division of Cancer Treatment, National Cancer Institute[4]

DOSAGE FORMS AND STRENGTHS: 300 mg vial[4]

STORAGE: Refrigerate.[4]

SOLUTION PREPARATION: Reconstitute with 10 ml of bacteriostatic sodium chloride injection, USP, or 5% dextrose injection, USP, to obtain a concentration of 30 mg/ml. It may further be diluted with 5% dextrose injection, USP, or 5% dextrose in sodium chloride injection, USP.[4]

STABILITY: Intact vials are stable for at least 12 months under refrigeration or at room temperature. Reconstitution with bacteriostatic sodium chloride injection, USP, results in stability of 30 days when refrigerated and 48 hours at room temperature. When pyrazofurin is reconstituted with a nonbacteriostatic solution, it is recommended that it be discarded after 8 hours.[4]

pH: Before reconstitution, 7.4; reconstituted solution, 7.0 to 8.0[4]

ROUTES OF ADMINISTRATION: IV[4]

COMPATIBILITY: Bacteriostatic sodium chloride injection, USP, sodium chloride injection, USP, 5% dextrose injection, USP, and 5% dextrose in sodium chloride injection, USP[4]

INCOMPATIBILITY: Further dilution in lactated Ringer's solution results in degradation of pyrazofurin within 24 hours.[4]

Pyrazolo imidazole

SYNONYMS: IMPY, NSC-51143[56]

MANUFACTURER: Division of Cancer Treatment, National Cancer Institute[4]

DOSAGE FORMS AND STRENGTHS: 500 mg vial[56]

STORAGE: Room temperature.[56]

SOLUTION PREPARATION: Reconstitute with 9.6 ml of sterile water for injection, USP, to produce a concentration of 50 mg/ml.[56]

STABILITY: The intact vials are stable for at least 18 months at room temperature. Shelf-life studies are ongoing. The reconstituted solution is stable for at least 7 days at room temperature. Further dilution of the reconstituted solution with 5% dextrose in sodium chloride injection, USP, does not affect solution stability. No preservative is present; therefore the solution should be discarded after 8 hours.[4]

pH: Reconstituted solution, 6.0 to 8.0[4]

ROUTES OF ADMINISTRATION: IV[56]

COMPATIBILITY: Sterile water for injection, USP, and 5% dextrose in sodium chloride injection, USP[56]

Razoxane

SYNONYMS: ICRF-159, NSC-129943[4,42]

MANUFACTURER: Division of Cancer Treatment, National Cancer Institute[4]

DOSAGE FORMS AND STRENGTHS: 50 and 500 mg tablets.[4,42]
STORAGE: Room temperature.[4,42]
STABILITY: The tablets are stable at least 4 years at room temperature.[4]
ROUTES OF ADMINISTRATION: Oral[4,42]

Semustine

SYNONYMS: Methyl-CCNU, MeCCNU, NSC-95441[4]
MANUFACTURER: Division of Drug Treatment, National Cancer Institute[4]
DOSAGE FORMS AND STRENGTHS: 10, 50, and 100 mg capsules[4]
STORAGE: Refrigerate. Can also be kept at room temperature for short-term storage. It does decompose.[4]
DRUG PREPARATION: No more than a single dose should be prepared for a patient. The dose should be to the nearest 10 mg. The patient should be cautioned to avoid exposing the drug to temperatures greater than 40° C and to moisture.[4]
STABILITY: Capsules in intact bottles refrigerated at 2° to 8° C are stable for 4 years. Capsules in intact bottles at room temperature (22° to 25° C) are stable for 1 year. Temperatures greater than 40° C result in decomposition of Methyl-CCNU capsules within 30 days. Methyl-CCNU is hygroscopic; therefore prolonged exposure to moisture should be avoided.[4]
DOSAGE: As a single agent the usual dose is 150 to 200 mg/m^2 orally every 6 to 8 weeks or in smaller doses every 4 weeks.[2] A reduction in dose is necessary with myelosuppression and liver impairment.[7]
ROUTES OF ADMINISTRATION: *Oral route only.* The drug should be administered to a patient with an empty stomach to minimize side effects.[2,4]
SPECIAL PRECAUTIONS: Semustine has delayed and cumulative bone marrow toxicity and should not be given any more frequently than every 6 weeks by an experienced individual. It should not be given until platelets and leukocytes have returned to acceptable levels (platelets ≥ 100,000/mm^3 and leukocytes ≥ 4,000/mm^3). More than one dose of semustine should note be dispensed at any one time because of its severe hematologic toxicities. Safe usage in pregnancy has not been established.[7,74]

Streptonigrin

SYNONYMS: NSC-45383, BA-163, PC-501[4]
MANUFACTURER: Division of Cancer Treatment, National Cancer Institute[4]
DOSAGE FORMS AND STRENGTHS: 0.2 mg capsules[4]
STORAGE: Room temperature.[4]
STABILITY: Stable at least 2 years at room temperature[4]
ROUTES OF ADMINISTRATION: Oral[4]

Streptozocin

SYNONYMS: Streptozotocin, U-9889, NSC-85998, Zanosar[2,4,9]

MANUFACTURER: Upjohn for the Division of Cancer Treatment, National Cancer Institute[4]

DOSAGE FORMS AND STRENGTHS: 1.0 g vial[4]

STORAGE: Refrigerate.[4]

SOLUTION PREPARATION: Reconstitute with 9.3 ml of sterile water for injection, USP, or sodium chloride injection, USP, to obtain a concentration of 100 mg/ml. This may be further diluted with 5% dextrose in sodium chloride injection, USP.[4]

STABILITY: Intact vials are stable 3 years when refrigerated and 1 year at room temperature. Both reconstituted and diluted solutions (up to 500 mg) are stable at least 48 hours at room temperature and 96 hours when refrigerated. Since no preservative is present, it is recommended that the solution be discarded after 8 hours.[4]

pH: 3.8 to 4.2[4]

DOSAGE: 400 to 500 mg/m^2 IV daily for 3 to 5 days; single doses up to 1.5 g/m^2; repeat every 3 weeks as blood count permits[2]

ROUTES OF ADMINISTRATION: IV. May be given IV push or by IV infusion in 50 ml of 5% dextrose in water[1]

COMPATIBILITY: Sterile water for injection, USP, sodium chloride injection, USP, 5% dextrose in sodium chloride injection, USP, and 5% dextrose in water injection, USP[4]

Tegafur

SYNONYMS: NSC-148958, FT-203, ftorafur[4,9]

MANUFACTURER: Division of Cancer Treatment, National Cancer Institute[4]

DOSAGE FORMS AND STRENGTHS: 500 mg vial and 2.0 g vial[4,39]

STORAGE: Room temperature.[4,39]

SOLUTION PREPARATION: Reconstitute the 500 mg vial with 9.7 ml of sterile water for injection, USP, resulting in a concentration of 50 mg/ml. Reconstitute the 2.0 g vial with 38.8 ml of sterile water for injection, USP, resulting in a concentration of 50 mg/ml also. These solutions may further be diluted with 5% dextrose injection, USP, or sodium chloride injection, USP.[4,39]

STABILITY: Intact vials are stable for at least 4 years at room temperature.[1] Reconstituted solutions are stable more than 30 days at room or refrigeration temperatures. Solutions that have been further diluted (up to 500 ml) are stable for 4 days at room and refrigeration temperatures. Since no preservative is present, it is recommended that the solutions be discarded after 8 hours.[4]

PH: Reconstituted solutions, 8.2 to 9.2[4,39]

DOSAGE: 2 g/m^2 per day for 5 days or single dose of 3 to 4 g/m^2; repeat every 2 to 4 weeks.[2]

ROUTES OF ADMINISTRATION: IV. May be given by slow IV infusion in 100 ml or more over 1 to 2 hours.[1]

SPECIAL PRECAUTIONS: Observe for possible hypotension.[2]

COMPATIBILITY: Sterile water for injection, USP, 5% dextrose injection, USP, and sodium chloride injection, USP[4,39]

Teniposide

SYNONYMS: VM-26, NSC-122819, Thenylidene-Liganan-P, PTG[4,9,60]

MANUFACTURER: Sandoz, Basle, Switzerland, distributed by Bristol in U.S., provided by the Division of Cancer Treatment, National Cancer Institute[4,60]

DOSAGE FORMS AND STRENGTHS: 50 mg ampule[4,60]

STORAGE: Room temperature.[4,60]

SOLUTION PREPARATION: Dilute the ampule solution with at least 5 volumes, and preferably 10 to 20 volumes, of sodium chloride injection, USP, or 5% dextrose in water, USP, before administration. It can also be further diluted with 50 to 100 volumes with the same solution. Discard solutions with a precipitate. A slight opalescence is due to surfactant in the preparation.[4]

STABILITY: The intact ampules are stable for approximately 4 years from date of manufacture. Solutions prepared in the manner above are physically stable for 4 hours at room temperature, except those diluted with 50 to 100 volumes. They are stable 6 hours.[4]

PH: 5.1[4,60]

DOSAGE: 100 mg/m^2 daily for 2 days or 40 mg/m^2 daily for 5 days, repeated every 3 to 4 weeks[2]

ROUTES OF ADMINISTRATION: IV. Give by IV infusion over 30 to 90 minutes.[1]

SPECIAL PRECAUTIONS: Patient should be recumbent. Give slowly to avoid hypotension.[2] If a precipitate is noted as the ampuled solution is being diluted as recommended above, do not administer the solution. A slight opalescence is due to the surfactant and does not make the solution unacceptable for use.[4,60]

COMPATIBILITY: Sodium chloride injection, USP, and 5% dextrose injection, USP[4,60]

α-TGdR

SYNONYMS: NSC-71851[4]

MANUFACTURER: Division of Cancer Treatment, National Cancer Institute[4]

DOSAGE FORMS AND STRENGTHS: 200 mg vial[4]

STORAGE: Room temperature.[4]

SOLUTION PREPARATION: Reconstitute with 19.6 ml of sterile water for injection, USP, or sodium chloride injection, USP, to produce a concentration of 10 mg/ml. This may further be diluted with 5% dextrose in sodium chloride injection, USP.[4]

STABILITY: Intact vials are stable for at least 48 months at room temperature. The reconstituted solution is stable for at least 24 hours at room temperature. Do not refrigerate, because a white precipitate will form within 2 hours. Further dilution in 500 ml of 5% dextrose in sodium chloride injection, USP, produces a solution that is stable for 8 hours at room temperature and 4 hours when refrigerated. After these time periods a precipitate will form. Since no preservative is present, it is recommended that the solutions be discarded within 8 hours.[4]

pH: Reconstituted solution, 9.8 to 10.8[4]

ROUTES OF ADMINISTRATION: IV[4]

COMPATIBILITY: Sterile water for injection, USP, sodium chloride injection, USP, and 5% dextrose in sodium chloride injection, USP[4]

3% Thymidine injection

SYNONYMS: NSC-21548[4,58]

MANUFACTURER: Division of Cancer Treatment, National Cancer Institute[4]

DOSAGE FORMS AND STRENGTHS: 15 g in 500 ml of 0.6% sodium chloride injection to produce a 3% injection solution[4,58]

STORAGE: Room temperature. Do not freeze or refrigerate thymidine infusion solutions. A precipitate is likely to occur.[4,58]

SOLUTION PREPARATION: None

STABILITY: 3% infusion solution is stable 24 months at room temperature. Shelf-life studies are continuing.[4]

pH: 4.5 to 7.5[4,58]

ROUTES OF ADMINISTRATION: IV infusion. Self-venting administration sets are required for infusion. In-line filters do not affect the potency of the drug.[4]

INCOMPATIBILITY: Do not add other medications to the 3% thymidine solution.[4]

TMCA

SYNONYMS: NSC-36354[4]

MANUFACTURER: Division of Cancer Treatment, National Cancer Institute[4]

DOSAGE FORMS AND STRENGTHS: 1 mg capsules[4]

STORAGE: Room temperature.[4]

STABILITY: Stable at least 2 years at room temperature[4]

ROUTES OF ADMINISTRATION: Oral[4]

Triflurothymidine

SYNONYMS: NSC-75520, F_3TDR, trifluridine[4]

MANUFACTURER: Division of Cancer Treatment, National Cancer Institute[4]

DOSAGE FORMS AND STRENGTHS: 200 mg vial[4]

STORAGE: Room temperature.[4]

SOLUTION PREPARATION: Reconstitute with 8 ml of sterile water for injection, USP, or sodium chloride injection, USP, to obtain a concentration of 25 mg/ml. Further dilution may be done with 5% dextrose injection, USP.[4]

STABILITY: Intact vials are stable at least 2 years at room temperature. The reconstituted solution (and with further dilution—up to 500 ml) is stable 24 hours at room temperature. Since it lacks a preservative, it is recommended that solutions be discarded after 8 hours.[4]

pH: Reconstituted solution, 4.5 to 5.5[4]

ROUTES OF ADMINISTRATION: IV[4]

COMPATIBILITY: 5% dextrose injection, USP, sterile water for injection, USP, and sodium chloride injection, USP[4]

Yoshi-864

SYNONYMS: NSC-102627, Japanese Cancer Institute No. 864[61]

MANUFACTURER: Division of Cancer Treatment, National Cancer Institute[4]

DOSAGE FORMS AND STRENGTHS: 100 mg vial[4]

STORAGE: Deep freeze temperatures (−20° to −10° C).[4]

SOLUTION PREPARATION: Reconstitute with 5 ml of sterile water for injection, USP, resulting in a concentration of 20 mg/ml. May further dilute with 5% dextrose in sodium chloride injection, USP.[4]

STABILITY: In deep freeze temperatures, intact vials are stable for 4 years and in refrigeration at least 2 months. Reconstituted and diluted solutions are stable (<10% decomposition) 6 hours at room temperature or when under refrigeration.[4]

pH: Reconstituted solution, 3.0 to 5.0[4]

ROUTES OF ADMINISTRATION: IV[61]

COMPATIBILITY: Sterile water for injection, USP, and 5% dextrose in sodium chloride injection, USP[4]

Zinostatin

SYNONYMS: NSC-157365, NCS, Neocarzinostatin[4,9]

MANUFACTURER: Bristol for the Division of Cancer Treatment, National Cancer Institute[4]

DOSAGE FORMS AND STRENGTHS: 2,000 units per ampule.[4,51] *Note:* NCS is assayed biologically with potency expressed as units of antibacterial activity. The expression of potency has been changed from the previously used "2 mg unit" to 2,000 units, which are equivalent.[4]

STORAGE: Intact ampules should be stored under refrigeration (2° to 8° C) and protected from light.[51]

SOLUTION PREPARATION: The ampule may be further diluted to a concentration of 2 to 5 units/ml in 5% dextrose injection, USP, or sodium chloride injection, USP.[4]

STABILITY: The intact ampules are stable for at least 2 years when refrigerated and protected from light. Biological potency is not affected by freezing. At room temperature the intact ampules are stable for 8 to 10 months with approximately 10% decomposition. Solutions are extremely light sensitive. Concentrations of 500 to 4,500 units/ml have a 50% to 70% decomposition in 2.5 minutes when exposed to direct sunlight. Further dilution to a concentration of 2 to 5 units/ml in 5% dextrose injection, USP, or sodium chloride injection, USP, results in a solution that is stable for 24 hours at room temperature when protected from light.[4]

pH: Intact ampules, 5.0. Optimal pH for stability, 4.5 to 5.5. pH 6.6 or greater, degradation increases significantly.[4]

ROUTES OF ADMINISTRATION: IV.[51] May be given by IV push or by 2-hour IV infusions, or by five 24-hour continuous infusions.[51]

SPECIAL PRECAUTIONS: Containers of infusion solutions should be wrapped in aluminum foil to protect them from light. Solutions for IV push administration should be given immediately or protected from light.[1]

COMPATIBILITY: 5% dextrose injection, USP, and sodium chloride injection, USP[51]

Zorubicin hydrochloride

SYNONYMS: Rubidazone (Rhodia), NSC-164011, daunorubicin benzoylhydrazone HCl, Rhodia 22,050[4,9]

MANUFACTURER: Division of Cancer Treatment, National Cancer Institute[4]

DOSAGE FORMS AND STRENGTHS: 50 mg vial of rubidazone base. A 4 ml ampule of solvent accompanies the drug; each milliliter of solvent contains glycine 37.2 mg, sodium glycinate 0.36 mg, and water for injection, USP, sufficient quantity for 1 ml.[4,57]

STORAGE: Room temperature.[4,57]

SOLUTION PREPARATION: Reconstituting with 4 ml of solvents results in a concentration of 12.5 mg/ml. This may be diluted with 5% dextrose in sodium chloride injection, USP.[4,57]

STABILITY: Intact vials have expiration dates on their labels. The reconstituted solution is stable 8 hours at room temperature and 24 hours under refrigeration. Further diluted solutions with 0.3 mg/ml concentration are stable at room and refrigeration temperatures with 9% decomposition for 5 hours. Since no preservative is present, it is recommended that solutions be discarded after 8 hours.[4]

DOSAGE: 100 to 300 mg/m² single dose for solid tumors or leukemia maintenance; up to 540 mg/m² single dose for leukemia induction, every 3 to 4 weeks.[2]

pH: Reconstituted solution, 6.8 to 7.8[57]

ROUTES OF ADMINISTRATION: IV. Give by IV infusion with a 1 to 2 mg/ml solution and infuse at approximately 500 mg/m² per hour. Normal saline solution is not recommended as an infusion solution because of the large volumes and rapid infusion rate required.[2]

SPECIAL PRECAUTIONS: Avoid extravasation.[2]

COMPATIBILITY: 5% dextrose in sodium chloride injection, USP

SELECTED REFERENCES*

1. Trissel, L. A.: Handbook on injectable drugs, Washington, D.C., 1980, American Society of Hospital Pharmacists.
2. Outlined guide for use of cancer chemotherapeutic agents, Houston, 1979, The University of Texas System Cancer Center, M. D. Anderson Hospital and Tumor Institute.
3. Dorr, R. T., and Fritz, W. L.: Cancer chemotherapy manual, New York, 1977, American Elsevier Publishing Co.
4. Davignon, J. P., et al.: Investigational drug—pharmaceutical data, Bethesda, Md., 1979, Pharmaceutical Resources Branch, National Cancer Institute.
5. Baker, C. E.: Physician's desk reference, Oradell, N. J., 1979, Medical Economics Co.
6. Kastrup, E. K., et al.: Facts and comparisons, 1977-79, St. Louis, Mo., 1979, Facts and Comparisons.
7. Carter, S. K., et al.: Chemotherapy of cancer, Toronto, Canada, 1977, John Wiley & Sons.
8. Reilly, M. J., et al.: American hospital formulary service, Washington, D.C., 1979, American Society of Hospital Pharmacists.
9. Griffiths, M. C., et al.: USAN and the USP dictionary of drug names, 1961-1979 cumulative list, Rockville, Md., 1979, United States Pharmacopeial Convention.
10. Jacobs, J.: Drug stability and compatibility in injections and intravenous infusions, Pharm. J. **205:**437-442, Oct. 17, 1970.
11. Rapp, R. P., et al.: Guidelines for the administration of commonly used intravenous drugs, Drug. Intell. Clin. Pharm. **10:**206-215, April, 1976.
12. Wolfert, R. R., and Cox, R. M.: Room temperature stability of drug products labeled for refrigerated storage, Am. J. Hosp. Pharm. **32:**585-587, 1975.
13. Notari, R. E., et al.: Arabinosylcytosine stability in aqueous solutions: pH profile and shelf life predictions, J. Pharm. Sci. **61:**1189-1196, 1972.

---

*References 1 through 16 are primary and secondary sources that provide information on antineoplastic drugs. The remaining references provide information on specific antineoplastic drugs and are listed in alphabetical order by common drug name.

14. Garnett, W.: Diluents for antineoplastic drugs, Drug Intell. Clin. Pharm. **5:**261, 1971.
15. Kirschenbaum, B. E., and Latiolais, C. J.: Stability of injectable medications after reconstitution, Am. J. Hosp. Pharm. **33:**767-791, 1976.
16. O'Bryan, R. M., et al.: Dose response evaluation of Adriamycin in human neoplasia, Cancer **30:**1940-1948, 1977.
17. L-Alanosine (NSC 153353) clinical brochure, Bethesda, Md., 1977, Investigational Drug Branch, Cancer Therapy Evaluation Program, Division of Cancer Treatment, National Cancer Institute.
18. Helman, L., et al.: Amino-thiadiazole (NSC-4728) clinical brochure, Bethesda, Md., 1976, Investigational Drug Branch, Cancer Therapy Evaluation Program, Division of Cancer Treatment, National Cancer Institute.
19. M-AMSA (NSC-249992) clinical brochure, Bethesda, Md., 1978, Investigational Drug Branch, Cancer Therapy Evaluation Program, Division of Cancer Treatment, National Cancer Institute.
20. Helman, L., et al.: Anguidine (NSC-141, 537) clinical brochure, Bethesda, Md., 1976, Investigational Drug Branch, Cancer Therapy Evaluation Program, Division of Cancer Treatment, National Cancer Institute.
21. Hrushesky, W.: Analysis of clinical studies of L-Asparaginase EC-2 (NSC-109929), Bethesda, Md., 1975, Investigational Drug Branch, Cancer Therapy Evaluation Program, Division of Cancer Treatment, National Cancer Institute.
22. Legha, S. S., et al.: Baker's Antifol (NSC-139105) clinical brochure, Bethesda, Md., 1975, Investigational Drug Branch, Cancer Therapy Evaluation Program, Division of Cancer Treatment, National Cancer Institute.
23. Patterson, W. E.: Preparing multiple doses of bleomycin sulfate, Am. J. Hosp. Pharm. **31:**631, July, 1974.
24. Bruceantin (NSC-165563) clinical brochure, Bethesda, Md., 1978, Md., Investigational Drug Branch, Cancer Therapy Evaluation Program, Division of Cancer Treatment, National Cancer Institute.
25. Livingston, R. B., et al.: Camptothecin sodium salt (NSC 100, 880) clinical brochure, Bethesda, Md., 1968, Investigational Drug Branch, Cancer Therapy Evaluation Program, Division of Cancer Treatment, National Cancer Institute.
26. Helman, L. J., et al.: Chlorozotocin (NSC-178, 248) clinical brochure, Bethesda, Md., 1976, Investigational Drug Branch, Cancer Therapy Evaluation Program, Division of Cancer Treatment, National Cancer Institute.
27. Earhart, R. H.: Instability of cis-dichlorodiammineplatinum in dextrose solution, Cancer Treat. Rep. **62:**1105-1106, 1978.
28. Handelsman, H., et al.: Cis-platinum (II) diamminedichloride (NSC-119875) clinical brochure, Bethesda, Md., 1974, Investigational Drug Branch, Cancer Therapy Evaluation Program, Division of Cancer Treatment, National Cancer Institute.
29. Strauss, G. M., et al.: Cyclocytidine (NSC 145668) clinical brochure, Bethesda, Md., 1975, Investigational Drug Branch, Cancer Therapy Evaluation Program, Division of Cancer Treatment, National Cancer Institute.
30. Brooke, D., et al.: Effect of briefly heating cyclophosphamide solutions, Am. J. Hosp. Pharm. **32:**44-45, January, 1975.
31. Brooke, D., et al.: Chemical stability of cyclophosphamide in parenteral solutions, Am. J. Hosp. Pharm. **30:**134-137, February, 1973.

32. Von Hoff, D. D., et al.: Daunomycin (NSC-82151) clinical brochure, Bethesda, Md., 1975, Investigational Drug Branch, Cancer Therapy Evaluation Program, Division of Cancer Treatment, National Cancer Institute.
33. Helman, L., et al.: Deazauridine (NSC-126,849) clinical brochure, Bethesda, Md., 1976, Investigational Drug Branch, Cancer Therapy Evaluation Program, Division of Cancer Treatment, National Cancer Institute.
34. Handelsman, H., et al.: Dibromodulcitol (NSC 104800) clinical brochure, Bethesda, Md., 1974, Investigational Drug Branch, Cancer Therapy Evaluation Program, Division of Cancer Treatment, National Cancer Institute.
35. Helman, L., et al.: Dichloroallyl lawsone (NSC-126, 771) clinical brochure, Bethesda, Md., 1976, Investigational Drug Branch, Cancer Therapy Evaluation Program, Division of Cancer Treatment, National Cancer Institute.
36. Clinical brochure for dichloromethotrexate (NSC 29630), Bethesda, Md., 1977, Investigational Drug Branch, Cancer Therapy Evaluation Program, Division of Cancer Treatment, National Cancer Institute.
37. Helman, L., et al.: Diglycoaldehyde (NSC-118, 994) clinical brochure, Bethesda, Md., 1976, Investigational Drug Branch, Cancer Therapy Evaluation Program, Division of Cancer Treatment, National Cancer Institute.
38. Goldsmith, M. A., et al.: 5-(3, 3-Dimethyl-1-triazeno) imidazole-4-carboxamide (DTIC, DIC) NSC-45388 clinical brochure, Bethesda, Md., 1972, Investigational Drug Branch, Cancer Therapy Evaluation Program, Division of Cancer Treatment, National Cancer Institute.
39. Handelsman, H., et al.: Ftorafur (FT-207) NSC-148958 clinical brochure, Bethesda, Md., 1974, Investigational Drug Branch, Cancer Therapy Evaluation Program, Division of Cancer Treatment, National Cancer Institute.
40. Helman, L. J., et al.: Gallium nitrate (NSC-15200) clinical brochure, Bethesda, Md., 1976, Investigational Drug Branch, Cancer Therapy Evaluation Program, Division of Cancer Treatment, National Cancer Institute.
41. Legha, S. S., et al.: Hexamethylmelamine (NSC 13875) clinical brochure, Bethesda, Md., 1974, Investigational Drug Branch, Cancer Therapy Evaluation Program, Division of Cancer Treatment, National Cancer Institute.
42. Wasserman, T. H., et al.: (+)1, 2-di (3,5-dioxopiperazin-1-yl) propane ICRF-159 (NSC-129943) clinical brochure, Bethesda, Md., 1973, Investigational Drug Branch, Cancer Therapy Evaluation Program, Division of Cancer Treatment, National Cancer Institute.
43. ICRF-187 (NSC-168780) clinical brochure, Bethesda, Md., 1978, Investigational Drug Branch, Cancer Therapy Evaluation Program, Division of Cancer Treatment, National Cancer Institute.
44. Indicine N-Oxide (NSC 132319) clinical brochure, Bethesda, Md., 1977, Investigational Drug Branch, Cancer Therapy Evaluation Program, Division of Cancer Treatment, National Cancer Institute.
45. Handelman, H., et al.: Isophosphamide (NSC-109724) clinical brochure, 1974, Bethesda, Md., Investigational Drug Branch, Cancer Therapy Evaluation Program, Division of Cancer Treatment, National Cancer Institute.
46. Investigator's brochure R 12,564 (Levamisole HCL) Film-Coated Tablets 50 mg, New Brunswick, N.J., 1977, Janseen R and D.
47. Legha, S. S., et al.: Nafoxidine (Pyrrolidine) NSC-70735 clinical brochure, Bethesda, Md., 1975, Investigational Drug Branch, Cancer Therapy Evaluation Program, Division of Cancer Treatment, National Cancer Institute.

48. Helman, L., et al.: Maytansine (NSC-153, 858) clinical brochure, Bethesda, Md., 1976, Investigational Drug Branch, Cancer Therapy Evaluation Program, Division of Cancer Treatment, National Cancer Institute.
49. Livingston, R. B., et al.: Methyl-GAG (NSC 32946) clinical brochure, Bethesda, Md., 1968, Investigational Drug Branch, Cancer Therapy Evaluation Program, Division of Cancer Treatment, National Cancer Institute.
50. Misonidazole (Ro 7-0582) clinical brochure, Bethesda, Md., 1977, Investigational Drug Branch, Cancer Therapy Evaluation Program, Division of Cancer Treatment, National Cancer Institute.
51. Neocarzinostatin (NSC 157365) clinical brochure, Bethesda, Md., 1978, Investigational Drug Branch, Cancer Therapy Evaluation Program, Division of Cancer Treatment, National Cancer Institute.
52. PALA (NSC 224131) clinical brochure, Bethesda, Md., 1977, Investigational Drug Branch, Cancer Therapy Evaluation Program, Division of Cancer Treatment, National Cancer Institute.
53. PCNU (NSC 95466) clinical brochure, Bethesda, Md., 1978, Investigational Drug Branch, Cancer Therapy Evaluation Program, Division of Cancer Treatment, National Cancer Institute.
54. Pentamethylmelamine (NSC 118742) clinical brochure, Bethesda, Md., 1978, Investigational Drug Branch, Cancer Therapy Evaluation Program, Division of Cancer Treatment, National Cancer Institute.
55. Strauss, G. M., et al.: Piperazinedione (NSC 135758) clinical brochure, Bethesda, Md., 1975, Investigational Drug Branch, Cancer Therapy Evaluation Program, Division of Cancer Treatment, National Cancer Institute.
56. Pyrazolo-imidazole (NSC 51143) clinical brochure, Bethesda, Md., 1977, Investigational Drug Branch, Cancer Therapy Evaluation Program, Division of Cancer Treatment, National Cancer Institute.
57. Henney, J. E., et al.: Rubidazone Clinical Brochure (NSC 164011), Bethesda, Md., 1976, Investigational Drug Branch, Cancer Therapy Evaluation Program, Division of Cancer Treatment, National Cancer Institute.
58. Thymidine 1-(2-deoxy-B-ribofuranosyl)-5-methyluracil (NSC 21548) clinical brochure, Bethesda, Md., 1978, Investigational Drug Branch, Cancer Therapy Evaluation Program, Division of Cancer Treatment, National Cancer Institute.
59. Handelsman, H., et al.: 4′-Demethyl-epipodophyllotoxin-B-D-ethylidene glucose (NSC 141540) VP 16-213 clinical brochure, Bethesda, Md., 1974, Investigational Drug Branch, Cancer Therapy Evaluation Program, Division of Cancer Treatment, National Cancer Institute.
60. Strauss, G. M., et al.: 4′-Demethyl-epipodophyllotoxin-B-D-thenylidene glucoside (NSC 122819) VM-26 clinical brochure, Bethesda, Md., 1975, Investigational Drug Branch, Cancer Therapy Evaluation Program, Division of Cancer Treatment, National Cancer Institute.
61. YOSHI 864 (NSC 102627), Annual Report To The Food And Drug Administration, Bethesda, Md., 1979, Investigational Drug Branch, Cancer Therapy Evaluation Program, Division of Cancer Treatment, National Cancer Institute.
62. Von Hoff, D., et al.: 5-Azacytidine—a new anticancer drug with effectiveness in acute myelogenous leukemia, Ann. Intern. Med. **85:**237-245, 1976.
63. Zafar, H. I., et al.: The disposition and pharmacokinetics in humans of 5-azacytidine administered intravenously as a bolus or by continuous infusion, Cancer Res. **36:**1453-1461, 1976.

64. Lomen, P., et al.: Phase I study of 5-azacytidine (NSC-102816) using 24-hour continuous infusion for 5 days, Cancer Chemother. Rep. **59**(6):1123, 1975.
65. Zackheim, H. S., et al.: Treatment of mycosis fungoides with topical nitrosourea compounds, Arch. Dermatol. **111:**1564-1570, 1975.
66. Shirkey, H. C.: Pediatric drug handbook, Philadelphia, Pa., 1977, W. B. Saunders Co.
67. Kremer, W. B., et al.: Cytarabine, Ann. Intern. Med. **82:**684-688, 1975.
68. Band, P. R., et al.: Treatment of central nervous system leukemia with intrathecal cytosine arabinoside, Cancer **32:**744-748, 1973.
69. Kleinman, L. M., et al.: Investigational drug information: dacarbazine, Drug Intell. Clin. Pharm. **10:**48-49, 1976.
70. Nixon, P. F., et al.: Effective absorption and utilization of oral formyltetrahydrofolate in man, N. Engl. J. Med. **286:**175-179, 1972.
71. Jaffe, N., et al.: Adjuvant methotrexate—citrovorum factor treatment of osteogenic sarcoma, N. Engl. J. Med. **291:**994-997, 1974.
72. Stoller, R., et al.: Use of plasma pharmacokinetics to predict and prevent methotrexate toxicity, N. Engl. J. Med. **297:**630-634, 1977.
73. Mishina, T., et al.: Mitamycin-C bladder instillation therapy for bladder tumor, J. Urol. **114:**217-219, 1974.
74. Sieber, S. M., et al.: Potential hazards associated with the use of 1-methyl-1-nitrosourea (NSC-23909), Cancer Chemother. Rep. **58:**617-618, 1974.

Section 6

ADVERSE REACTIONS TO ANTICANCER DRUGS

COMPLICATIONS OF CANCER CHEMOTHERAPY

As new antineoplastic agents become available each year, it can be expected that new toxicities unique to these drugs will occur. These adverse effects, which usually fall into the group of long-term or delayed complications, can also be categorized into expected or unexpected toxicities (Table 6-1 and Table 6-2). The first part of this section will delineate the reported incidence, onset, clinical presentation, and current management of several of the known toxicities to major organ systems. The second part will give guidelines on dose modification in renal or hepatic disease. The latter part of the section will end with a list of the individual agents and their respective adverse effects. This information will allow the clinician to outline a plan for the monitoring of patients receiving a particular combination of drugs.

ORGAN SYSTEM TOXICITY

Bone marrow suppression

The dosage of most drugs is determined by their effects on the bone marrow production of leukocytes, platelets, or erythrocytes. If a drug is used in a moderate or large dose, the nadir (lowest value) blood count may be expected to occur 7 to 14 days after the drug is administered, with recovery by 21 to 28 days. Some agents, such as the nitrosoureas, busulfan, melphalan, chlorambucil, and mitomycin C, produce a more delayed pattern of bone marrow toxicity (see Fig. 6).[1] In addition to these general patterns of toxicity, some classes (alkylating agents and nitrosoureas) have cumulative effects on the bone marrow elements, which manifest as more profound cytopenias requiring major decrements in dosage. The unique pattern for each drug is delineated in Table 6-3, (p. 252-253).

Not all anticancer drugs produce dose-limiting myelotoxicity.[2] Both vincristine and bleomycin are devoid of significant bone marrow suppression.

Table 6-1. Adverse effects from antineoplastic agents

Expected toxicity	Drug or class	Unexpected toxicity	Drug or class
Congestive heart failure	Daunorubicin, doxorubicin	Fever	See Table 6-2
Emesis	Cisplatin, mechlorethamine, dacarbazine, dactinomycin, cyclophosphamide, cytarabine, doxorubicin, daunorubicin	Hepatitis	Cytarabine, daunorubicin, mercaptopurine, methotrexate, nitrosoureas, thioguanine
		Hypersensitivity	L-asparaginase, bleomycin, cisplatin
Mucositis	Cytarabine, daunorubicin, fluorouracil, methotrexate	Ileus	Vinblastine, vincristine
		Jaw pain	Vinblastine, vincristine
Myelosuppression	All agents except: bleomycin, prednisone, vincristine	Photosensitivity	Actinomycin, fluorouracil, methotrexate
Neuropathy	Methotrexate, vincristine, vinblastine	Neuropathy	Cisplatin, cytarabine, dacarbazine, fluorouracil, hexamethylmelamine
Renal and urinary dysfunction	Cyclophosphamide, cisplatin, methotrexate, streptozocin		
Respiratory	Bleomycin, alkylating agents		
Tissue necrosis after extravasation	Vesicants (see Table 7-21)		

Table 6-2. Antineoplastic drugs associated with fever

Asparaginase	Cytosine arabinoside	Methotrexate
Azathioprine	Dacarbazine	Mithramycin
Bleomycin	Daunorubicin	Procarbazine
Chlorambucil	Doxorubicin	Vinblastine
Cyclophosphamide	Mercaptopurine	Vincristine

From Prince, R. A., and Klainer, A. S.: Drug Intell. Clin. Pharm. **9**:126-128, 1975.

Drugs such as cisplatin, L-asparaginase, streptozocin, and high-dose methotrexate with leucovorin rescue have mild myelosuppressive toxicity. Some agents spare toxicity on one hematopoietic element, such as in the case of cyclophosphamide's platelet-sparing effect. These exceptions make these drugs useful in combination therapy.

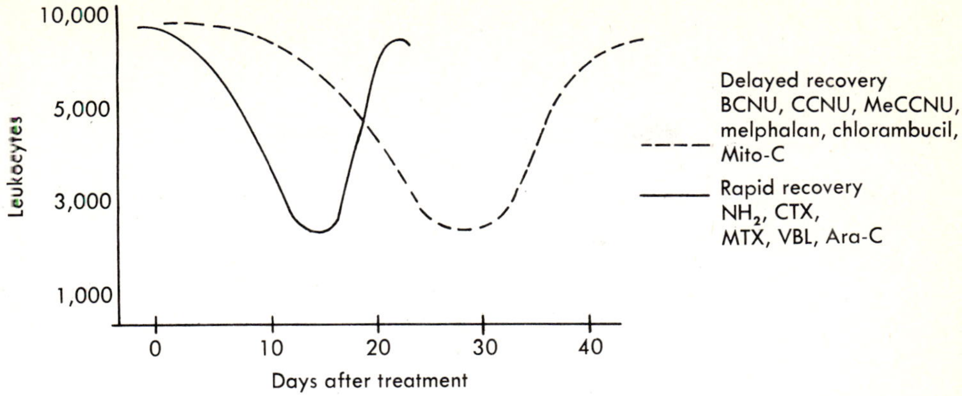

Fig. 6. Patterns of myelotoxicity from anticancer drugs. *NH_2*, nitrogen mustard; *CTX*, cyclophosphamide; *MTX*, methotrexate; *VBL*, vinblastine; *Ara-C*, cytarabine; *BCNU*, carmustine; *CCNU*, lomustine; *MeCCNU*, semustine; and *Mito-C*, mitomycin C.

Cardiac toxicity

The agents most commonly associated with cardiac damage are the anthracycline antibiotics (daunomycin and Adriamycin) and cyclophosphamide.

Cardiotoxicity by daunomycin and Adriamycin is manifested by two types of reactions: (1) transient electrocardiographic (ECG) abnormalities and (2) congestive heart failure (CHF).[4] ECG abnormalities include tachycardia, extrasystoles, and ST-t wave changes and occur in 2% to 30% of patients usually within 1 week of drug administration.[6,7] ST-t wave abnormalities reverse within 1 to 2 weeks and arrhythmias within a few hours of a single intravenous dose.[4] ECG changes do not appear to be associated with the development of congestive heart failure and do not preclude the use of further therapy. Cardiomyopathy can be severe and rapidly progressive. It manifests as congestive heart failure with the usual signs of cardiomegaly, hepatomegaly, and tachypnea. The incidence of CHF from Adriamycin is dose related, occurring in 0.5% of patients given total doses less than 550 mg/m^2 in both adults and children and 30% and 12% at doses of 600 mg/m^2 or greater in adults and children respectively.[5,6] Thus doses of 550 mg/m^2 should not be exceeded.

Several risk factors have been identified which appear to be associated with the development of ECG changes and CHF. Patients with a 30% or greater decrease in limb-lead QRS voltage have a significantly higher incidence of ECG abnormalities.[6] Radiation therapy that encompasses the heart,

Table 6-3. Myelosuppression of antineoplastic agents

Drugs	Dose	Route and schedule	Degree of suppression*	Major element†	Onset (days)	Nadir (days)	Recovery (days)	Comment
Asparaginase	200 units/kg	IV, IM, SC daily for 28 days	0	L	3-5	7-10	14	Peripheral leukopenia
Azacitidine	100-200 mg/m^2	IV for 5-7 days	4+	G+L+P	10	14-17	28	
Bleomycin	1-10 units/m^2	IV, IM, SC every week	1+	G	7	10	14	Marrow-sparing
	30 units	IV infusion	1+	G	7	10	14	
Busulfan	2-6 mg	PO daily	3+	G	14	21-28	42-56	Cumulative
Carmustine	200 mg/m^2	IV every 4-6 weeks	4+	G+P	14	21	35-42	Cumulative, especially platelets
Chlorambucil	2-6 mg	PO daily	3+	G+L	14	21-28	42-56	Cumulative
Cisplatin	100 mg/m^2	IV every 3 weeks	1+	G	10	14	21	
Cyclophosphamide	1-1.5 g/m^2	IV every 3-4 weeks	3+	G	7-10	14	21	Cumulative
	50-100 mg	PO daily	2+	G	7-10	14	21	Cumulative
	100 mg/m^2 (CMF)	PO daily for 14 days	3+	G	7-10	14	21	Cumulative
	400 mg/m^2 (CVP)	PO daily for 5 days	3+	G	7-10	14	21	Cumulative
Cytarabine	100-200 mg/m^2	IV for 5-7 days	4+	G+L+P	4-7	10	21	
	500 mg/m^2	IV for 5-7 days	4+	G+L+P	4	7-10	21	
	3000 mg/m^2	IV for 5 days	4+	G+L+P	4	7-10	21	
Dacarbazine	1,000 mg/m^2	IV every 3 weeks	2+	G	10	14	21	
	200 mg/m^2	IV for 5 days every 3 weeks	2+	G	10	14	21	
Dactinomycin	0.3 mg/m^2 (max. 0.5 mg)	IV for 3 days	4+	G+P	10	14	21-28	
	0.4 mg/m^2	IV every 3 weeks	4+	G+P	10	14	21-28	
Daunorubicin	45 mg/m^2	IV for 3 days	4+	G+P	7	10	21-28	
Doxorubicin	40 mg/m^2	IV every 3 weeks	2+	G+P	10	14	21	
	60 mg/m^2	IV every 3 weeks	3+	G+P	10	14	21	
	80 mg/m^2	IV every 3 weeks	4+	G+P	10	14	21	
Etoposide	250 mg/m^2	IV every 3 weeks	2+	G+P	7-10	14	21	25% incidence
	175 mg/m^2	PO daily for 3 days every week	2+	G+P	7-10	14	21	25% incidence
	170 mg/m^2	PO daily for 5 days every 3 weeks	2+	G+P	7-10	14	21	25% incidence

Fluorouracil	12-15 mg/kg	IV for 5 days every 3 weeks	3+	G	7	10-14	21	
	500-1,000 mg/m²	IV infusion for 5 days	2+	G	7	10-14	21	
Hexamethylmelamine	75-100 mg/m²	PO daily	2+	G	10	14	21	
Hydroxyurea	25 mg/kg	PO daily	3+	G	4	7	14	
Lomustine	130 mg/m²	PO every 4-6 weeks	4+	G+P	14	21-28	42	Cumulative
Mechlorethamine	0.4 mg/kg	IV days 1 & 8 (MOPP)	3+	G+P	10	14	21-28	Cumulative
Melphalan	0.2 mg/kg	PO daily	3+	G+P	14	21	28-40	Cumulative
Mercaptopurine	2.5 mg/kg	PO daily	2+	G+L	7	10-14	21-28	
Methotrexate	40 mg/m²	IV, IM every week	2+	G+P	7	10	14	
	2.5-5 mg	PO every day	2+	G	7	10	14	
	100 mg/m²	IV	3+	G+P	7	10	21	
	1-10 g/m² with citrovorum rescue	IV	2+	G+P	4-7	10	14	
Mithramycin	50 μg/m²	IV every other day for 8 doses	3+	P	10	14	21	
Mitomycin C	2 mg	IV every day for 10 days	4+	P+G	10	21-28	40-55	Cumulative, especially platelets
	10-20 mg/m²	IV every 8 weeks	3+	P+G	10	21-28	40-55	
Mitotane	8-10 g	PO daily	0	—	—	—	—	
Procarbazine	100 mg/m²	PO daily for 14 days	3+	G+P	10	14	21-28	
Pyrazofurin	200 mg/m²	IV weekly	2+	L+G+P	7	10	21	
Razoxane	1,000 mg/m²	PO weekly	2+	G+P	7	10	14	
Semustine	200 mg/m²	PO every 4-6 weeks	4+	G+P	14	30	60	Cumulative, especially platelets
Streptozocin	1000 mg/m²	IV weekly	1+	L+G	7	10	14	
Teniposide	30 mg/m²	IV daily	2+	G+P	7-10	14	21	25% incidence
	100 mg/m²	IV weekly	2+	G+P	7-10	14	21	25% incidence
Thioguanine	2 mg/kg	PO daily	2+	G+P	7	10	21	
Thiotepa	0.2 mg	IV every day for 5 days	3+	P+G	14	21	40-50	
	25 mg/m²	IV every 6 weeks	3+	P+G	14	21	40-50	
Vinblastine	0.1-0.3 mg/kg	IV every week	3+	G+P	4-7	10	21	WBCs > platelets
Vincristine	1.4 mg/m²	IV every week	1+	G	4-7	10	21	Marrow-sparing

*0, none; 1+ and 2+, mild; 3+, moderate; 4+, severe.

†G, granulocytes; L, lymphocytes; P, platelets. The order of element listed indicates the severity of toxicity. For example, G+P indicates that granulocytes are depressed more than platelets.

uncontrolled hypertension, aortic stenosis, and concurrent cyclophosphamide all increase the incidence of CHF.[6,11,12] Under such conditions the dose of Adriamycin should be limited to 450 mg/m^2 [6,9,10] in adults and 350 mg/m^2 in children.[5,7]

Several techniques have been investigated to assist the clinician in predicting patients at risk for impending CHF. Echocardiography provides a measurement of ventricular ejection fraction and systolic time intervals.[7a,8] However, these tests are too sensitive and thus not predictive of toxicity. Serial endomyocardial biopsies have shown that progressive myocardial damage occurs even at doses less than 300 mg/m^2, but this technique has limited practical usefulness.[8]

Daunorubicin produces cardiotoxicity similar to that of Adriamycin but its overall incidence appears to be slightly lower than Adriamycin when given at the same relative doses.[7] There also is a higher incidence of CHF in children than adults, 1.6% versus 0.69%.[5] The higher incidence may reflect the lower performance status (in children) in this study.[5] As in adults, concurrent radiotherapy to heart or concurrent administration of cyclophosphamide increase the cardiotoxicity of daunorubicin.[9,10]

The pathobiology of the anthracyclines is not totally defined but appears to be related to ability of these agents to bind strongly to DNA within the myocardial cell. The biochemical alterations that subsequently develop suggest that these agents inhibit mitochondrial function and promote lipid peroxidation.[4,13] Histologically, the myocardial lesion is nonspecific and consists of nuclear degeneration, loss of myofibrils, and mitochondrial changes.[3]

In most cases of ECG abnormalities treatment is unnecessary. In congestive heart failure induced by anthracyclines, however, treatment is frequently ineffective, especially if the diagnosis is not made early in the course of therapy. The best available treatment is prevention by observing these accepted guidelines[9]:

1. Limit total dosage

	Adult	**Pediatric**
Doxorubicin	550 mg/m^2	450 mg/m^2
Doxorubicin + Cyclophosphamide	450 mg/m^2	350 mg/m^2
Doxorubicin + Mediastinal XRT	450 mg/m^2	350 mg/m^2
Doxorubicin + Cardiac disease	450 mg/m^2	350 mg/m^2
Daunorubicin	550 mg/m^2	450 mg/m^2

2. Baseline ECG or echocardiogram or both every 3 months.
3. If QRS voltage is decreased by 40% or the ejection fraction is decreased by 20%, therapy should be withheld.

Pulmonary toxicity

Several antineoplastic agents are associated with pulmonary toxicity[14,15,16,16a] (Table 6-4). Several risk factors such as age (over 60), concurrent lung irradiation, and preexisting pulmonary disease appear to enhance the effect of these drugs on the lung parenchyma.[14] In addition, other conditions may complicate the diagnosis of chemotherapy-induced pulmonary toxicity (Table 6-5).

The radiologic features of chemotherapy-induced pulmonary toxicity are similar among the various drugs implicated and show a diffuse interstitial infiltrate that is usually basilar in location and not unlike the interstitial pneumonitis or fibrosis from other noxious stimuli such as radiation, oxygen, or infectious organisms.[15] However, the onset of symptoms and radiologic changes vary among the different classes of agents (Table 6-4).

The *alkylating agents,* busulfan, cyclophosphamide, chlorambucil, and melphalan, when used in low-dose continuous therapy, can produce symptoms of respiratory insufficiency that consist of dyspnea, cough, fever, and rales.[16] The *nitrosoureas* produce a similar clinical pattern when used in high-dose intermittent regimens.[2] The *antimetabolites* methotrexate, mercaptopurine, and azathiprine have been reported to produce pulmonary toxicity, but the symptomology is more abrupt in onset compared to that of the alkylating agents or nitrosoureas.[17] Recovery from the pulmonary effects of the antimetabolites is rapid and complete, which is in contrast to the other agents.

Bleomycin is the antineoplastic drug most frequently associated with pulmonary toxicity. Approximately 10% of patients treated with this drug may experience pneumonitis, and in 10% of these patients the complication may be fatal.[18] Symptoms include bibasilar rales and dyspnea that are indistinguishable from the symptoms of infectious pneumonia. Unfortunately, there are no pulmonary function tests, symptoms, or radiologic findings that can be used to warn clinicians of impending toxicity.

Bleomycin pulmonary toxicity appears to be related to the age of the patient and the total dose of drug.[19,20] Patients over 70 years of age who have received doses exceeding 400 mg (units) have an incidence of 15% compared to 5% in younger patients. Characteristic lung toxicity has been seen at all dose levels, even as low as 50 mg (1 mg = 1 unit).

After pulmonary toxicity is evident, arterial hypoxemia is usually present, lung diffusing capacity (DCO) is diminished, and a restrictive lung component may be present. If bleomycin is stopped at the first sign of pulmonary toxicity, approximately 50% of patients will recover within 1 to 2 months without development of x-ray findings.[21] The other half may develop radio-

Table 6-4. Antineoplastic drugs associated with pulmonary toxicity

Drug	Incidence	Symptoms	Pathology	Drug schedule
Asparaginase[14]	22%	SOB,* hives	Uncertain	Daily
Azathioprine[16]	Rare	SOB, DOE†	Alveolitis	Daily
Bleomycin[20,21]	10%	SOB	Pneumonitis	Weekly
Busulfan[15,16a]	Uncommon	DOE, cough, fever	Interstitial fibrosis	Daily
Carmustine[15]	Rare	DOE, cough	Interstitial fibrosis	Monthly
Chlorambucil[49]	Uncommon	DOE, cough	Interstitial fibrosis	Daily
Cyclophosphamide[14,16a]	Uncommon	DOE	Interstitial fibrosis	Daily
Melphalan[50]	Rare	DOE	Interstitial fibrosis	Daily
Mercaptopurine[16]	Rare	DOE	Interstitial fibrosis	Daily
Methotrexate[16,25]	Uncommon	Headache, malaise, dyspnea, cough, fever, rales	Alveolitis, nodular x-ray, hilar lymphadenopathy	Daily, biweekly
Mitomycin C[16a]	Rare	Dyspnea, cough, occasional fever	Alveolar cell hypertrophy, interstitial infiltrates	Intermittent (4-6 weeks)
Procarbazine[14,27]	Rare	Fever, cough, dyspnea, pleurisy	Alveolitis	Daily
Semustine[16a]	Rare	Dyspnea, cough	Interstitial fibrosis	Intermittent

*Shortness of breath.
†Dyspnea on exertion.

Mechanism of action	Onset	Revers-ibility	Comment
Hypersensitivity	Rapid (days)	+	IV therapy, urticaria (65%), hypotension, control with antihistamines
Hypersensitivity	Moderate (weeks)	+	Steroids lead to rapid improvement
Direct pulmonary damage	Delayed (months)	+/−	Dose dependent >200 mg/m² 10% (1% fatal), <200 mg/m² 5% Avoid doses >100 mg/m² with concurrent chest irradiation; steroids usually of no benefit
Direct pulmonary damage	Delayed (years)	−	Corticosteroids ineffective; 24 case reports up to 1978
Direct pulmonary damage	Delayed (years)	−	Eleven cases reported after total doses of 0.58-2.1 g/m² over six months to 3 years
Direct pulmonary damage	Delayed (months)	−	Four cases reported; no mention of steroid use
Direct pulmonary damage	Delayed (years)	−	Two cases reported
Direct pulmonary damage	Delayed (years)	−	Two cases reported
Direct pulmonary damage	Rapid (days)	+	Discontinuation of treatment leads to rapid recovery
Probable hypersensitivity	Rapid (days)	+	Eosinophilia (50%), cyanosis (50%), skin eruptions (16%); leucovorin ineffective; acute illness lasts 10-40 days; if treated with steroids, defervescence decreased to 4-8 days; prednisone 30 mg daily required as an effective dose; continued therapy does not worsen condition; over 30 case reports; not related to dose or route of administration—30-80 mg per week or several grams per week with leucovorin rescue; has occurred after IV, IM, PO, IT
Direct pulmonary damage	Moderate (8-30 weeks)	+/−	Steroids appear to be effective; 12 case reports
Hypersensitivity	Delayed (months)	+	Two case reports; rechallenge of drug reproduces symptom complex; recovery complete after discontinuation of treatment
Direct pulmonary damage	Delayed	?	One case report after 4.1 g over 2 years

Table 6-5. Factors associated with pulmonary toxicity

Factor	Effect
Age	Increased risk
Concurrent chemotherapy	Increased risk
Concurrent or recent radiation therapy	Increased risk
Prior pulmonary disease	Increased risk
Metastatic lung disease	Complicates diagnosis
Pulmonary infection	Complicates diagnosis
Connective tissue disease of the lung	Complicates diagnosis
Pulmonary emboli	Complicates diagnosis
Pulmonary edema	Complicates diagnosis

logic changes but will subsequently improve their respiratory status, although at a slower rate than those without radiologic findings.[21]

Concurrent chest irradiation and bleomycin has been reported by Einhorn and Samuels to act synergistically in producing pulmonary injury.[22,23] In a combination chemotherapy-radiotherapy protocol for small cell carcinoma of the lung, 6 of 13 patients (35%) who had received 90 mg total dose (15 mg weekly for six doses) developed pulmonary toxicity. In five of six patients, biopsy revealed severe interstitial pulmonary fibrosis. Three patients died of respiratory failure.

Once bleomycin toxicity is present, treatment of the pulmonary symptoms is not usually beneficial. Some investigators report that corticosteroids may be beneficial if started at the first sign of toxicity.[18] More frequently, the mere discontinuation of the drug leads to improved respiratory function.

Pulmonary toxicity from *methotrexate* has occurred in patients treated both for nonmalignant disorders, such as psoriasis or renal transplantation, as well as for malignant diseases.[24] It appears that this toxicity is not associated with dose or route of administration as has been previously suggested.[15] Methotrexate given either on a weekly or daily basis or in low or high doses can produce pulmonary toxicity.

The toxicity is a relatively benign interstitial pneumonitis with peripheral eosinophilia, which is readily reversible even with persistent exposure to methotrexate.[14,26] Corticosteroids shorten the recovery period from 8 to 10 days to 3 to 4 days. Thus it appears that the pneumonitis from methotrexate is a hypersensitivity reaction. However, rechallenge often does not reproduce the reaction.

Busulfan is commonly used in the long-term management of chronic myelogenous leukemia. The onset of pulmonary toxicity is approximately 4 years.[26,27] The true incidence of "busulfan lung" is unknown but appears to be uncommon since only 24 cases have been reported despite the widespread use of this agent.

Symptoms of toxicity develop insidiously, but once present, they lead to irreversible pulmonary fibrosis. After symptoms develop, mean survival is approximately 5 months. Diagnosis can be made on sputum cytology with the presence of type II pneumocytes.

Treatment is purely symptomatic and includes bronchodilators and corticosteroids. Successful treatment has been reported, but reversal of the pathologic lesion has not been proven.

Hepatotoxicity

Hepatic effects from cancer chemotherapeutic agents can range from transient enzyme elevation to fibrosis with or without jaundice (Table 6-6).[2,27]

It is often difficult to incriminate an antineoplastic drug alone as a cause of liver dysfunction because one or several factors may contribute to development of this condition. Table 6-7 lists the clinical situations frequently encountered in patients in which hepatic dysfunction is evident.

ANTIMETABOLITES

Methotrexate (MTX).[52,53,54] Several reports of hepatotoxicity have been documented for methotrexate. The prevalence of cirrhosis and fibrosis appears to be significantly higher in those patients receiving small daily doses of MTX than in those receiving larger doses intermittently.[52,55] Also, the incidence of hepatic damage appears to be directly proportional to the duration of treatment. Hepatic damage is not usually seen after only 1 year of MTX; fibrosis can occur after 33 months, and cirrhosis is evident by 4 years. In contrast, cirrhosis is not observed in patients who receive intermittent weekly therapy. Hepatic enzyme tests do not appear to predict subsequent damage in patients. The bromsulphalein (BSP) retention appears to be the most sensitive indication for future toxicity.

High doses of MTX frequently produce mild-to-moderate elevations of serum transaminases and occasional elevations of bilirubin.[54] In most cases, these abnormalities reverse to normal within 1 month after treatment.

While MTX is considered a true hepatotoxin, its mechanism of producing damage has not been completely elucidated either in animals or humans.

6-Mercaptopurine (6-MP). Several reports of 6-MP liver toxicity have been described, but its incidence is not well established.[51,56] Jaundice has been reported in 40% to 50% of leukemic patients. However, this incidence may be overestimated because of other contributing factors such as infectious

Table 6-6. Hepatic toxicity from antineoplastic drugs

Drug	Dosing schedule	Occurrence rate*	Histopathology	Clinical presentation†	Reversibility	Comment
Antimetabolites						
Methotrexate[52,53,54]	Daily (psoriatics)	Common	Fibrosis (27%) Cirrhosis (19%) Fatty metamorphosis (46%)	Normal bilirubin Enzyme elevation Jaundice	Recovery in 14-28 days	Dose related; 2-4 grams cumulative dose
	Weekly (25 mg PO)	Rare	Fibrosis (5.6%) Cirrhosis (6.8%)	Elevated transaminases	Recovery in 14 days	Duration related
	High-dose with leucovorin rescue	Rare	Fibrosis (50%) Cirrhosis (uncommon)	Normal bilirubin Elevated transaminases (75%) Hyperbilirubinemia (7%)	Recovery in 14 days	Liver damage related to duration of treatment
Mercaptopurine[56,57]	Daily	Common	Cholestasis (primarily) Hepatocellular necrosis	Elevated alkaline phosphatasc and bilirubin Normal transaminases Jaundice	Recovery in 14-28 days; some cases irreversible	
Azathioprine[58,59]	Daily	Uncommon	Cholestasis (primary) Hepatocellular necrosis	Elevated alkaline phosphatase and bilirubin Normal transaminases	Recovery in 14-28 days	
Cytarabine[62,63]	Daily for 5-7 days every 3-4 weeks	Uncommon	None demonstrated	Elevated LFTs†	Recovery in 14 days	Case reports often associated with sepsis
Alkylating agent[64,65] Cyclophosphamide	Intermittent	Two case reports	Hepatocellular necrosis	Jaundice Elevated LFTs	No	Not well documented

Nitrosoureas[69,70]	Intermittent	Common	Hepatocellular necrosis	Elevated LFTs No jaundice Mild course	Recovery in 14-28 days	Prior transaminase elevations do not preclude further use of drug
Carmustine						
Streptozocin						
Antitumor antibiotics						
Doxorubicin or daunorubicin[72,73]	Intermittent	Uncommon	No data	Elevated LFTs	Recovery in 14 days	Not well documented
Bleomycin[75]	Intermittent	Uncommon	Not demonstrated	Elevated LFTs	Recovery in 14 days	
Mitomycin C[76,77]	Intermittent	Rare	Centrilobular stasis	Bilirubin Alkaline phosphatase BSP retention	Recovery in 14-28 days	
Mithramycin[78]	Daily for 10 days	Very common	Centrilobular stasis, fatty metamorphosis	Transaminases Alkaline phosphatase	Recovery in 14-28 days	
	Alternate day	Uncommon	Centrilobular stasis, fatty metamorphosis	Transaminases Alkaline phosphatase	Recovery in 14-28 days	
Miscellaneous						
Dacarbazine[71]	Intermittent	Uncommon	No data	Elevated LFTs	Recovery in 14-28 days	
L-Asparaginase[79,80,81]	Daily for 3-7 days	Very common	Fatty metamorphosis, steatosis	Elevated LFTs Prothrombin time Cholesterol Fibrinogen	Recovery in 14 days	
Vinca alkaloids[51]	Intermittent	No reports				
Etoposide and teniposide[51,82]	Intermittent	Uncommon	No data	Transaminases	Recovery in 7-14 days	

*Very common, 75% incidence; common, 20-75% incidence; uncommon, 5-20% incidence; rare, 5% incidence.
†LFTs, liver function tests (alkaline phosphatase, transaminases, bilirubin).

Table 6-7. Conditions associated with hepatic dysfunction in patients receiving antineoplastic drugs

Hepatic metastases
Viral hepatitis
Abdominal irradiation with or without concurrent chemotherapy
Concurrent hepatotoxic drugs (e.g., phenothiazines, isoniazid, oral contraceptives)
Graft-versus-host disease
Blood product transfusions

hepatitis or other drugs[57] (Table 6-7). Biochemically, bilirubin and alkaline phosphatase are abnormally elevated while transaminases remain normal. Histologically, either cholestasis and hepatocellular necrosis are seen. In most cases the hepatic abnormalities regress, but some are irreversible. Since 6-MP characteristically produces similar lesions in animals, it is believed to be a direct hepatotoxic.

Azathioprine (AZ). AZ produces hepatotoxicity in both animals and man. The incidence of this adverse effect in cancer patients (or renal transplant recipients) is unknown.[58,59] Biochemically, serum bilirubin and alkaline phosphatase are elevated. Recovery occurs rapidly in most cases. The hepatic lesion looks similar to 6-MP liver toxicity with cholestasis with or without parenchymal damage. There have been a few reports of hepatic veno-occlusive disease and peliosis of the liver following AZ.

Fluorouracil (5-FU). While there are a few reports of 5-FU liver toxicity after both IV infusion and arterial hepatic infusion, the investigators do not provide sufficient data regarding the hepatic abnormalities to convince toxicologists.[60,61]

Cytarabine (Ara-C). There are several reports of Ara-C induced hepatotoxicity, primarily in leukemic patients.[62,63] However, most of the cases were associated with sepsis during the period of severe myelosuppression. Biochemically, hyperbilirubinemia and slight elevations of transaminases and alkaline phosphatase were observed in 15% to 46% of the cases. Histologic abnormalities have not been demonstrated on autopsy. When true Ara-C induced hepatotoxicity was observed, it was usually mild and readily reversible after discontinuation of therapy.

ALKYLATING AGENTS

Cyclophosphamide (CTX). While there is some suggestion of hepatotoxic effects of CTX in animals, there are few reports of its occurrence in humans.[64,65,66] One case of fulminant hepatic necrosis and another case with transient transaminase elevation have been reported. A study by Ylostalo[66] found no significant elevation of liver function tests in 41 patients.

Reports of hepatotoxicity caused by other alkylating agents (mustard derivatives) have not been well documented.[51]

NITROSOUREAS

Most reports of nitrosourea-induced hepatotoxicity pertain to BCNU and streptozocin.[51] BCNU has been shown to transiently elevate serum transaminases and/or alkaline phosphatase and/or bilirubin in approximately one fourth of patients.[67] These abnormalities return to normal by the next course of treatment.

Streptozocin. From 30% to 67% of patients may develop elevated liver function tests (bilirubin, alkaline phosphatase, and transaminases) occurring usually 2 to 3 weeks into the course of therapy.[68,69] In all cases these abnormalities regressed rapidly to normal in a few days after treatment.[70] Histologically, a few biopsy reports showed hepatocellular necrosis, but the material was obtained 3 months after cessation of therapy. No animal models for streptozocin hepatotoxicity have been developed.

ANTITUMOR ANTIBIOTICS

Anthracyclines (Adriamycin and daunorubicin). Sparse reports of modest elevations of liver function tests have been observed after administration of both Adriamycin and daunorubicin, but sufficient substantial data is lacking.[72,73]

Bleomycin. Hepatotoxicity in animals and man has been reported.[74,75] Moderate and transient hyperbilirubinemia has been observed in 30% of patients, but hemolysis may have been involved in these cases. Two other large clinical studies have reported liver function test abnormalities in only a few subjects.[18,19] No liver abnormalities have been reported on autopsy cases.

Mitomycin C. Only a few cases of documented hepatotoxicity in the use of mitomycin C are reported.[76,77] Biochemically, abnormal BSP retention occurred in 23% and elevated bilirubin and alkaline phosphatase occurred in 10%. Histologically, the lesion was described as "centrilobular stasis."

Mithramycin. Transaminase and alkaline phosphatase elevation are very common in patients receiving mithramycin.[78] These abnormalities occur most frequently (50%) with a daily dosage schedule of the drug and less so (10%) with alternate day schedules of the same total dose. These biochemical alterations regress within 30 days after treatment. Histologically, the lesion consists of fatty changes and centrilobular stasis.

MISCELLANEOUS

Dacarbazine (DTIC). Elevations of liver function tests (bilirubin, transaminases, and alkaline phosphatase) occur in a small number of patients and are rapidly reversible.[71] There have been no histopathologic reports in man.

L-Asparaginase. Hepatotoxicity is very common after L-asparaginase.[79,80,81] Some form of liver function abnormality occurs in approximately 75% of patients. The incidence of toxicity appears to be greater in adults than children. Serum albumin levels decrease in 70% to 80% of patients. Serum transaminase levels and bilirubin and alkaline phosphatase are increased in 50% to 60% and 30% to 50% of patients respectively. Hypocholesterolemia occurs in 85% of patients. Clotting abnormalities are common: fibrinogen levels are decreased in over 90% and prothrombin time prolonged in 20% of patients studied. Bleeding, however, is an uncommon clinical finding (6%). Histologically, L-asparaginase induces a diffuse fatty metamorphosis with marked steatosis in 40% to 85% of biopsy specimens. The liver function abnormalities rapidly regress within 14 days after stopping therapy.

• • •

It has been hypothesized that the mechanisms of hepatotoxicity are: (1) allergic hypersensitivity, (2) bacterial endotoxin from contaminated preparations, and (3) protein-synthesis inhibition of clotting factors and other proteins vital to hepatic synthesis.

Gastrointestinal toxicity

EMESIS

Many but not all of the antineoplastic drugs produce either nausea or vomiting.[2] Emesis begins from 2 to 6 hours after drug administration and is mediated through the cytotoxic effect of the chemotherapy in the vomiting center located in the central nervous system (medulla), not through direct action on the gastrointestinal mucosa. In some cases, psychological influences may play a role in the development of emesis, especially when previous vomiting episodes have been severe. Such patients may recall the previous "bad" experience and have a vomiting episode at the mere sight of the needle or syringe. Other patients may develop nausea, sweating, and even elicit feelings of lightheadedness while receiving chemotherapy, which are signs of a vaso-vagal reaction. The practitioner should be able to discern the most likely cause for a patient's emetic episode by observing its onset and pattern. Table 6-8 outlines the differences between vomiting induced by chemotherapy, vasovagal reactions, or psychological factors.

The clinician should also know which agents are likely to produce nausea and vomiting. Table 6-9 provides a list of agents that induce severe, moderate, and mild emesis. The treatment and prevention of this problem has

Table 6-8. Emesis associated with chemotherapy

Course	Patterns of emesis
Psychological	Occurs prior to or within 5 minutes of drug administration; anti-anxiety drugs may be helpful
Vasovagal	Occurs during or after drug administration; sweating with or without dizziness usually accompanies the episode
Chemotherapy	Occurs 2 to 6 hours after drug administration; antiemetics may be helpful

Table 6-9. Emetic potential of antineoplastic drugs*

Severe	Moderate	Mild-to-none
Azacitidine (rapid injection)	Azacitidine (slow infusion)	Bleomycin
Carmustine	Cytarabine	Busulfan
Cisplatin	Etoposide	Chlorambucil
Cyclophosphamide (high-dose parenteral)	Hexamethylmelamine	Fluorouracil
Dacarbazine	Mitotane	Hydroxyurea
Dactinomycin	Procarbazine	L-Asparaginase
Daunorubicin	Razoxane	Melphlan
Doxorubicin	Teniposide	Mercaptopurine
Lomustine	Thiotepa	Methotrexate
Mechlorethamine	Vinblastine	Mitomycin C
Mithramycin		Thioguanine
Semustine		Vincristine
Streptozocin		

*The listing of agents is based on the frequency and severity of nausea and vomiting. That is, severe includes a frequency of >75% incidence of vomiting usually with retching; moderate is between 25% and 75% vomiting; and mild is either nausea or less than 25% vomiting.

not been overwhelmingly successful and is discussed in Section 7, Ancillary Therapy.

MUCOSITIS

Because antineoplastic drugs are cytotoxic to rapidly dividing cells, gastrointestinal toxicity is a common adverse effect. Mucositis presents clinically in several forms: oral stomatitis, esophagitis, gastritis, and colitis. The most frequent manifestation is stomatitis.[28] Table 6-10 lists those agents most commonly associated with gastrointestinal toxicity. In most cases, drugs that most effectively kill cells in S-phase will most frequently produce gastrointestinal toxicity. The treatment of mucositis is empirical and supportive. Several institutions have developed mixtures containing several pharmacologic agents: local anesthetics, antacids, antibiotics, anti-inflammatory agents, and analgesics.[29] No controlled trials or anecdotal experiences have been reported in the literature. A rationale preparation might

Table 6-10. Antineoplastic agents associated with gastrointestinal toxicity

Drug	Site in the GI tract	Mani-festation	Onset and recovery	Complication
Bleomycin	Mouth	Stomatitis	Onset by day 7 Recovery by day 14	Difficulty in eating
Cytarabine	Mouth	Stomatitis	Onset by day 7 Recovery by day 14-21	Difficulty in eating
	Gut	Diarrhea	Onset by day 7 Recovery 3-5 days after therapy discontinued	Weight loss
	Anus	Tissues		Infection
Daunorubicin	Mouth	Stomatitis	Onset 7-10 days Recovery by day 14	Difficulty in eating
Doxorubicin	Mouth	Stomatitis	Onset 7-10 days Recovery by day 14	Difficulty in eating
Fluorouracil	Mouth	Stomatitis	Onset 4-7 days Recovery by day 10-14	Difficulty in eating
	Gut	Diarrhea	Onset by day 5-7 Recovery by day 10-14	Weight loss
	Anus	Perianal		
Mercaptopurine	Mouth	Stomatitis	Onset by day 7-10 Recovery by day 14	Difficulty in eating
Methotrexate	Mouth	Stomatitis	Onset by day 4-7 Recovery by day 10	Difficulty in eating
Thioguanine	Mouth	Stomatitis	Onset by day 7-10	Difficulty in eating
Vinblastine	Intestine	Constipation	After high doses (>15 mg)	Ileus
Vincristine	Intestine	Constipation	After 8-10 mg total dose	Ileus

include a local anesthetic in a soothing oral mouthwash or hygienic solution, such as hydrogen peroxide. These are applied just prior to meals to assist with oral feeding. Treatment of oral mucositis is discussed in Section 7, Ancillary Therapy.

Dermatologic toxicity

Several types of dermatologic reactions commonly occur after the administration of cancer chemotherapeutic agents.[2,30] These include hypersensitivity, which is manifested by generalized urticarial rashes or maculopapular rashes, petechiae from antileukemia treatment with cytarabine and daunorubicin, acute anaphylaxis from the antitumor antibiotics, especially bleomycin and L-asparaginase, photosensitivity from the radiomimetic antineoplastic agents (actinomycin D, methotrexate, bleomycin), radiation "recall' phenomena from doxorubicin and actinomycin, local necrosis from paravenous extravasation of vesicant agents, and nail changes. Table 6-11

Table 6-11. Dermatologic reactions associated with antineoplastic agents

Type of reaction	Drug	Incidence	Management or prevention
Hypersensitivity (urticarial or petechial rash)	Cytarabine	30%-50%	Discontinue therapy if platelets <20,000; treat with antihistamines
	Daunorubicin	25%	
	Mercaptopurine	10%	
	Methotrexate	10%	
Anaphylaxis	L-Asparaginase		Administer test dose of 0.1 ml subcutaneously; give asparaginase IM, treat with adrenalin and antihistamine
	Intravenous	5%	
	Intramuscular	<1%	
	Bleomycin	0.01%-0.1%	Have adrenalin and antihistamines readily available
Photosensitivity	Actinomycin D	25%	Avoid excessive sunlight for 1-2 days after therapy; sunscreens that inhibit ultraviolet light may prevent the reaction
	Bleomycin	10%	
	Methotrexate	30%-40%	
	Fluorouracil	10%-20%	
Radiation recall	Actinomycin D	30%	This reaction probably cannot be prevented but may be treated with local anti-inflammatory agents
	Doxorubicin	10%-20%	
	Mechlorethamine	10%	
Local necrosis	Vesicants	1%-5%	See section on ancillary therapy, Table 7-21
Nail banding	Bleomycin	20%-40%	None
	Cyclophosphamide		None
	Doxorubicin	30%-50%	None
Keratopathy	Fluorouracil	5%-10%	Emollient creams (e.g., Eucerin)
	Bleomycin	10%	
Onycolysis	Doxorubicin	Rare	None

lists the type of reaction associated with the particular drug and provides guidelines for the prevention or management of these reactions.

The hypersensitivity reactions from most antineoplastic drugs are usually self-limiting and associated with morbidity only in patients at high risk for hemorrhagic diathesis into urticarial or petechial lesions.[31] An example of such a situation is the patient with acute leukemia who is receiving aggressive induction therapy (for example, cytarabine plus daunorubicin) with consequential thrombocytopenia to less than 20,000 platelets. Supportive platelet transfusions are essential in this situation.

Anaphylaxis from asparaginase was initially reported with the early preparations that were cultured from *E. coli* and given by intravenous infusion. With better purification techniques, a significantly lower incidence of anaphylaxis has been reported and is even lower when the drug is given by the intramuscular route.[32] Asparaginase derived from *Erwinia corotovoro* is not cross reactive with the *E. coli* preparation and can be substituted if necessary.[33]

Anaphylactoid reactions from bleomycin are well documented in the literature.[19] The preparation consists of thirteen bleomycin homologues derived from streptomyces bacteria. It is unknown which species is responsible for the reaction. Fortunately, the overall incidence is very low, less than 1%. However, nine of ten reported cases occurred in lymphoma patients (6% in this group).[19]

Photosensitivity is caused by several anticancer drugs through their radiosensitizing properties. This effect is most prominent during the first few days after chemotherapy. The agents most commonly associated are actinomycin D, doxorubicin, and mechlorethamine.

Radiation recall phenomena has occurred when local radiation to the skin is "reactivated" after administration of a radiomimetic drug.[30,34] Most antineoplastic drugs are radiomimetic, but not all of them appear to be associated with this phenomena (see Table 6-11).

Local necrosis from extravasation of vesicant anticancer drugs frequently produces a severe skin reaction.[35,36] Because this problem may be minimized with good phlebotomy technique, a separate section on this and other treatment measures for cancer patients is provided (see Section 7, Ancillary Therapy).

Keratopathy of the nail is frequently caused by anticancer drugs.[37] Nail change consists of either horizontal or vertical binding, which usually occurs 5 to 10 weeks after the patient has received chemotherapy. The most frequently associated drugs are bleomycin and doxorubicin, but several other agents have been anecdotally reported. *Horizontal* banding phenomena is most commonly seen in black or dark-skinned patients because the mechanism appears to be related to melanocyte-stimulating hormone.[38] *Longitudinal* banding from bleomycin, cytoxan, and doxorubicin is thought to result from ACTH stimulation[39] or a melanocyte-stimulating hormone.[39a] No morbidity is associated with banding.

Another type of nail change is oncolysis and skin keratopathy. These changes have been seen with fluorouracil or doxorubicin.[40]

Neurologic toxicity

The expected toxic effects on the nervous system from chemotherapy consist of peripheral, autonomic, or central nerve dysfunction. Vincristine frequently produces damage to the myelin sheaths of peripheral nerves, which leads to numbness and tingling in the finger tips and toes and loss of deep-tendon reflexes (ankle and knee jerk).[41] This adverse effect can disable the patient to the point of severe weakness in the lower extremities if therapy is continued after the onset of moderate to severe peripheral symptoms. It is recommended that vincristine be discontinued when patients exhibit signs of proximal muscle weakness. Vinblastine can also produce a

Table 6-12. Neurotoxic syndrome associated with intrathecal methotrexate*

Reaction	Incidence	Onset	Signs or syndromes	Comments
Arachnoiditis	Common with doses of 12 mg/m^2 every 2-3 days; uncommon with weekly doses	2-4 hours	Fever, back pain, dizziness, meningismus, vomiting, headache, CSF pleocytosis; may last 12-72 hours	Depends on MTX dose and frequency; arachnoiditis more common in patients with *overt* CNS leukemia; reversible
Weakness or paralysis	Rare—can occur in MTX prophylaxis but more common in overt CNS leukemia; multiple doses required	Delayed; earliest occurrence after 5 doses (range, 5-23 doses)	Leg pain, hemiplagia, spinal nerve damage	May be related to high or prolonged concentrations of MTX; usually reversible
Encephalopathy, transient or progressive	Rare—can occur in either MTX prophylaxis or treatment	Early or late	Often associated with arachnoiditis symptoms: headache, vomiting, irritability, and CSF pleocytosis	Usually occurs with concurrent radiotherapy; toxicity related to a demyelinating process

*Modified from Pochedly, C.: Med. Ped. Oncol. **3**:101-115, 1977.

Table 6-13. Renal and urinary toxicity from antineoplastic drugs*

Drug	Site	Incidence	Pathology	Onset	Recovery	Management
Cisplatin	Kidney	10%-40%	Tubular necrosis	1-4 weeks	2-4 weeks	Prehydration with saline with or without mannitol and furosemide
Cyclophosphamide	Bladder, ureter	5%	Cystitis	2-3 days	3-5 days	Hydration with 1-2 liters of fluid
Methotrexate (1-10 gm/m^2)	Renal pelvis	5%	Tubular obstruction from drug precipitation	6-12 hours	1-7 days	Prevention: prehydration with saline; alkalinization of urine with sodium bicarbonate or acetazolamide
Mithramycin (daily doses)	Kidney	20%	Tubular necrosis	7-14 days	1-4 weeks	Alternate-day therapy produces much lower incidence of nephrotoxicity
Semustine (>1500 mg total dose)	Kidney	50%	Tubular necrosis	14-18 months	Months	General supportive care dose related
Streptozocin	Kidney	30%-40%	Tubular necrosis	7-14 days	1-4 weeks	Dosing every 3-4 weeks may allow greater recovery

*Data from Garnick, M. B., and Mayer, R. J.: Semin. Oncol. **5**:155-165, 1978.

similar neuropathologic consequence, but the incidence is much lower and also requires much higher doses than vincristine.

Both vincristine and vinblastine paralyze the autonomic nerves that control bladder and intestinal motility.[42] This effect is most troublesome in the elderly patient (over 60 years) and is manifested as urinary retention or constipation. As in incidence of peripheral neuropathy, vincristine is much more potent in this regard. It is recommended that patients receiving vincristine be given stool-softening agents or mild laxatives to ensure proper bowel function.

Methotrexate is frequently administered by the intrathecal route. High concentration of methotrexate in the cerebral spinal fluid has been associated with CNS toxicity.[43] Three types of syndromes have been observed: (1) arachnoiditis, (2) delayed central inflammation, and (3) leukoencephalopathy.[44] The characteristics of each of these reactions is outlined in Table 6-12. The most severe form is leukoencephalopathy, which fortunately is rare, but when present leads to substantial morbidity. Concurrent cranial irradiation in combination with intrathecal methotrexate has been associated with all case reports of leukoencephalopathy.

Renal and urinary toxicity

Several antineoplastic agents are toxic to the kidneys and urinary tract and include cisplatin, cyclophosphamide, methotrexate (high-dose), semustine (methyl CCNU), mithramycin, and streptozocin.[45] Table 6-13 lists the specific location of the toxicity, the incidence, recovery period, and management recommendation for each drug.

Other chemotherapeutic drugs are excreted by the kidney but are not necessarily toxic to parenchymal tissue.[45] These include bleomycin, hydroxyurea, dacarbazine (DTIC), mitomycin C, and thioguanine. Since the effect of renal failure on the body clearance of many of these drugs is unknown, there are few established guidelines for their use in this setting.

DOSE MODIFICATION IN RENAL OR HEPATIC DISEASE

In the presence of renal or hepatic disease, anticancer drugs may produce serious toxicities, such as leukopenia, thrombocytopenia, and mucositis. Unfortunately, guidelines for dosage adjustment exist for only a small number of anticancer drugs, namely Adriamycin, daunomycin, cisplatin, and methotrexate. In order to calculate a dose modification for most drugs, sites of drug detoxification and excretion must be known. By determining the degree of drug clearance by the liver, kidney, or tissues, one can calculate a reasonable estimate of the dose with the use of simple pharmacokinetic principles. Table 6-14 lists the pharmacokinetic parameters and major sites of elimination for most of the available antineoplastic agents.

Table 6-14. Pharmacokinetics of anticancer drugs

Drug	Plasma T½	Metabolism and excretion	Condition requiring dose reduction
L-Asparaginase[100a]	T½ = 8-30 hours	Intracellular sequestration; excretion unknown	
Azacitidine[91]	T½ = 3.4-6.2 hours	Hepatic metabolism and renal excretion of parent compound (20%) and metabolites	Hepatic dysfunction
Bleomycin[87,92,105]	T½ = 2-4 hours (IV) T½ = 6 hours (intraperitoneal)	Hepatic, kidney, tissue metabolism; renal excretion of 20%-60% of active drug	Renal failure, creatinine clearance <40 ml/min
Busulfan[100a]	Rapid, 90% in 3 minutes	Hepatic; metabolites unknown; renal excretion of 25%-35% methanesulfonic acid	
Carmustine[100a]	T½ = 5 minutes for BCNU T½ = 27-72 hours for metabolites	Hepatic metabolism to active compounds; renal excretion of 80% metabolites in 24 hours	Renal dysfunction; guidelines uncertain
Chlorambucil[84]	T½ = 1.5 hours	Hepatic metabolism and renal excretion of 50% unchanged drug	Guidelines uncertain
Chlorozotocin[101]	T½ = 13 minutes	Probably hepatic metabolism and renal excretion of metabolites (unknown) + active drug	Renal dysfunction; guidelines uncertain
Cisplatin[93,100]	T½α = 30-77 minutes T½β = 61-96 hours	Unknown metabolism; metabolites not detected; renal excretion of 20% and 30% in 24 and 48 hours, respectively	Renal dysfunction, oliguria; avoid if creatinine clearance less than 50 ml/min
Cycloleucine[95]	T½ = 3 days	Unknown metabolism; renal excretion of 20% in 24 hours	
Cyclophosphamide	T½ = 4-6.5 hours	Hepatic metabolism to active metabolites (88%); renal excretion of 50%-75% in 48 hours, 12% of unchanged drug	Renal dysfunction: decrease dose proportionate to decrease in creatinine clearance
Cytarabine[100a]	T½α = 10 minutes T½β = 140 minutes	Hepatic and blood deamination to inactive uracil arabinoside; renal excretion of 90% metabolite and 4%-10% unchanged drug	None
Dacarbazine	T½ = 30-45 minutes	Hepatic demethylation to active aminoimidazole carboximide; renal excretion of 50% metabolite and 50% unchanged drug in 6 hours	Renal dysfunction; decrease dose proportionate to decrease in creatinine clearance

Table 6-14. Pharmacokinetics of anticancer drugs—cont'd

Drug	Plasma T½	Metabolism and excretion	Condition requiring dose reduction
Dactinomycin	Rapid (85% in 2 minutes)	Unknown metabolism; biliary excretion of 50%-90% in 24 hours; renal excretion of 12%-20% in 24 hours	Elevated bilirubin (>3.0 g%)
Daunorubicin[111]	T½ = 30-50 hours	Hepatic metabolism to daunorubicinol; renal excretion of 25% of unchanged drug in 5 days; biliary excretion of 75% of of unchanged drug in 5 days	Elevated bilirubin
Deazauridine[106]	T½ = 4.6 hours (bolus) T½ = 23 hours (infusion)	Unknown metabolism; renal excretion of 90%-100% unchanged	Avoid in severe renal failure
Doxorubicin[85,86]	T½α = 12 minutes T½β = 3 hours T½λ = 28 hours	Hepatic metabolism to adriamycinol and conjugated metabolites; biliary excretion of 85% active drug in 24 hours; renal excretion of 5% in 24 hours	Elevated bilirubin 1.5-2.9 g%, give 50% of dose; >3.0 g%, give 25% of usual dose
Etoposide[100a]	Unknown	Hepatic metabolism; less than 16% biliary excretion; renal excretion 30% unchanged	
Fluorouracil[102,108]	T½ = 10-20 minutes	Hepatic metabolism to inactive uracils and urea; renal excretion of 10%-20% unchanged drug	None
Hydroxyurea[100a]	T½ = 2-5 hours	Hepatic metabolism and renal excretion of 80% of parent compound in 12 hours	Renal dysfunction; no definite guideline
Lomustine[100a]	T½α = 5 minutes T½β = 72 hours T½ (metabolites) = 24-36 hours	Hepatic metabolism to active metabolites; renal excretion of 50% and 75% in 1 and 4 days respectively.	Renal dysfunction probably would increase toxicity
Mechlorethamine[100a]	T½ = 15 minutes	Hydrolysis by plasma or cellular water to inactive products; renal excretion <0.01% of drug	None
Melphalan[84,107]	T½ = 2-4 hours	Hepatic metabolites to unknown products; renal excretion of 11% of parent compound	Unknown

Continued.

Table 6-14. Pharmacokinetics of anticancer drugs—cont'd

Drug	Plasma T½	Metabolism and excretion	Condition requiring dose reduction
Mercaptopurine[100a]	T½ = 6-8 hours	Xanthine oxidase; renal excretion of 20%-40% unchanged drug and 20%-60% metabolites	Concurrent allopurinol; renal dysfunction of creatinine clearance <20 ml/minute
Methotrexate[94,109]	T½ = 45 minutes T½ = 2-4 hours T½ = 10-27 hours	Hepatic metabolism 10% to 7-hydroxy methotrexate; renal excretion 90% at low doses and 50%-80% at high doses	Renal dysfunction; avoid at less than 50 ml/minute; decrease dose proportionate to decrease in creatinine clearance
Misonidazole	T½ = 10 hours	Hepatic metabolism to desmethyl misonidazole; renal excretion of 10% of unchanged drug in 36 hours and 40%-60% metabolites in 36 hours	Avoid with hepatic dysfunction
Mithramycin[100a]	Rapid, 85% in 3 hours (1 patient)	Unknown; renal excretion of 27% of unchanged drug in 2 hours	Renal dysfunction
Mitomycin C[100a]	T½ = 10-20 minutes	Hepatic metabolism to active agents; renal excretion of 6% unchanged drug	
Procarbazine[100a]	T½ = 7 minutes	Hepatic and erythrocyte metabolism to active metabolites; renal excretion of 20%-70% of inactive metabolites	None
Pyrazolo-imidazole (IMPY)	T½α = 25 minutes T½β = 7.1 hours	Unknown metabolism; renal excretion of unchanged drug	Severe renal dysfunction
Semustine (MeCCNU)[100a]	Rapid	Hepatic metabolism to active metabolites; renal excretion of 60% inactive metabolites in 48 hours	None
Streptozocin[100a]	T½ = 15 minutes	Hepatic metabolism to unknown metabolites; insufficient data on activity; renal excretion of 10%-20% unchanged drug	Renal dysfunction; nephrotoxic agent
Tamoxifen[99]	T½α = 16 hours T½β = 35 hours	Unknown; renal excretion of unknown products	
Tegafur[90]	T½ = 6-16 hours	Hepatic activation to 5-FU and FU metabolites; renal excretion of 5-FU and metabolites less than 2%	None

Table 6-14. Pharmacokinetics of anticancer drugs—cont'd

Drug	Plasma T½	Metabolism and excretion	Condition requiring dose reduction
Thioguanine[100a]	Unknown	Hepatic metabolism to S-methylated inactive product; renal excretion of 40% S-methyl derivative	Hepatic and renal dysfunction
Thiotepa[100a]	Rapid	Hepatic to inactive metabolite and renal excretion of metabolites	None
Vinblastine[100a]	T½ = 15 hours (bolus) T½ = 78 hours (infusion)	Hepatic metabolism and primary biliary excretion; renal excretion of 5%-20% unchanged drug in 96 hours	Elevated bilirubin
Vincristine[100a]	T½α = 1.5 minutes T½β = 2.6 hours	Hepatic metabolism and biliary excretion of 40% in feces; renal excretion of 10% unchanged in 24 hours	Elevated bilirubin
Vindesine[100a]	T½α = 4 minutes T½β = 99 minutes T½λ = 20 hours	Hepatic metabolism; renal excretion of 13% in 24 hours	Elevated bilirubin

Renal dysfunction

It has been recommended that drugs that are both excreted by and toxic to the kidney (methotrexate, cisplatin, and streptozocin) should not be given to patients with renal dysfunction. However, the severity of the renal dysfunction often determines whether these agents should be completely avoided or merely decreased slightly. As a general guide, in patients with creatinine clearances of less than 30 ml/minute, methotrexate, cisplatin, and streptozocin should probably not be administered. However, the decision to withhold therapy should also depend upon the clinical setting. If the drug is one of the above and represents the patient's best chance for response, the clinician and patient may accept this risk. Table 6-15 lists those anticancer drugs requiring dose reduction. Those agents for which there are specific guidelines for dose modification are discussed below.

METHOTREXATE (MTX)

In patients with moderate renal dysfunction (30 to 50 ml/min), MTX can probably be administered but at decreased doses. The nomogram by Tozer[46] can be used to modify dosage in renal failure:

$$Q = 1 - (f_e)(1 - K_f)$$

Table 6-15. Anticancer drugs requiring dose modification in patients with renal dysfunction

Definite modification of dose	Potential modification of dose
Cisplatin	Carmustine
Cyclophosphamide	Chlorozotocin
Deazauridine	Cycloleucine
Hydroxyurea	Dacarbazine
Methotrexate	Daunorubicin
Pyrazolo-imidazole	Lomustine
Streptozocin	Mercaptopurine
	Mitomycin C
	Procarbazine
	Thioguanine

Table 6-16. Aqueous solubility (mM/L) of methotrexate and 7-hydroxymethotrexate and pH change

Compound	pH 5.0 (mM/L)	pH 6.0 (mM/L)	pH 7.0 (mM/L)
MTX	0.97	3.52	19.6
7-OH MTX	0.29	0.81	3.4

Table 6-17. Guidelines for the prevention of methotrexate nephrotoxicity

Procedure	Comment
1. Hydration	*Goal:* Increase urine output to >120 ml/hr and dilute tubular concentration of MTX *Use:* Dextrose and saline (¼, ½, 1 NS); add potassium salts 3-6 liters over 24 hours; prehydrate for 6-24 hours
2. Alkalinization	*Goal:* Increase urine pH to 7 or greater *Use:* $NaHCO_2$ IV/PO; IV—give 100-150 mEq over 4 hours; test urine pH each void; PO—give 1 g every 6 hours for 4 doses; test urine pH every 6 hours; use acetazolamide (Diamox) if sodium is contraindicated; dose is 250 mg every 6 hours starting 24 hours prior to MTX continuing for 24 hours after therapy
3. Monitoring of MTX levels	*Goal:* Levels should fall below 1 μM at 24 hours and 0.1 μM at 48 hours

where Q = dosage reduction factor; f_e = fraction of renal excretion; K_f = fraction of normal renal function.

For example, a patient has a creatinine clearance of 30 ml/min and is to receive MTX (f_e = 90%). The Q factor is 0.43. Thus the patient should receive about 40% of the usual dose.

Whenever MTX is administered to a patient with decreased renal function, serum levels of the drug should be monitored, and if elevated at 24 or 48 hours, leucovorin should be increased to 50 mg/m^2 and continued until the serum level falls to below 0.1 μM (1×10^{-7} M).[47]

Besides decreased MTX clearance in patients with renal dysfunction, methotrexate has been associated with nephrotoxicity, usually after high-dose therapy (>1 g/m^2).[48] In most instances this toxicity has been the result of renal precipitation of MTX. The mechanism of precipitation has been attributed to the low aqueous solubility of MTX and its 7-hydroxymetabolite (7-OH MTX), the latter accounting for 10% of the dose administered. The solubility of MTX and 7-OH MTX is pH dependent (Table 6-16). Vigorous hydration and urinary alkalinzation have sharply reduced the incidence of nephropathy from high-dose MTX therapy.[47] Table 6-17 provides guidelines for the prevention of renal precipitation of MTX when used in high-dose therapy.

CISPLATIN

Because cisplatin is nephrotoxic, it has been suggested that this drug be avoided in patients with renal dysfunction.[49] However, damage to kidney tissue is dose or concentration related, and so mere dilution of the drug may be all that is necessary to prevent or minimize the nephrotoxic effects of this drug. Thus, unless anuria is present, patients with mild to moderate renal dysfunction should be able to tolerate cisplatin therapy. In fact, at the University of California at San Francisco cisplatin has been used in patients with creatinine clearances between 50 to 80 ml/min without undue nephrotoxic effects. The critical factor appears to be the administration of adequate hydration and diuresis (>120 ml/hr). These researchers do not recommend cisplatin in patients with creatinine clearances of less than 50 ml/min, because they are uncertain of its safety in this situation.

Controversy exists as to whether cisplatin is less nephrotoxic when administered as a slow or continuous infusion or with prior mannitol or furosemide.[50] It appears that slow infusions are associated with a lower incidence of renal toxicity. A plausible explanation is that lower peak drug levels result in a decreased accumulation of cisplatin into renal tissue. Studies are currently being directed toward this question.

The use of mannitol or furosemide alone does not appear to lower the

Table 6-18. Guidelines for the prevention of cisplatin nephrotoxicity

Procedures
1. a. 5 hours prior to cisplatin infusion give D_5W ½ NS 1,000 ml IV at 200 ml/hour b. Just prior to cisplatin infusion give 25 g mannitol IV bolus and 40 mg furosemide IV c. Continue D_5W ½ NS 5 hours after cisplatin infusion
2. Combine cisplatin with 40 mEq of KCl, 37.5 g of mannitol and 40 mg of furosemide in D_5W ½ NS 2,000 ml and give over a 6-hour period; replace fluid losses from emesis and diuresis with subsequent hydration
3. a. Prehydrate with D_5W ½ NS over 12-24 hours prior to cisplatin b. Maintain IV fluids for a minimum of 24 hours after administering cisplatin
4. In patients with severe CHF disease: a. Give cisplatin in 200 ml D_5W ½ NS or in 10% mannitol solution followed by an additional 200 ml of 10% mannitol

incidence of renal toxicity. The role of diuretics is in the setting of decreased urine output (<100 ml/hr). These agents are definitely useful to the clinician, especially in the elderly patient. It is uncertain whether furosemide, a known nephrotoxin, exacerbates the nephrotoxic effects of cisplatin. However, other nephrotoxic drugs, cephalothin and aminoglycoside antibiotics, have been shown to increase the risk of renal toxicity to cisplatin. Table 6-18 gives four different procedures for the prevention of renal toxicity of cisplatin administration.

STREPTOZOCIN

The major dose-limiting effect of streptozocin is renal toxicity. Toxicity is dose related, occurring with doses greater than 1.5 mg/m^2 given weekly or 500 mg/m^2 given daily for 5 consecutive days. The site of renal damage is the proximal renal tubule, where the drug is concentrated and may release an active methylating agent. The drug should be discontinued at the earliest sign of renal damage, which is proteinuria or aminoaciduria.

In the presence of prior renal dysfunction, the general recommendation is to avoid streptozocin in patients with a creatinine clearance of less than 50 ml/min.

CYCLOPHOSPHAMIDE

Most of the administered drug (88%) is metabolized in the liver; 17% is in the form of active metabolites, phosphoramide mustard, and acrolein, which are excreted in urine within 30 hours.[88] These metabolites are toxic and possibly carcinogenic to the bladder mucosa. Although cyclophosphamide is not nephrotoxic per se, its metabolites can produce both chemical and hemorrhagic cystitis. Thus, it would seem advisable to reduce the dose of cyclophosphamide in patients with renal dysfunction. The degree of dos-

Table 6-19. Drug modification in patients with hepatic dysfunction

Definite adjustment	Condition	Modification
Daunorubicin	Bilirubin 1.5-2.9 mg/100 ml	Decrease by 50%
Doxorubicin	Bilirubin 3.0 mg/100 ml	Decrease by 75%
	Potential adjustment	
Asparaginase	Fluorouracil	Thioguanine
Azacitidine	Melphalan	Vinblastine
Chlorambucil	Mercaptopurine	Vincristine
Cytarabine	Tegafur	Vindesine
Dactinomycin		

age reduction can be calculated from the equation, $Q = 1 - (f_e)(1 - K_f)$, as in MTX adjustments (see page 275).

MISCELLANEOUS

Several other anticancer drugs such as azathioprine, bleomycin, pyrazolo imidazole (IMPY), melphalan, 6-mercaptopurine, daunorubicin, procarbazine, and thioguanine are partially excreted by the kidney, but no definitive guidelines are reported for their use in patients with renal dysfunction. However, enhanced toxicity may occur in patients who are anuric or oliguric, so the clinician should be aware of the possibility of such developments in these patients.

Of note is the fact that the half-life of bleomycin increases dramatically in patients with creatinine clearances less than 40 ml/min.[92] However, enhanced toxicity was not observed in these patients and therefore dosage adjustment is probably not indicated.

Only 10% of melphalan is excreted as the parent compound in the urine.[84] No documented cases of enhanced toxicity have been reported in patients with severe renal dysfunction. However, Alberts reported that the drug was threefold more toxic in dogs after they were made anephric and that several of them died of marrow failure. Therefore dose adjustment may be necessary in the human.

Hepatic dysfunction

There are even fewer guidelines for anticancer drugs in patients with hepatic dysfunction than with renal dysfunction. Only two drugs, Adriamycin and daunorubicin, have definite dosage adjustments. Several other agents are metabolized in the liver, but it is uncertain if they will be more toxic in the presence of hepatic dysfunction. These agents are listed in Table 6-19.

COMPLICATIONS OF CHEMOTHERAPY

Antineoplastic drugs

Over thirty drugs are commercially available to the oncologist for the treatment of human malignancy. In addition, several investigational agents are available from the National Cancer Institute for use in research studies. All of these agents must by definition cause toxicity. Since combination chemotherapy is common to most investigational protocols, the clinician must titrate drug dosage in order to avoid serious toxicity. Most agents have several adverse effects that can be classified into acute and delayed toxicities. Acute toxicities are usually observed within 24 hours of drug administration, whereas delayed toxicities may appear several days to months after continuous drug administration.

With regard to bone marrow depression, most antineoplastic drugs are limited in their doses and schedule by their effect on hematopoietic cells. Those agents that have little or no bone marrow toxicity include bleomycin, cisplatin, L-asparaginase, vincristine, and streptozocin. Thus in Table 6-20 a special note will be made in the comment section for those toxicities considered to be dose limiting. Table 6-20 lists in alphabetical order most of the commonly used antineoplastic drugs and their toxicities.

Table 6-20. Antineoplastic drug toxicities

Toxicity	Incidence	Onset	Comment
L-Asparaginase			
Clotting abnormalities	60%	10-14 days	Monitor prothrombin time, hemogram, and signs of bleeding; if present, treat with fresh frozen plasma
Decrease in factors V, VII, VIII, IX, X, prothrombin, fibrinogen			
Severe bleeding	1%	14 days	
CNS dysfunction			
Somnolence, lethargy	33%	7 days	Reversible
Confusion	10%	7 days	Reversible
Personality changes	60%	7 days	Reversible
Encephalopathy	Uncommon	24 hours to several days	Rapid recovery if rapid onset, slow recovery if slow onset
Gastrointestinal			
Nausea and vomiting	30%	1-3 hours	Usually mild
Anorexia	30%	24 hours	
Weight loss	25%	2-3 weeks	5%-10% loss
Hepatotoxicity			
Increase in liver function tests	50%	3-7 days	Mild and transient; severe transaminase elevation is rare
Fatty metamorphosis	42%-87%	Months	Reversible
Hyperglycemia	Common	7-10 days	Control with insulin; more common in patients over 10 years of age and doses over 6,000 units
Hypersensitivity reactions			
Mild allergic: urticaria, fever, chills	25%	3-6 hours	Pretreat with acetaminophen plus diphenhydramine
Anaphylaxis	3.3% (after 1-4 doses) 32% (after 5 doses or more)	Immediate	Epinephrine (0.5 mg) and hydrocortisone (100 mg) at the bedside
Hematologic			
Granulocytopenia	100%	4-7 days	Bone marrow not affected
Thrombocytopenia	30%	5-10 days	

Continued.

Table 6-20. Antineoplastic drug toxicities—cont'd

Toxicity	Incidence	Onset	Comment
L-Asparaginase—cont'd			
Hypocholesterolemia	85%	7 days	Reversible after treatment
Renal			
Azotemia	30%	4-7 days	Reversible
Proteinuria or cylinduria	15%		Increased urea production; not toxic to renal parenchyma
Pancreatitis	5%	14-21 days	Reversible in 14 days; hemorrhage, hyperglycemia, and shock are associated
Azacitidine			
Bone marrow depression			
Leukopenia	100%	14-17 days	Recovery by day 28
Thrombocytopenia	100%	14-17 days	
Anemia	100%	14-21 days	
Gastrointestinal			
Nausea and vomiting	70% (bolus)	2-4 hours	Give by slow infusion over 4-6 hours
	25% (continuous infusion)	2-4 hours	
Diarrhea	30%-50%	7-14 days	Recovery by day 21-28
Hepatotoxicity			
Increased transaminases	15%	14-21 days	Reversible
Hepatic coma	5%		
Hypersensitivity reaction			
Fever	10%	6-12 hours	Treat with acetaminophen and diphenhydramine
Neuromuscular			
Weakness, lethargy, confusion	Rare	14-21 days	Reversible
Bleomycin			
Gastrointestinal			
Nausea and vomiting	15%	3-6 hours	
Anorexia, weight loss		7-14 days	In high doses (30 units or more)

Hypersensitivity reactions			
Anaphylaxis	Rare	5-15 minutes	Most often occurs in lymphoma
Fever and chills	30%	4-6 hours	Treat with acetaminophen and diphenhydramine
Pulmonary			
Pneumonitis	8%	6-8 months	Dose related 200 mg/m^2
Fibrosis	1%		Exacerbated by prior irradiation or pulmonary disease or in patients over 60 years of age
Skin and mucous membrane			
Hyperpigmentation	25%	4-8 weeks	Slowly reversible
Ulceration and severe tenderness	10%	3-4 months	Usually after twice weekly dosage of 10 units or more
Skin peeling	10%	3-4 months	
Nail banding (horizontal)	10%	3 months	Especially in blacks; associated with MSH release
Stomatitis	15%	2-3 days	Treat with lidocaine 2% mouthwash
Alopecia	50%	4-6 weeks	Reversible
Leukopenia	20%	7-10 days	Mild, usually only after high-dose 24-hour infusion
Hypertension	17%	2-4 days	After high-dose regimens of 25 units per day for 5 days
Hyperbilirubinemia	30%	14 days	After high-dose regimens of 25 units per day for 5 days
Busulfan			
Bone marrow depression			
Leukopenia	100%	7 days	Delayed recovery
Thrombocytopenia	70%	14 days	
Pulmonary toxicity			
Fibrosis	20%	3 years	Only with continued use
Miscellaneous			
Addison's disease	Rare	2-3 years	Prolonged daily therapy
Porphyria cutanea tarda	Rare		
Cataracts	Rare	2 years	
Gynecomastia	Rare		
Amenorrhea	Common	3-4 months	
Carmustine			
Bone marrow depression			
Leukopenia	100%	21 days	Delayed recovery (40-50 days)
Thrombocytopenia	100%	28 days	Cumulative toxicity

Continued.

Table 6-20. Antineoplastic drug toxicities—cont'd

Toxicity	Incidence	Onset	Comment
Carmustine—cont'd			
Gastrointestinal			
Nausea and vomiting	80%	2-6 hours	Use prophylactic antiemetics
Anorexia		24 hours	
Hepatotoxicity			
Bilirubinemia	5%-25%	21-30 days	Reversible; SGOT, alkaline phosphatase usually normal
Pulmonary			
Respiratory failure	Uncommon	9 days to 32 months	Dose related; total cumulative dose of 400-2,075 mg/m^2 (mean 720); 30% of cases reversible
Skin and mucous membrane			
Alopecia	Uncommon		
Phlebitis	Common	During infusion	Slow infusion (60-90 min) in at least 250 ml of IV fluid decreases incidence
Stomatitis	Uncommon	14-21 days	Reversible
Chlorambucil			
Bone marrow depression			
Leukopenia	100%	7-10 days	Recovery in 21 days
Thrombocytopenia	100%	14 days	Cumulative toxicity
Gastrointestinal			
Nausea and vomiting	10%	2-3 days	Mild
Hepatotoxicity			
Increased liver function tests	Rare	14-21 days	Reversible
Hypersensitivity reactions			
Exfoliative dermatitis	Rare	2-4 days	
Fever	Rare	6-12 hours	Treat with antipyretics
Pulmonary			
Fibrosis	Uncommon	Months to years	Long-term continuous treatment
Cisplatin			
Bone marrow depression			
Leukopenia	20%	7-10 days	Mild and transient; worsens in presence of renal dysfunction
Thrombocytopenia			
Gastrointestinal			
Nausea and vomiting	100%	3-6 hours	May be decreased by 24-hour infusions
Hypersensitivity reactions			
Anaphylaxis	Rare	Immediate	Treat with epinephrine and corticosteroids

Neuropathy			
Peripheral neuritis	10%	4-8 weeks	Reversible upon discontinuation of drug
Ototoxicity	30%	4-8 weeks	High frequency hearing loss; irreversible
Renal damage			
Acute tubular necrosis	25%	1-4 weeks	Irreversible; incidence is decreased with forced diuresis; monitor creatinine clearance
Cyclophosphamide			
Bladder toxicity			
Cystitis	4%-35%	3-7 days	Associated with dehydration; prevent with 1-2 liters of fluid on the day of therapy with frequent urination; severe bleeding must be treated with bladder instillation with formalin or fulgaration
Hemorrhagic cystitits	5%	3-7 days	
Fibrosis	Uncommon	Months	Associated with prolonged therapy
Bone marrow depression			
Leukopenia	100%	10-14 days	Dose limiting; recovery in 21 days
Thrombocytopenia	20%	14 days	Mild
Gastrointestinal			
Nausea and vomiting	90% with doses >1 g/m^2	4-6 hours	Divided oral doses associated with a lower incidence; use prophylactic antiemetic prior to parenteral cyclophosphamide (CTX)
	50% with 0.5 g/m^2	4-6 hours	
Cardiac			
CHF	Rare and only with doses >50 mg/kg	2 weeks	May or may not be irreversible; exacerbates anthracycline cardiomyopathy
Pulmonary			
Fibrosis	Rare, occurs with chronic, long-term therapy	6 months to 5 years	Irreversible
Skin and mucous membrane			
Alopecia	70%-80%	1-3 months	Reversible
Syndrome inappropriate ADH			
Hyponatremia	20% in high doses (>1 g/m^2)	12-24 hours	Reversible
Other			
Amenorrhea	90%	7 months	Some cases irreversible
Azospermia	90%-100%	6 months	Most patients sterile after 6 months of CTX; 20% of patients recover spermatogenesis after 2 years
Teratogenic	Common	1-2 months	Spontaneous abortion

Continued.

Table 6-20. Antineoplastic drug toxicities—cont'd

Toxicity	Incidence	Onset	Comment
Cytarabine			
Bone marrow toxicity			
Leukopenia	100%	4-7 days	Therapeutic effect
Thrombocytopenia	100%	4-7 days	Platelet support usually required for 30%-50% of hospital days post-therapy
Gastrointestinal			
Nausea and vomiting	15%-20%	6-12 hours	
Diarrhea	20%-25%	3-4 days	Usually requires antidiarrheals such as diphenoxylate
Hepatotoxicity			
Abnormal liver function tests	30%-50%	7-10 days	Reversible
Hypersensitivity reactions			
Fever and chills	10%-20%	24 hours	
Skin rashes	20%	2-3 days	May have to discontinue if hemorrhagic petechial rash develops
Skin and mucous membrane			
Stomatitis	30%-50%	7-10 days	Nystatin topical mouthwash and swallow
Dacarbazine			
Bone marrow depression			
Leukopenia (mild)	30%-50%	7-10 days	Recovery by day 24
Thrombocytopenia (mild)	30%-50%	7-10 days	
Gastrointestinal			
Nausea and vomiting	90%	2-4 hours	Often dose limiting; total dose given in one large infusion is no more emetogenic than divided 5-day schedule
Anorexia			
Flu-like syndrome			
Malaise, myalgias, fever	10%-20%	7 days	Recovery 1-3 weeks
Hepatotoxicity			
Transaminasemia	Uncommon	3-4 days	Reversible
Bilirubinemia			
Other			
Photosensitivity	Rare		
Facial flushing	Uncommon		
Facial paresthesias	Uncommon		

Azotemia	Uncommon		
Phlebitis	Common		Dilution and slow IV infusion
Dactinomycin			
Bone marrow depression			
Leukopenia	55%	7-10 days after 5-day course	Dose limiting
Thrombocytopenia	44%	1-7 days after 5-day course	Usually more severe than leukopenia
Anemia	50%	7-14 days after 5-day course	
Gastrointestinal			
Nausea and vomiting	Mild (90%)		
	Moderate-severe (20%)	3-6 hours	Dose related recovery in 24 hours
Diarrhea	3%-5%	3-5 days	Reversible in 7-10 days; mild laxatives for treatment
Proctitis	20%-25%	5-7 days after completion of course	Dose limiting; therapy should be discontinued until pain has subsided
Skin and mucous membrane			
Stomatitis	30% at 0.015 mg/day for 5 days, 1% at 0.010 mg/day for 5 days	3-5 days after completion of course	Dose limiting
Glossitis and tongue erythema	5%-10%	7-10 days after completion of 5-day course	
Dermal reactions	Common	7 days-3 months	Site of previous irradiation is most vulnerable
Follicular acne (on face and trunk)	80%-90% at doses of 0.015 mg/day for 5 days	7-14 days following chemotherapy	Associated with a follicular body rash
Alopecia	47% (children)	7-10 days following chemotherapy	Reversible after chemotherapy is discontinued

Continued.

Table 6-20. Antineoplastic drug toxicities—cont'd

Toxicity	Incidence	Onset	Comment
Daunorubicin			
Bone marrow depression			
Leukopenia	90%	7-10 days	Therapeutic effect; platelet transfusions required for 30%-50% of hospital days post-therapy
Thrombocytopenia	90%	7-10 days	
Cardiotoxicity			
CHF	2%-5%	7-9 months	>700 mg/m²; symptomatic treatment
Cardiomyopathy	1%	7-9 months	>700 mg/m²; symptomatic treatment
Arrhythmias	30%	24 hours	Transient; reversible
Gastrointestinal			
Nausea and vomiting	50%	2-6 hours	Premedicate with antiemetics
Diarrhea	25%	3-5 days	
Hypersensitivity reactions			
Fever, chills	33%	6-12 hours	Prophylaxis with acetaminophen
Skin rash	6%	3-4 days	Reversible
Skin and mucous membranes			
Alopecia	90%	2-4 weeks	Reversible
Vesicant	2%	5-10 days	See section on treatment and prevention of extravasation reactions
Other			
Red urine	90%	12-24 hours	20% of drug excreted in urine
Doxorubicin			
Bone marrow depression			
Leukopenia	100%	10 days	Dose limiting
Thrombocytopenia	30%-40%	10-14 days	Recovery by 21 days
Anemia		14 days	
Cardiotoxicity			
Arrhythmias and ECG changes	33%	12-24 hours	Not dose related; recovery in 3-7 days; not an indication to discontinue therapy
Heart failure	1% at doses <550 mg/m² 11% between 550-600 mg/m² 31% at doses >600 mg/m²	1-6 months	Dose limiting; avoid drug in patients with prior myocardial disease

Gastrointestinal			
Nausea and vomiting	45%	4-6 hours	Duration of 6 hours
Hypersensitivity reactions			
Fever and chills	Rare	4-8 hours	Duration of 2-4 hours
Anaphylaxis	Rare	Immediate	Treat with epinephrine and antihistamines
Skin and mucous membrane			
Rashes	Rare	24-48 hours	Reversible
Erythema and hyperpigmentation	Common at previous irradiated areas	24 hours	Treat with topical corticosteroids
Phlebitis	5%-10%	1-24 hours	
Vesication	Common upon extravasation	4-7 days	See Section 7, Ancillary Therapy, for local treatment
Stomatitis	75%	3-7 days	
Alopecia	80%-90%	7-14 days	
Urine changes			
Red urine	100%	With first few voidings	Between 5%-10% of the drug is rapidly excreted in the urine
Etoposide and *teniposide*			
Bone marrow depression			Dose related
Leukopenia	100% in large doses, 16% in divided doses over 5 days	5-7 days	Reversible
Thrombocytopenia	100% in large single dose, 7% in divided doses	7-10 days	
Gastrointestinal			
Nausea and vomiting	25%	3-8 hours	
Stomatitis	Uncommon	4-7 days	
Hypersensitivity reactions			
Fever, chills	Uncommon	3-6 hours	
Generalized erythemia	Uncommon	12-24 hours	
Bronchospasm and anaphylaxis	Rare	Immediate	
Hypotension	Common with rapid drug administration	5-10 minutes	Administer drug over 30 minutes or more
Skin toxicity			
Alopecia		14-21 days	
Vascular phlebitis	Common	12-24 hours	Dilute in large volume

Continued.

Table 6-20. Antineoplastic drug toxicities—cont'd

Toxicity	Incidence	Onset	Comment
Fluorouracil			
Bone marrow depression			
Leucopenia	100% in high-dose (HD) regimens 50% in weekly dose (WD) therapy		Dose limiting; 5-day continuous infusion less myelosuppression
Gastrointestinal			
Nausea and vomiting	50%-90% (HD) 20% (WD)	3-6 hours 3-6 hours	Dose limiting
Stomatitits	60%-75% (HD) 4%-8% (WD)	4-7 days	
Diarrhea	30%-80% (HD) 5% (WD)	5-7 days	
Anorexia	30%-50%	2-5 days	
Hypersensitivity reaction			
Maculopapular rash	5%	2-5 days	
Neurotoxicity			
Cerebellar ataxia	5% 21% with concurrent hydroxyurea	8-12 months	Long-term therapy
Skin and mucous membrane			
Alopecia	5%-50% (HD) 5%-10% (WD)	3-4 weeks 3-4 weeks	Usually not total; often regrows during therapy
Dry scaling dermatitis	10%-20%	4-6 weeks	Nasal mucosa can be affected leading to epistaxis
Hexamethylmelamine			
Bone marrow depression (1,000-2,000/mm^3)			
Leukopenia	10%	7-10 days (in high doses of 8 mg/kg/day; 2 months in low dose of 4 mg/kg/day (applies to both leukopenia and thrombocytopenia)	
Thrombocytopenia	8%		

Gastrointestinal			
Nausea and vomiting	55%	3-6 hours	May be decreased with divided dosage
Diarrhea			
Neurologic			
Peripheral neuropathy, ataxia	3%	3 months	Long-term high-dose therapy for at least 3 months; reversible when treatment is stopped or managed with pyridoxine (100 mg three times daily) and dosage decreased to 4-6 mg/kg/day
Insomnia	10%	3 months	
Hallucinations	3%	3 months	
Skin and mucous membrane			
Rashes	3%	2-4 days	
Alopecia	1%	7-14 days	
Hydroxyurea			
Bone marrow depression			
Leukopenia	70%	3-5 days	Recovery in 4-6 days
Thrombocytopenia	20%	4-7 days	Recovery in 4-6 days
Anemia	34%	2-3 weeks	
Megaloblastosis	90%	30 days	
Gastrointestinal			
Nausea and vomiting	25%	6-12 hours	Doses of 25-50 mg/kg/day
Diarrhea	10%	3-4 days	
Stomatitis	Common	7-10 days	Usually occurs with high doses
Ulceration	Uncommon	10-21 days	Usually occurs with high doses (40 mg/kg/day)
Dermatologic reactions			
Maculopapular rash	Uncommon	7-14 days	Reversible
Facial erythema	Uncommon	30-60 days	Occurs with long-term therapy
Pigmentation	Common	30-60 days	Occurs with long-term therapy
Neurotoxicity			
Hallucinations	Rare		Potentiates 5-FU neurotoxicity
Headache, dizziness, disorientation	Rare		
Convulsions	Rare		
Renal dysfunction	Rare	12-24 hours	Mild, reversible, high dose (40 mg/kg/day)
Skin and mucous membrane			
Alopecia (partial)	Rare	7-14 days	
Stomatitis	Rare	5-7 days	

Continued.

Table 6-20. Antineoplastic drug toxicities—cont'd

Toxicity	Incidence	Onset	Comment
Lomustine			
Bone marrow depression			
Leukopenia	75%	14 days	Delayed recovery
Thrombocytopenia	90%	14 days	Usually more severe than leukopenia; 30% systemic absorption after intrapleural injection can lead to myelosuppression
Gastrointestinal			
Nausea and vomiting	90%	4-12 hours	Dose limiting
Stomatitis	Uncommon	10-14 days	
Hepatotoxicity			
Increased transaminases	35%	14-21 days	Reversible
Renal dysfunction			
Increased BUN and creatinine	1%		Reversible
Mechlorethamine			
Bone marrow depression			
Leukopenia	100%	7-10 days	Leukopenia
Thrombocytopenia	100%	10-14 days	Thrombopenia
Gastrointestinal			
Nausea and vomiting	95%	1-4 hours	Duration of 6-24 hours
Diarrhea	10%	5-7 days	
Hypersensitivity reactions			
Fever, chills	30%-40%	4-6 hours	Premedicate with acetaminophen and antihistamines if necessary
Rash	Uncommon	3-4 days	
Anaphylaxis	Rare	Immediate	Antihistamines and sympathomimetics
Skin and mucous membrane			
Alopecia	75%	14-28 days	Reversible
Vesicant	100%		Avoid extravasation (see Section 7 for management)
Dermatitis	Rare		
Other			
Amenorrhea	75%	30 days	
Azospermia	40%	30-60 days	Recovery may occur in 2 years

Melphalan			
Bone marrow depression			Dose limiting, cumulative
Leukopenia	65%	21-28 days	Slow recovery may necessitate dosing every 6-8 weeks
Thrombocytopenia	75%	21-28 days	
Anemia	75%	36-48 days	
Gastrointestinal			
Nausea and vomiting	30% (in large doses)	6-12 hours	Suggest divided dosage; oral absorption varies from 40%-70% of parenteral dose
	10% (in divided doses)	6-12 hours	
Pulmonary toxicity			
Respiratory failure	Rare	8-18 months	Daily low-dose therapy
Skin and mucous membrane			
Alopecia	Rare	21-28 days	Reversible
Other			
Second malignancies	Uncommon	3-5 years	Increased risk in long-term survivors
Mercaptopurine			
Bone marrow depression			
Leukopenia	Common	7-10 days	Dose limiting
Thrombocytopenia	Uncommon	7-10 days	Usually high dose
Anemia	Uncommon	14-21 days	
Gastrointestinal			
Nausea and vomiting	25%	4-8 hours	Antiemetics if needed
Anorexia	25%	1-2 days	
Stomatitis	Rare	4-6 days	
Hepatotoxicity			
Jaundice	33%	21-30 days	Usually reversible
Transaminase elevation	15%	10-17 days	Usually reversible
Hepatic necrosis	Rare	14-30 days	
Reactions			
Dermatitis	5%-10%	2-4 days	Reversible
Drug fever	5%	3-5 days	Reversible
Eosinophilia	Uncommon		
Renal dysfunction			
Acute tubular necrosis	Rare	Immediate	Only after large single doses
Hematuria and crystaluria	Uncommon	Immediate	Dehydration and acidic urine predispose to crystaluria; decrease dose in patients with decreased creatinine clearance

Continued.

Table 6-20. Antineoplastic drug toxicities—cont'd

Toxicity	Incidence	Onset	Comment
Methotrexate			
Bone marrow depression			
Leukopenia and thrombocytopenia	30% (without leucovorin)	5-10 days	Reversible; use leucovorin rescue with doses >100 mg/m^2
	10% (with leucovorin)	5-10 days	
Anemia	Uncommon	10-17 days	
Gastrointestinal			
Nausea and vomiting	10% (with conventional doses)	4-12 hours	Duration of 3-12 hours
	65% (with high doses)	4-12 hours	
Diarrhea	5%-10%	4-7 days	Recovery by 10 days
GI ulceration	5%	7 days	
Glossitis	10%	10-14 days	
Pharyngitis	5%		
Stomatitis	10%-40%	4-7 days	More common with high-dose regimens
Hepatotoxicity			
Transaminasemia	20%	5-10 days	Reversible
Portal fibrosis	1%	1-2 years	More common in alcoholic patients; most cases occur after long-term daily treatment
Hypersensitivity reactions	10%	24-48 hours	More common after high-dose therapy
Neurotoxicity (intrathecal methotrexate only)			
Peripheral neuropathy	Rare	1-24 hours	Related to high CSF concentrations and delayed drug clearance
Dementia	Rare		
Seizures	Rare		Limit total dosage to 12 mg
Quadriplegia or paraplegia	Rare		Life threatening
Headache, blurred vision, and meningismus	20%-60%	2-4 hours	Due to drug irritation; reversible in about 5 days
Leucoencephalopathy	1%	24 hours	Associated with high CSF concentrations, delayed drug clearance, and cranial irradiation

Pulmonary			
Pneumonitis	1%	2 weeks-3 months	Allergic reaction; not dose-related; reversible in 2-3 days; corticosteroids may shorten the course of toxicity
Renal dysfunction			
Anuria	5% with doses of 1-10 g/m^2	6-12 hours	Prehydration $NaHCO_3$ (see pp. 276, Renal Toxicity)
Skin and mucous membrane			
Alopecia	5%-10%	14-21 days	Reversible
Other reactions			
Osteoporosis	Rare	Years	Occurs after long-term daily therapy
Mithramycin			
Bone marrow depression			
Leukopenia	Uncommon		
Thrombocytopenia	Common	7-10 days after a 5-10 day course	Usually occurs only after 10-day course
	Uncommon after 1 dose of 25 μg/kg		
Dermatologic reactions			
Facial flushing	3%	1-2 days	Recovery 5-10 days
Skin rash	2%	1-2 days	Recovery 3-6 days
Electrolyte disturbances (daily dosage)			
Hypocalcemia	Common	1-3 days	Used to treat hypercalcemia secondary to malignancy
Hypokalemia	Common	1-3 days	
Hypophosphatemia			
Gastrointestinal			
Nausea and vomiting	90%	4-6 hours	Duration of 12-24 hours
Stomatitis	3%	7-10 days	Reversible
Diarrhea	2%	5-7 days	
Hemorrhage	5% (doses of 10-30 μg/kg for 4-10 daily doses)	7-10 days	Life threatening; results from effects on platelets, fibrinolysis, depression of clotting factor II, V, VII, X

Continued.

Table 6-20. Antineoplastic drug toxicities—cont'd

Toxicity	Incidence	Onset	Comment
Mithramycin—cont'd			
Hepatotoxicity			
Increased hepatic enzymes	90%	3-5 days after a 4-10 day course	Reversible in 14 days
Hypersensitivity reactions			
Fever	15%-83%	6-12 hours	Duration of 2-4 hours; prophylactic acetaminophen
Neurotoxicity			
Irritability	6%-75%	3-5 days post-therapy	Time- and dose-related; 75% at 50 μg/kg daily; 50% at 50 μg/kg every other day; 6% at 30 μg/kg daily
Lethargy, akathisia		3-5 days post-therapy	
Headache		3-5 days post-therapy	
Renal toxicity			
Proteinuria	20%-40%	5-7 days post-therapy	
Increased BUN and creatinine			40% increased BUN at doses of ≥25 μg/kg/day for 5 days; several deaths from renal failure; 20% increased BUN but not >45 mg% and no deaths at doses ≥50 μg/kg/day every other day for 3 days
Skin and vascular toxicity			
Phlebitis	Common	6 hours	
Vesication	Common if extravasated	2-7 days	See Section 7 for management of extravasation
Mitomycin C			
Bone marrow depression			Dose limiting; cumulative bone marrow damage; thrombocytopenia > leukopenia
Leukopenia	100%	Delayed 10-14 days	
Thrombocytopenia	100%	10-14 days	
Dermatologic reactions			
Rash	5%-10%	3-4 days	

Vesication	Common if extravasated	1-7 days	Severe, may require surgical debridement
Gastrointestinal			
Nausea and vomiting	75%	4-6 hours	
Diarrhea	20%	5-7 days	Mild
Stomatitis	20%	5-7 days	Mild
Neurologic			
Headache	Rare		
Blurred vision	Rare		
Confusion	Rare		
Syncope	Rare		
Pulmonary	Uncommon	8-30 weeks	Usually reversible
Renal dysfunction			
Glomerular sclerosis	Rare	Delayed	Associated with high doses
Increased creatinine	10%	6-7 months	
Procarbazine			
Bone marrow depression			Dose limiting
Leukopenia	100%	10 days	Reversible
Thrombocytopenia	100%	10 days	Reversible
Dermatologic reactions			
Maculopapular rash	5%	24 hours	Reversible upon discontinuation of drug
Urticaria	5%	24 hours	
Gastrointestinal			
Nausea and vomiting	75%-95%	1-3 days	Dose related; divided dosage may decrease incidence
Anorexia	75%	1-3 days	
Diarrhea	Uncommon	5-7 days	
Stomatitis	6%	5-7 days	
Hypersensitivity reactions			
Fever	Rare	1-3 days	After parenteral use only
Eosinophilia	Rare	1-3 days	Associated with pleuropulmonary infiltration

Continued.

Table 6-20. Antineoplastic drug toxicities—cont'd

Toxicity	Incidence	Onset	Comment
Procarbazine—cont'd			
Neurologic	10% overall		
Sedation, lethargy	Rare	3-5 days	After high doses only (>300 mg/day); may be related to decreased pyridoxyl phosphate; treat with pyridoxine 50 mg/day
Psychosis	Rare	3-5 days	
Ataxia	Rare		
Stupor	Rare	7-14 days	
Paresthesias	5%	7-14 days	
Orthostatic hypotension	Uncommon	5-10 days	Reversible on discontinuation of drug
Alcoholic intolerance	Uncommon	6-12 hours	Avoid strong alcoholic beverages
CNS depression with barbiturates, narcotics, sedatives	Uncommon	12-24 hours	Drug interaction contraindicates
Miscellaneous			
Hypertension from concurrent catecholamine and tyramine containing foods	Uncommon	12-24 hours	Mild effect; avoid sympathomimetics, tricyclic-antidepressants, cheese, red wine, beer, and yogurt
Skin reactions			
Alopecia	Uncommon	14-21 days	Reversible
Semustine			
Bone marrow depression			Dose-limiting
Leukopenia	80%	21-28 days	Thrombocytopenia > leukopenia; cumulative bone marrow damage
Thrombocytopenia	100%	20-28 days	
Anemia	20%	30 days	
Gastrointestinal			
Anorexia	70%	24 hours	
Nausea and vomiting	90%	12-24 hours	Premedicate with antiemetics
Hepatotoxicity			
Increased SGOT, SGPT, LDH	20%	30 days	Transient, reversible
Renal toxicity			
In children	Uncommon		
Glomerular sclerosis	40%	17 months	Dose related
Interstitial fibrosis	30%	17 months	>1500 mg/m^2 total dose
Tubular necrosis	30%	17 months	Monitor with IVP
Decreased renal size	40%		Renal dysfunction occurs only with long-term treatment
Increased BUN and creatinine	80%	24 months	

Streptozocin			
Bone marrow depression			
Leukopenia	0%-5%	7-10 days	Not dose limiting
Thrombocytopenia	0%-5%	7-10 days	
Anemia	20%	14-21 days	Reversible
Gastrointestinal			
Nausea and vomiting	90%	3-6 hours	Dose limiting; dose related
Hepatotoxicity			
Increased SGOT, SGPT	67%	1-3 days	Reversible in 3-5 days; no pathologic damage occurs
Renal dysfunction	65% (total)		Dose limiting
Tubular necrosis	25%		
Proteinuria	28%		Earliest manifestation; discontinue drug at this point until renal function recovers
Decreased creatinine clearance	28%		
Renal tubular acidosis with hypophosphatemia	25%		
Death from renal failure	10%		
Teniposide (see *etoposide*)			
Thioguanine			
Bone marrow depression			Dose limiting
Leukopenia	100%	7-10 days	
Thrombocytopenia	100%	7-10 days	
Gastrointestinal			
Nausea and vomiting	Uncommon	4-8 hours	
Stomatitis	Rare	4-7 days	Reversible
Thiotepa			
Bone marrow depression			
Leukopenia	40%	14-21 days	
Thrombocytopenia	80%	14-21 days	Dose limiting
Anemia	50%	21 days	
Gastrointestinal			
Nausea and vomiting	10%-15%	6-12 hours	
Miscellaneous			
Local pain at injection site	10%-20%	Immediate	Not reported to be vesicant

Continued.

Table 6-20. Antineoplastic drug toxicities—cont'd

Toxicity	Incidence	Onset	Comment
Vinblastine			
Bone marrow depression			Dose limiting
Leukopenia	100% at doses >0.3 mg/kg	4-7 days	
Thrombocytopenia	100% at doses >0.3 mg/kg	4-7 days	
Anemia	50%	10-14 days	
Gastrointestinal			
Nausea and vomiting	20%	4-8 hours	
Anorexia	20%	4-8 hours	
Neurologic			Dose related
Paresthesia	10%	6-8 weeks	Cumulative
Footdrop	10%	6-8 weeks	Much less than vincristine
Ataxia	1%	10-12 weeks	
Constipation	20%	2-3 weeks	Slowly reversible
Motor weakness	75% in high doses (0.3 mg/kg)	10-12 weeks	Reversible
Slapping gait	Rare	10-12 weeks	
Jaw pain	10%	6-24 hours	
Cranial nerve abnormalities VI and VII, diplopia, vocal paralysis	Rare	6-8 weeks	
Confusion, depression	Rare	6-8 weeks	
Vincristine			
Bone marrow depression			
Mild leukopenia	5%	4-7 days	Can be used in combination in full dosage
Gastrointestinal			
Nausea and vomiting	Uncommon	4-8 hours	
Stomatitis	Uncommon	4-7 days	
Neurotoxicity			
Peripheral neuropathy	100%	4-6 weeks	
Decreased reflexes	50%-100%	4-6 weeks	

Motor weakness	25%-30%	4-6 weeks	Distal muscle groups such as those of the fingers and feet
Paresthesia	50%		
Autonomic dysfunction	40%	4-6 weeks	
Severe constipation	35%	3-4 weeks	Most severe in patients over 60 years of age
Ileus	5%-10%	3-4 weeks	
Cranial nerve toxicity III, V, VI, VII	50% (in children) Uncommon (in adults)	6-8 weeks	Slowly reversible
Confusion, depression	Occasional cases	4-6 weeks	Reversible
Other			
Arthralgias, myalgias	Uncommon	12-24 hours	Usually occurs in older patients after the first or second injection
Jaw pain		6-24 hours	Apparently more common in head and neck cancer
Orthostatic hypotension	Rare	6-24 hours	
Headache	Occasional	1-3 days	
Skin toxicity			
Alopecia	90%-100%	14-21 days	
Vesication	100%	1-24 hours	See section on treating drug extravasation
STEROID HORMONES			
Estrogens			
Diethylstilbestrol			
Ethinyl estradiol			
Electrolyte disturbances			
Hypercalcemia	10%	2-5 days	In patients with bone metastases
Sodium and fluid retention	90%	4-7 days	Exacerbates heart failure
Gastrointestinal			
Nausea and vomiting	50%-70%	1-2 days	May subside in 1-2 weeks even with continued therapy
Hormonal changes			
Breast engorgement	80%	2-3 weeks	
Endometrial hypertrophy	Common	21-28 days	
Uterine bleeding	Common when drug discontinued	2-3 days	

Continued.

Table 6-20. Antineoplastic drug toxicities—cont'd

Toxicity	Incidence	Onset	Comment
STEROID HORMONES—cont'd			
Estrogens—cont'd			
Diethylstilbestrol—cont'd			
Ethinyl estradiol—cont'd			
Psychological changes			
Anxiety, depression	Uncommon	1-2 weeks	
Thromboembolic complications			
Thrombophlebitis	Increased risk especially in predisposed patients		Avoid estrogens if possible
Pulmonary embolism			
Stroke			
Antiestrogens			
Tamoxifen			
Bone marrow depression			
Leukopenia (mild)	10%	7-14 days	Mechanism unknown
Thrombocytopenia (mild)			
Gastrointestinal			
Nausea and vomiting	10%-20%	12-24 hours	Usually improves during therapy
Electrolyte disturbances			
Hypercalcemia	Unknown	3-7 days	Most common in patients with bone metastases
Sodium and fluid retention	80%-90%	2-5 days	Mild diuretics will reverse this problem
Hypersensitivity reactions			
Erythematous skin rash	Uncommon	24-48 hours	
Ocular toxicity			
Decreased visual acuity	Rare	12-16 months	Common with very high doses
Lens opacities	Rare	12-16 months	Common with very high doses
Retinopathy	Rare	12-16 months	Common with very high doses

Progestins			
Hydroxyprogesterone caproate			
Gastrointestinal			
Mild nausea and vomiting	Uncommon	1-2 days	Decreases after 7 days of therapy
Electrolyte disturbance			
Mild sodium and fluid retention	20%-30%	7-14 days	Mild diuretic if needed
Miscellaneous			
Sterile abscess at site of IM injection	Uncommon	4-7 days	
Medroxyprogesterone acetate			
Gastrointestinal			
Mild nausea	10%-20%	2-3 days	Decreases after 7 days of therapy
Mild weight gain	30%	7-14 days	Mild diuretic if needed
Electrolyte disturbance			
Fluid retention	30%	7-14 days	Mild diuretic if needed
Megestrol acetate			
Gastrointestinal			
Weight gain	10%-20%	7-14 days	Treat with mild diuretics
Electrolyte disturbance			
Fluid retention	10%-20%	7-14 days	Treat with mild diuretics
Androgens			
Testosterone propionate			
Fluoxymesterone			
Dromostanolone			
Testolactone			
Electrolyte disturbance			
Hypercalcemia	10%	3-7 days	Most common in patients with bone metastases
Sodium and fluid retention	50%	2-4 days	Mild diuretics will reverse this problem
Gastrointestinal			
Mild nausea and vomiting	30%-40%	2-5 days	Usually improves during continued therapy
Hepatotoxicity			
Cholestatic jaundice	Uncommon	30-60 days	Discontinue therapy

REFERENCES

1. Bergsagel, D. E., et al.: An assessment of massive-dose chemotherapy of malignant disease, Can. Med. Assoc. J. **104:**31, 1971.
2. Cadman, E.: Toxicity of chemotherapeutic agents. In Becker, F. F.: Cancer, vol. 5, New York, 1977, Plenum Press, pp. 59-111.
3. Billingham, M. E., et al.: Anthracycline cardiomyopathy monitored by morphologic changes, Cancer Treat. Rep. **62:**865-872, 1978.
4. Lenaz, L., et al.: Cardiotoxicity of adriamycin and related anthracyclines, Cancer Treat. Rev. **3:**111-120, 1976.
5. Von Hoff, D. D., et al.: Daunomycin-induced cardiac toxicity in children, Ann. Intern. Med. **62:**200-208, 1977.
6. Minow, R. A., et al.: Adriamycin cardiomyopathy—an overview with determination of risk factors, Cancer Chemother. Rep. **6:**195-201, 1975.
7. Gilladoga, A. C., et al.: The cardiotoxicity of adriamycin and daunomycin in children, Cancer **37:**1070-1078, 1976.

7a. Rinehart, J., et al.: Adriamycin cardiotoxicity in man, Ann. Intern. Med. **81:** 475-478, 1974.

8. Bristow, M. R., et al.: Doxorubicin cardiomyopathy: evaluation by phonocardiography, endomyocardial biopsy, and cardiac catheterization, Ann. Intern. Med. **88:**168-175, 1978.
9. Minow, R. A., et al.: Adriamycin cardiomyopathy—risk factors, Cancer **39:** 1397-1402, 1977.
10. Von Hoff, D. D.: Risk factors for doxorubicin-induced congestive heart failure, Ann. Int. Med. **91:**710-717, 1979.
11. Mulvin, G. M., et al.: Intensive cyclophosphamide therapy for solid tumors, part 1, Cancer Chemother. Rep. **59:**411, 1975.
12. Santos, G. W., et al.: Marrow transplant in man utilizing cyclophosphamide: summary of the Baltimore experience, Exp. Hematol. **20:**78, 1970.
13. Myer, C. E., et al.: Adriamycin: the role of lipid peroxidation in cardiac toxicity and tumor response, Science **197:**165, 1977.
14. Green, M. R.: Pulmonary toxicity of antineoplastic agents, West. J. Med. **127:** 292-298, 1977.
15. Willson, J. K.: Pulmonary toxicity of antineoplastic drugs, Cancer Treat. Rep. **62:**2003-2008, 1978.
16. Sostman, H. D.: Cytotoxic drug-induced lung disease, Am. J. Med. **62:**608-615, 1977.

16a. Weiss, R. B., and Muggia, F. M.: Cytotoxic drug-induced pulmonary disease: update 1980, Am. J. Med. **68:**259-266, 1980.

17. Bailey, C. C., et al.: Fatal pulmonary fibrosis following 1,3-bis (2-chloroethyl)-1-nitrosourea (BCNU) therapy, Cancer **42:**74-76, 1978.
18. Yagoda, A., et al.: Bleomycin, an antitumor antibiotic: clinical experience in 274 patients, Ann. Intern. Med. **77:**861, 1972.
19. Blum, R. H., et al.: A clinical review of bleomycin—a new antineoplastic agent, Cancer **31:**903, 1973.
20. Crooke, S. T., et al.: Bleomycin, a review, J. Med. **7:**333, 1976.
21. DeLena, M., et al.: Clinical radiologic and histopathologic studies on pulmonary toxicity induced by treatment with bleomycin, Cancer Chemother. Rep. **56:** 343-356, 1972.

22. Einhorn, L. H., et al.: Enhanced pulmonary toxicity with bleomycin and radiotherapy in oat cell lung cancer, Cancer **37**:2414, 1976.
23. Samuels, M. L., et al.: Large-dose bleomycin therapy and pulmonary toxicity. A possible role of prior radiotherapy, J.A.M.A. **235**:117, 1976.
24. Rosenow, E.: The spectrum of drug induced pulmonary disease, Ann. Intern. Med. **77**:977-991, 1972.
25. Sostman, H. D., et al.: Methotrexate induced pneumonitis. Medicine **55**:371-388, 1976.
26. Podoll, L.: Busulfan lung, Ann. Surg. **120**:151-156, 1974.
27. Schein, P., et al.: Immunosuppressive and cytotoxic chemotherapy: long-term complications. Ann. Intern. Med. **82**:84-94, 1975.
28. Dreizen, S.: Stomatotox manifestations of cancer chemotherapy, J. Prosthet. Dent. **40**:650-655, 1978.
29. Beck, S.: Impact of a systemic oral care protocol on stomatitis after chemotherapy, Cancer Nurs. **2**:185-199, June, 1979.
30. Levine, N., et al.: Side effects from cancer chemotherapy, Cancer Treat. Rev. **5**:67-84, 1978.
31. Killander, D., et al.: Hypersensitivity reactions and antibody formation during L-asparaginase treatment of children and adults with acute leukemia, Cancer **37**:220, 1976.
32. Jones, B. J., et al.: Optimal use of L-asparaginase in acute lymphocytic leukemia. Med. Ped. Oncol. **3**:387-400, 1977.
33. Dellinger, C. T., et al.: Comparison of anaphylactic reactions to asparaginase derived from E. coli and from Erwinia cultures, Cancer **38**:1843, 1976.
34. Donaldson, S. S., et al.: Adriamycin activating a recall phenomenon after radiation therapy, Ann. Intern. Med. **81**:407-408, 1974.
35. Rudolph, R., et al.: Skin ulcers due to adriamycin, Cancer **38**:1087, 1976.
36. Ignoffo, R. J., et al.: Therapy of local toxicities caused by extravasations of cancer chemotherapeutic drugs, Cancer Treat. Rev., March, 1980.
37. Levine, N., and Greenwald, E. S.: Mucocutaneous side effects of cancer chemotherapy, Cancer Treat. Rev. **5**:67-84, 1978.
38. Pratt, C. B., and Shanks, E. C.: Hyperpigmentation of nails from doxorubicin, J.A.M.A. **228**:460, 1974.
39. Shetty, M. R.: Case of pigmented banding of the nail caused by bleomycin, Cancer Treat. Rep. **61**:501-502, 1977.
39a. Morris, D., et al.: Horizontal pigmented banding of the nails in association with Adriamycin chemotherapy, Cancer Treat. Rep. **61**:499-500, 1977.
40. Heidelberger, C.: Pyrimidines and their nucleosides. In Sartorelli, A. C., and Johns, D. G., editors: Antineoplastics and immunosuppressive agents. Part II, Berlin, 1975, Springer-Verlag, p. 219.
41. Weiss, H. D., et al.: Neurotoxicity of commonly used antineoplastic agents, part 2, New Engl. J. Med. **297**:127, 1974.
42. Holland, J. F., et al.: Vincristine treatment of advanced cancer: a cooperative study of 392 cases, Cancer Res. **33**:1258, 1973.
43. Bleyer, W. A., et al.: Neurotoxicity and elevated cerebrospinal fluid methotrexate concentration in meningeal leukemia, New Engl. J. Med. **289**:770-773, 1973.

44. Pochedly, C.: Neurotoxicity due to CNS therapy for leukemia, Med. Ped. Oncol. **3**:101-115, 1977.
45. Garnick, M. B., and Mayer, R. J.: Acute renal failure associated with neoplastic diseases and its treatment, Semin. Oncol. **5**:155-165, 1978.
46. Tozer, T. N.: Nomogram for modification of dosage regimens in patients with chronic renal function impairment, J. Pharmacokinet. Biopharm. **2**:13-28, 1974.
47. Nirenberg, A., et al.: High dose methotrexate with citrovorum factor rescue: predictive value of serum methotrexate concentrations and corrective measures to avert toxicity, Cancer Treat. Rep. **61**:779-783, 1977.
48. Stoller, R. G., et al.: Use of plasma pharmacokinetics to predict and prevent methotrexate toxicity, New Engl. J. Med. **297**:630-634, 1977.
49. Rubio, F. A.: Possible pulmonary effects of alkylating agents, New Engl. J. Med. **287**:1150, 1972.
50. Codling, B. W., and Chakera, T. M.: Pulmonary fibrosis following therapy with melphalan for multiple myeloma, J. Clin. Path. **25**:668-673, 1972.
51. Menard, D. B., et al.: Antineoplastic agents and the liver, Gastroenterology **78**: 142-164, 1980.
52. Dahl, M. G., et al.: Liver damage due to methotrexate in patients with psoriasis, Br. Med. J. **1**:625-630, 1971.
53. Nyfors, A., et al.: Liver biopsies from psoriatics related to methotrexate therapy. 2. Findings before and after methotrexate therapy in 88 patients. A blind study, Acta Pathol. Microbiol. Scand. **84**:262-270, 1976.
54. Jaffe, N., et al.: Toxicity of high-dose methotrexate and citrovorum factor in osteogenic sarcoma, Cancer Chemother. Rep. **6**:31-36, 1975.
55. Poldurgiel, B. J.: Liver injury associated with methotrexate therapy for psoriasis, Mayo Clin. Proc. **48**:787, 1973.
56. Shorey, J., et al.: Hepatotoxicity of mercaptopurine, Arch. Int. Med. **122**:54-58, 1968.
57. Minow, R. A., et al.: Clinico-pathologic correlation of liver damage in patients treated with 6-mercaptopurine and adriamycin, Cancer **38**:1524-1528, 1976.
58. Sparberg, M., et al.: Intrahepatic cholestasis due to azathioprine, Gastroenterology **57**:439-441, 1969.
59. Sopko, J., et al.: Liver disease in renal transplant recipients, Am. J. Med. **64**: 139-146, 1978.
60. Massey, W. H., et al.: Hepatic artery infusion for metastatic malignancy using percutaneously placed catheters, Am. J. Surg. **121**:160-164, 1971.
61. Bateman, J. R., et al.: 5-Fluorouracil given once weekly: comparison of intravenous and oral administration, Cancer **28**:907-913, 1971.
62. Ellison, R. R., et al.: Arabinosyl cytosine: a useful agent in the treatment of acute leukemia in adults, Blood **32**:507-523, 1968.
63. Goodell, B., et al.: Cytosine arabinoside in acute granulocytic leukemia, Clin. Pharmacol. Ther. **12**:599-606, 1971.
64. Hill, D. L.: A review of cyclophosphamide, Springfield, Ill., 1975, Charles C Thomas, Publisher.
65. Aubrey, D. A.: Massive hepatic necrosis after cyclophosphamide, Br. Med. J. **3**:588, 1970.
66. Ylostalo, P., et al.: Hepatic and adrenocortical function during cyclophosphamide therapy, Acta Obstet. Gynecol. Scand. **52**:299-302, 1973.

67. DeVita, V. T., et al.: Clinical trials with 1,3-bis (2-chloroethyl)-1-nitrosourea, NSC-409962, Cancer Res. **25**:1876-1881, 1965.
68. Schein, P. S., et al.: Clinical antitumor activity and toxicity of streptozotocin (NSC-85998), Cancer **34**:993-1000, 1974.
69. Broder, L. E., et al.: Pancreatic islet cell carcinoma: II. Results of therapy with streptozotocin in 52 patients, Ann. Intern. Med. **79**:108-118, 1973.
70. Lokick, J. J., et al.: Hepatic toxicity of nitrosourea analogues, Clin. Pharmacol. Ther. **16**:363-367, 1974.
71. Luce, J. K.: Clinical trials with the antitumor agent 5-(dimethyltriazeno) imidazole-4-carboximide (NSC-45388), Cancer Chemother. Rep. **54**:119-124, 1970.
72. Penta, J. S., et al.: Hepatotoxicity of combination chemotherapy for acute myelocytic leukemia, Ann. Intern. Med. **87**:247-248, 1977.
73. Benjamin, R. S., et al.: A phase 1 and 2 trial of rubidazone in patients with acute leukemia, Cancer Res. **37**:4623-4628, 1977.
74. Ishizuka, M., et al.: Activity and toxicity of bleomycin, J. Antibiot. (Tokyo) **20**:15-24, 1967.
75. Samuels, M. L.: Continuous intravenous bleomycin (NSC-125066) therapy with vinblastine (NSC-49842) in stage III testicular neoplasia, Cancer Chemother. Rep. **59**:563-570, 1975.
76. Robert, J., et al.: Hepatotoxicity of cytostatic drugs evaluated by liver function tests and appearance of jaundice, Digestion **1**:229-232, 1968.
77. Crooke, S. T., et al.: Mitomycin C: a review, Cancer Treat. Rev. **3**:121-139, 1976.
78. Kennedy, B. J.: Metabolic and toxic effects of mithramycin during tumor therapy, Am. J. Med. **49**:494-503, 1970.
79. Capizzi, R. L., et al.: L-Asparaginase, Ann. Rev. Med. **21**:433-444, 1970.
80. Haskell, C. M., et al.: L-Asparaginase. Therapeutic and toxic effects in patients with neoplastic disease, New Engl. J. Med. **281**:1028-1034, 1969.
81. Oettgen, H. F., et al.: Toxicity of E. Coli L-asparaginase in man, Cancer **25**: 253-278, 1970.
82. Muggia, F. M.: Clinical studies with a new podophyllotoxin derivative 4-demethyl-9-(4,6,0,2-thenylidene-B-D-glucopyranoside) (NSC-122819), Cancer Chemother. Rep. **55**:575-581, 1971.

Dose adjustment in renal and hepatic disease

83. Cohen, J. L., et al.: Pharmacokinetics of cyclophosphamide in man, Br. J. Pharmacol. **43**:677, 1971.
84. Alberts, D. S., et al.: Comparative pharmacokinetics of chlorambucil and melphalan in man, 1979. To be published in Cancer Research.
85. Benjamin, R. S., et al.: Plasma pharmacokinetics of adriamycin and its metabolites in humans with normal hepatic and renal function, Cancer Res. **37**:1416-1420, 1977.
86. Benjamin, R. S., et al.: Pharmacokinetics and metabolites of adriamycin in man, Clin. Pharmacol. Ther. **14**:592, 1973.
87. Kramer, W. G., et al.: The pharmacokinetics of bleomycin in man, J. Clin. Pharmacol. **18**(7):346-352, 1978.
88. Juma, F. D., et al.: Pharmacokinetics of intravenous cyclophosphamide in man, estimated by gas-liquid chromatography, Cancer Chemother. Pharmacol. **1**: 229-231, 1978.

89. Owellen, R. J., et al.: Pharmacokinetics of Vindesine in humans, Cancer Res. **37**:2603-2607, 1977.
90. Au, J. L., et al.: Pharmacokinetics and metabolism of ftorafur in man, Cancer Treat. Rep. **63**(3):343, 1979.
91. Troetel, W. M., et al.: Absorption, distribution and excretion of 5-azacytidine in man, Cancer Chemother. Rep. part 1, vol. 56, No. 3, 1972.
92. Crooke, S. T., et al.: Bleomycin serum pharmacokinetics as determined by a radioimmunoassay and a microbiologic assay in a patient with compromised renal function, Cancer **39:**1430, 1977.
93. Ostrow, S., et al.: High dose cis-dichlorodiamine platinum therapy: pharmacokinetic analysis and toxicity using furosemide vs. mannitol diuresis, Proc. Am. Assoc. Cancer Res. **20:**88, No. 353, 1978.
94. Smith, D., et al.: Preliminary clinical pharmacology of intermediate dose oral methotrexate, Proc. Am. Assoc. Cancer Res. **70:**100, No. 402, 1978.
95. Fraile, R. J., et al.: Pharmacokinetics of cycloleucine, Proc. Am. Assoc. Cancer Res. **20:**108, No. 438, 1978.
96. Strong, J. M., et al.: Pharmacokinetic studies of parenteral misonidazole in monkeys and man, Proc. Am. Assoc. Cancer Res. **200:**200, #809, 1978.
97. Fong, K. L. L., et al.: Clinical pharmacology of 2,-3 Di hydro-IH-imidazole (2,3-6)-pyrazole (IMPY) using immunoassay, Proc. Am. Assoc. Cancer Res. **20:** 204, No. 826, 1978.
98. Abelson, H. T., et al.: Serum and cerebrospinal fluid–pharmacokinetic studies of high-dose methotrexate-carboxy peptidase G, Proc. Amer. Assoc. Cancer Res. **20:**213, No. 861, 1978.
99. Wilkinson, P., and Ribeiro, G.: Tamoxifen citrate pharmacokinetics in patients with metastatic breast cancer, Proc. Amer. Assoc. Cancer Res. **20:**209, C-71, 1978.
100. Williams, C. J., and Stevenson, K. E.: Pharmacokinetics and toxicity of cis diammine dichloro platinum given by IV bolus, 24 or 48 infusion, Proc. Am. Assoc. Cancer Res. **20:**317, C-108, 1978.

100a. Spreafico, F., and Rossi, M. S.: Antineoplastic agents. In Morselli, P. L., editor: Drug disposition during development, New York, 1977, Spectrum Publications, p. 101.

101. Pamasci, L., et al.: The effects of glucose infusion on chlorozotocin pharmacokinetics and toxicity, Proc. Am. Assoc. Cancer Res. **20:**340, C-205, 1978.
102. Cano, J. P., et al.: Pharmacokinetic studies of 5-fluorouracil in cancer patients using GC/MS and HPLC methods, Proc. Am. Assoc. Cancer Res. **20:**356, C-270, 1978.
103. Kerr, T. A., et al.: Pharmacokinetics of pyrazolo-imidazole (IMPY) in humans, Proc. Am. Assoc. Cancer Res. **20:**366, C-311, 1978.
104. Luk, K., et al.: Comparative clinical pharmacology of vinblastine in patients with advanced breast cancer: single vs continuous infusion. Proc. Am. Assoc. Cancer Res. **20:**271, C-333, 1978.
105. Alberts, D., et al.: Systemic absorption of bleomycin after intracavitary administration, Proc. Am. Assoc. Cancer Res. **19:**77, No. 305, 1978.
106. Benvenuto, J. A., et al.: Clinical pharmacokinetics of 3-deazauridine (3-DAU), Proc. Am. Assoc. Cancer Res. **19:**78, No. 310, 1978.
107. Alberts, D. S., et al.: Variability of melphalan absorption in man, Proc. Am. Assoc. Cancer Res. **19:**334, No. C-112, 1978.

108. Gudauskas, G., and Goldie, J. H.: The pharmacokinetics of high-dose continuous-5-fluorouracil infusions, Proc. Am. Assoc. Cancer Res. **19**:364, No. C-230, 1978.
109. Stoller, R. G., et al.: Pharmacokinetics of high dose methotrexate (NSC-740), Cancer Chemother. Rep. **6**(3):25-29, 1975.
110. Prince, R. A., and Klainer, A. S.: Antineoplastic agents as a cause of fever, Drug Intell. Clin. Pharm. **9**:126-128, 1975.

Section 7

ANCILLARY THERAPY

INTRODUCTION

In addition to the primary cancer chemotherapy used to control neoplasms, there is a second group of drugs used in oncology for the supportive treatment of cancer patients. These drugs include those agents used for the treatment of paraneoplastic syndromes and toxicities of anticancer drugs. The paraneoplastic syndromes and therapeutic approaches discussed in this chapter are those for *malignant effusions* (encompassing pleural effusions, ascites, and pericardial effusions), *electrolyte abnormalities* (encompassing hyponatremia and SIADH, hypokalemia, hyperkalemia, hyperphosphatemia and hypocalcemia, and hypercalcemia), and *CNS metastases* (encompassing intracerebral and leptomeningeal metastases). In addition to the above, this section discusses pain due to infiltration of nerves, blood vessels, and tissue by neoplastic cells and the management of pain.

The toxicities of antineoplastic agents and therapeutic approaches discussed are those for nausea and vomiting, hyperuricemia, methotrexate toxicity with leucovorin rescue, extravasation, and mucositis.

This area of therapeutics in oncology is in its early development. In recent years, more attention has been paid to its importance in the successful treatment plan for neoplastic diseases.

MANAGEMENT OF PARANEOPLASTIC SYNDROMES

Malignant effusions[1-9]

PLEURAL EFFUSION

Many malignancies cause fluid accumulation in the pleural space. Effusions develop in almost 50% of all patients with disseminated breast or lung cancer and less frequently with lymphoma, mesothelioma, sarcoma, and ovarian or gastric cancer. Malignant effusions can be chemically distinguished from transudative effusions on the basis of the following criteria:

	Exudate	Transudate
Appearance	Cloudy or blood tinged	Clear
WBC/mm^3	>1,000	<1,000

	Exudate	Transudate
RBC/mm^3	>100,000	<100,000
Specific gravity	>1.016	<1.016
Total protein	>3 g/100 ml	<3 g/100 ml
Fluid protein to serum protein ratio	>0.6	<0.6

The primary goal of treatment of pleural effusions is palliation (symptomatic control of dyspnea, cough). Long-lasting control of pleural effusion can prolong survival as well as improve the patient's quality of life, especially when effusions are caused by tumors that are highly responsive to chemotherapy such as lymphoma or breast cancer. Response of effusions approaches 100% in patients who have responded to systemic chemotherapy and only 60% in those who have failed to respond to chemotherapy.

The control of *recurrent* effusions includes closed thoracentesis techniques with suction, instillation of sclerosing agents, and in severe cases, surgical procedures such as pleurectomy or pericardiectomy.

Thoracentesis employs placement of a thoracostomy tube or catheter into pleural space. Repeated needle thoracentesis alone is rarely effective in recurrent effusions whereas continuous drainage thoracentesis is successful in about 40% of cases and is considered the initial treatment of choice because of its minimal morbidity. Pleurectomy is always effective but is associated with major morbidity in 6% to 10% of patients. Several sclerosing agents have been used in the treatment of recurrent effusion. Their therapeutic effect is related to their irritant properties and not their cytotoxic activity. In all cases, thoracostomy with continuous suction drainage enhances the effect and response rates of these agents. Table 7-1 gives the overall response rates for the various agents that have been employed.

Table 7-1. Sclerosing agents in the treatment of pleural effusions

Therapy	Dosage	Response	Toxicity	Comments
Nitrogen mustard	8-40 mg (average 20 mg)	97/210 (47%)	Fever, nausea, vomiting, leukopenia, local pain	Vesicant
5-FU	2-3 mg	23/35 (65%)	Minimal	
Bleomycin	15-240 mg (average 120 mg)	24/38 (63%)	None	Expensive—$150/120 mg
Quinacrine	300-1200 mg over 3-5 days	55/83 (66%)	Daily fever (90%) Local pain (50%)	No longer commercially available
Tetracycline	500 mg	45/52 (86%)	Pain (40%) Fever (10%)	

Table 7-2. Technique for intrapleural administration of sclerosing agents

1. Use closed thoracostomy drainage until fluid is less than 100 ml over 12 hours.
2. Dilute sclerosing agent in 50 ml of normal saline solution.
3. Stop suction apparatus and administer sclerosing agent (flush with 20 ml of normal saline) and clamp tube for 1-2 hours.
4. Rotate patient in various positions every 10 minutes for 60 minutes.
5. After 2 hours unclamp tube and resume suction.
6. If tetracycline or nitrogen mustard are to be used, premedicate the patient with analgesics or antipyretics or both.

Until recently, nitrogen mustard was the most frequently used sclerosing agent. Its primary disadvantage, however, is that approximately 30% of the dose is absorbed into the systemic circulation, which frequently produces bone marrow suppression and compromises concurrent systemic chemotherapy. It also produces severe pain and fever after administration. In contrast, tetracycline has shown an improved response rate with no myelosuppression and only mild to moderate local pain. Fluorouracil and bleomycin are not as effective as tetracycline and are therefore infrequently used. The method of drug instillation is important for effective drug distribution. Our current technique for instillation is modified after Wallach and is shown in Table 7-2.

ASCITES

Ascites results from the implantation of tumor cells on the surface of the peritoneum. The malignancies most frequently associated with ascites formation are ovarian carcinoma and lymphoma.

Control of malignant ascites is usually best accomplished by successfully treating the underlying disease. However, patients with severe distention and abdominal discomfort often are managed by paracentesis in addition to systemic therapy. Refractory cases are treated with abdominal irradiation or drug instillation of either nitrogen mustard and tetracycline, but these agents frequently produce complications of adhesions and bowel obstruction and are not generally recommended. The only drug which appears to have some reasonable chance of response is bleomycin. In doses of 60 to 120 mg (units), it has produced beneficial responses in 4 of 14 patients with a median duration of 180 days and has the advantage of minimal side effects.

PERICARDIAL EFFUSION

Malignant pericardial effusion (250 to 1,000 ml) results from neoplastic infiltration of the pericardial sac or mediastinal radiation therapy. It mani-

Table 7-3. Treatment of pericardial effusions

Procedure	Indication	Dose	Comment
Local therapy			
Radiotherapy	Rapid, progressive effusion	2,000-4,000 rads	Treatment of choice
Surgery	Radiation pericarditis or prior cardiac x-ray therapy		Patient must be surgical candidate
Intracavitary	Prior cardiac irradiation		
Fluouracil		0.5-1.0 g at time of pericardiocentesis	Agent of choice, least toxic Cardiac arrhythmias; mechanism of action = cytotoxic
Nitrogen mustard		10-22 mg	Severe initial serositis and effusion; transient arrhythmias; systemic absorption
Thiotepa		10-15 mg	Little experience; systemic absorption
Systemic therapy	High response tumors		Lymphoma, Hodgkin's, breast cancer, leukemia

fests as cardiac tamponade with as little as 200 ml of pericardial fluid. The malignant diseases usually associated with this complication are carcinomas (breast or lung), acute leukemia, and lymphomas.

Two mechanisms of pericardial effusion have been proposed: (1) tumor implantation on serosal surfaces with fluid exudation and (2) lymphatic obstruction by hilar or mediastinal neoplastic infiltration with fluid transudation.

Control of pericardial effusions involves either (1) local therapy or (2) systemic therapy. Local therapy includes radiotherapy, surgery, or intracavitary chemotherapy. The current initial treatment of choice is radiotherapy (2,000 to 4,000 rads). Systemic therapy is indicated only when pericardial effusion is not life threatening, and the cancer is usually responsive to chemotherapy (for example, lymphoma). Intracavitary therapy is infrequently used because of the high incidence of transient cardiac arrhythmias and the worsening of cardiac output caused by the initial reactive effusion of the sclerosing agent. Surgical management (pericardiectomy or a pleural-pericardial window) is reserved for patients with severe radiation-induced pericarditis or patients who have received previous cardiac irradiation. The most effective intracavitary drugs are fluorouracil or nitrogen mustard. The treatment of pericardial effusion is outlined in Table 7-3.

Electrolyte abnormalities

HYPONATREMIA AND SIADH[10-15]

Hyponatremia has been reported in several malignant diseases. The most common cause has resulted from the syndrome of inappropriate secretion of antidiuretic hormone (SIADH). Small cell (oat cell) lung cancer and acute myeloblastic leukemia are frequently associated with SIADH while thymoma, lymphoma, and gastrointestinal carcinoma are less frequent.

Two chemotherapeutic agents are associated with SIADH, namely cyclophosphamide (CTX) and vincristine. The pattern and mechanism of toxicity is different for each of these drugs. Cases of SIADH from CTX have appeared to be dose related, occurring usually with high doses (>1.5 g as a single dose). Because forced diuresis is critical in the prevention of CTX-induced cystitis, an increased risk of SIADH is expected. The onset of this complication occurs from 24 to 48 hours after administration of CTX. In contrast, vincristine-induced SIADH is not dose related and takes 3 to 7 days to manifest as hyponatremia (125 mEq/liter or less). In all cases, lethargy and severe neurotoxicity (absent reflexes or ileus) occur. However, SIADH is not observed after initial use of vincristine.

In preliminary trials vindesine, a semisynthetic derivative of vinblastine, has also produced two cases of SIADH.

The treatment of SIADH should include fluid restriction and the discontinuation of any offending agent. If hyponatremia persists after an appropriate trial of fluid restriction, control can be achieved with demeclocycline (13 to 15 mg/kg/day). Response usually occurs within 5 days. Demeclocycline is more effective and less toxic than lithium carbonate.

HYPOKALEMIA[16-19]

There is a strong relation between hypokalemia and acute leukemias. It occurs in almost 60% of the cases of acute myeloblastic leukemia. The decrease in serum potassium results from renal tubular losses of the cation owing to either lysozymuria or renal tubular damage. In any case, potassium loss may reach as high as 350 mEq per day. The antibiotics carbenicillin and ticarcillin both produce renal potassium loss and are frequently used in the empiric therapy of fever in the leukopenic leukemic patient. Similarly, aminoglycosides such as gentamicin can exacerbate renal potassium losses secondary to nephrotoxicity. With repeated aminoglycoside therapy (dose >8 g total) cumulative nephrotoxicity and attendant kaluresis can result.

The management of severe hypokalemia from hyperkaluria during induction therapy presents a difficult therapeutic problem to both clinician and nurse. The replace 300 to 400 mEq of potassium is no easy maneuver because of the large number of concurrent parenteral drugs so often used in the leukemic patient. However, one can decrease the amount of potassium replacement significantly by administering spironolactone 100 to 200 mg per day in 2 to 3 divided doses, because it is felt that hyperaldosteronism is present in the leukemic patient with large renal tubular losses. Another approach would be to substitute ticarcillin for carbenicillin because its lower recommended dose (18 g/day) produces one-third less kaluresis.

Once a patient recovers from induction chemotherapy, renal potassium losses diminish and frequently revert to normal.

HYPERKALEMIA[20-22]

Hyperkalemia is occasionally observed in acute leukemic patients following induction chemotherapy. Therapy can lead to rapid cell lysis with release of intracellular potassium and/or uric acid, the latter of which can lead to acute renal failure and resultant hyperkalemia. Irradiation of the spleen in patients with chronic myelocytic leukemia has also been associated with hyperkalemia.

Hyperkalemia has occurred in other rapidly proliferating neoplasms as well as in leukemias, such as Burkitt's lymphoma and Hodgkin's disease.

The treatment involves potassium exchange anions, alkalinization, glucose, and insulin. Occasionally dialysis may have to be used in refractory cases.

HYPERPHOSPHATEMIA AND HYPOCALCEMIA[23,24]

Elevated phosphate may result from rapid cell lysis in rapidly proliferating neoplasms such as acute leukemia or lymphoma. An outpouring of intracellular phosphate and concurrent renal dysfunction leads to subsequent binding of calcium ions. Severe hypocalcemia frequently results in tetany or myoclonic contractions.

HYPERCALCEMIA[25-28]

The exact incidence of hypercalcemia in malignancy is not known, but certain tumors, such as breast cancer, multiple myeloma, hypernephroma, epidermoid carcinoma of the head and neck, and esophagus, squamous cell carcinoma of the lung, and lymphomas are especially likely to cause hypercalcemia. It is a serious complication that must be treated rapidly because of the pathologic effects of ionized calcium on the myocardium and the kidney. Hypercalcemia frequently decreases glomerular filtration and tubular function leading to a diabetes-insipidus-like clinical picture. Renal function frequently improves with fluid replacement.

The treatment of hypercalcemia depends on the clinical setting. Unless the patient is having signs of myocardial arrhythmias, hydration and volume

Table 7-4. Drugs useful in the treatment of hypercalcemia

Drug	Dose	Route	Onset of effect	Contraindications
Furosemide and	40-100 mg	IV	3-4 hours	Severe dehydration
normal saline solution	3-5 liters	IV	3-4 hours	Pulmonary edema
Mithramycin	25 μg/kg every 48 hours	IV	24-48 hours	Renal dysfunction Thrombocytopenia
Calcitonin	2-8 μ/kg	IV infusion over 24 hours	2-3 hours	Allergic reactions
Sodium phosphate	1.5 g	IV infusion over 6 hours	8-12 hours	Renal dysfunction
Glucocorticoids				
Hydrocortisone	100-150 mg	IV	2-4 days	History of psychiatric disease, peptic ulcer disease
Prednisone	40-60 mg	Oral	2-4 days	
Oral phosphate				
Neutrophos (250 mg capsule)	0.5 g 4 times daily	Oral	2-4 days	Renal dysfunction, contains ~30 mEq/potassium per g phosphate
Phosphosoda (750 mg/5 ml liquid)	5 ml 3 times daily	Oral	2-4 days	Renal dysfunction Diarrhea, dilute liquid to reduce diarrhea

replacement is the first therapeutic maneuver. Intravenous saline solution is the best fluid electrolyte to administer. Concurrent calciuretic drugs are usually administered after hydration is begun and are listed in Table 7-4.

Therapy of central nervous system metastases[29-33a]

Central nervous system (CNS) complications of systemic cancer are common, as high as 20% of cases. The majority of CNS effects result from metastases, although metabolic encephalopathy, infection, or vascular disorders are not uncommon. Signs of CNS metastases are usually headache, paralysis, dementia, incontinence, convulsion, or loss of cranial nerves. Metastases usually are classified into intracerebral, leptomeningeal, and spinal types.

INTRACEREBRAL METASTASES

In intracerebral metastases, symptoms are usually associated with inflammation and edema surrounding the lesion(s). The initial therapy of choice is glucocorticoids, which ameliorate symptoms in about 70% of patients. It is believed that glucocorticoids decrease edema surrounding the tumor rather than having a direct antitumor effect. Both methylprednisolone and dexamethasone have been used in high doses. Most clinicians use

Table 7-5. Treatment of intracerebral metastases

Acute cerebral herniation	Stable patients
1. Mannitol 1.5 g/kg IV over 30 minutes	1. Dexamethasone 4 mg every 4 hours orally
2. Dexamethasone 10 mg IV, then 4 mg every 6 hours	2. RT (after 3 days of RT) 300 rad/day for 10 days
	3. Taper steroids after 10-14 days

dexamethasone because of its lower salt retention; the initial dose is 16 mg in four divided doses. If the patient does not respond in 24 hours, 32 and 64 mg of dexamethasone may be used for several days. Survival in patients who respond to glucocorticoids is 2 months compared to 1 month for those who fail to respond. Osmotic agents, mannitol or glycerol, may be combined with glucocorticoids if a patient is refractory to steroids alone.

The use of anticonvulsants for seizure prophylaxis is controversial in the patient with intracerebral metastases. Occasionally phenytoin will complicate corticosteroid effectiveness by enhancing its hepatic metabolism. Posner recommends anticonvulsants only when seizures are evident.

Whole brain radiotherapy is the most beneficial of all therapies, increasing survival from 1 month to 6 months. It is most effective in radiosensitive tumors (breast carcinoma, histiocytic lymphoma, and small cell lung carcinoma).

Chemotherapy with either systemic or intrathecal administration is usually ineffective. Even the highly lipid-soluble nitrosoureas, which are active against primary brain tumors, are not effective against cerebral metastases. Only in metastatic lymphoma does high-dose systemic methotrexate or intrathecal methotrexate appear to any substantial effect. The treatment of intracerebral metastases is outlined in Table 7-5.

LEPTOMENINGEAL METASTASES

Neurologic dysfunction, as with intracerebral tumors, is usually more widespread and severe than symptoms indicate. Symptoms are manifested as increased intracranial pressure, hydrocephalus, seizures, hemiparesis, incontinence, or lower motor neuron signs. The diagnosis is made by spinal fluid analysis and cytology.

Treatment is directed to the entire neuronal axis. Radiation therapy is directed to the major site of symptoms. If headache and papilledema are prominent, cranial irradiation is instituted. Conversely, if a cauda syndrome is evident, lumbosacral irradiation is preferred. The nonirradiated neuraxis is sterilized with methotrexate or cytarabine or both.

Methotrexate 12 mg (adult dose) and cytabarine 30 mg/m² may be administered either via lumbar injection or an Ommaya device. The Ommaya device has several advantages: (1) improved drug distribution into the ventricles, (2) lack of subdural or epidural injection (5% to 10% occurrence after lumbar injection), and (3) ease of administration. The disadvantages are surgical morbidity (rare) and infection.

The major complications from intrathecal therapy are chemical arachnoiditis, subacute neuritis, and rare toxic encephalopathy from methotrexate. Table 7-6 delineates the characteristics of various forms of MTX neurotoxicity. It is clear that neurotoxicity is associated with elevated CSF MTX concentration as well as the frequency of MTX dosing. Weekly intrathecal therapy is rarely neurotoxic. Thus CSF MTX determination should be performed when intrathecal MTX is repeated at intervals of less than 7 days. Bleyer suggests dosing guidelines for intrathecal MTX (Table 7-7). The dose of MTX recommended by Bleyer is based on the amount of brain extracellular fluid, which is less in children (under 3 years of age) than in adults. This dosage schedule provides much more consistent CSF concentrations than when MTX is dosed by body surface area and may lead to a lower incidence of neurotoxicity.

Table 7-6. Methotrexate neurotoxicity

Neurotoxicity	Symptoms	Onset	Causative factors
Chemical arachnoiditis	Headache, fever, vomiting, meningismus, meningeal pleocytosis	4-12 hours	Peak MTX concentration
Subacute motor neuritis	Paraplegia, quadriplegia, cerebellar ataxia, seizures, cranial palsies	14 days	Continuous high MTX levels
Leukoencephalopathy	Dementia, dysarthria, dysphagia, spasticity, seizures, coma	Months	XRT >2,000 rads plus MTX >50 mg/m² or frequent MTX >40 mg/m² twice weekly

Table 7-7. Guidelines to CNS methotrexate

Age (years)	MTX dose
<1	6 mg
1	8 mg
2	10 mg
>3	12 mg

If a patient's CSF MTX concentration is higher than 1×10^{-7} molar prior to a dose, accumulation in the CSF and potential neurotoxicity may result. Dosage may have to be lowered to avoid drug accumulation.

Pain management[34-49c]

Pain has been described as a sensory experience similar to hunger and thirst. Each is caused by internal events that are difficult to describe and that are affected strongly by emotions. Like thirst and hunger, pain causes one to seek relief; if he does not find it, his efforts become more intense and he experiences greater stress. Emotional responses of fear, anger, anxiety, and concern are a part of the overall pain response. Chronic pain is characterized by the patient focusing more and more on his condition and less and less on his surroundings. If pain is not appropriately treated, depression deepens, complaining becomes constant, and the search for treatment begins to dominate life.

Pain had been thought of as a simple sensory message that signaled the body of tissue damage. We now know that it is much more complex. Ideally pain functions instead to signal the body to take action. It has been found that there may be no correlation between the amount of pain a patient is experiencing and the amount of tissue damage present.

Since the emotions are part of the overall pain response, such factors as the patient's attitudes toward life and his disease, and his interpersonal relationships with his doctor, nurse, family, and friends can all have a profound influence on the pain response. These relationships and attitudes can either increase his fear, anxiety, and depression, thereby accentuating the pain response, or they can minimize these emotions, resulting in less pain and better pain control with analgesics.

Cancer and pain are often viewed synonymously. However, only about 50% of the patients who have cancer ever experience pain. Of those 50%, 10% have mild pain and 40% will have severe chronic pain that will need the attention of a skilled health professional.

Pain in cancer can be caused by a number of pathologic conditions such as the following:

1. Compression of nerve roots, trunks, or plexus by a tumor
2. Metastatic fracture of bone adjacent to nerves
3. Infiltration of the nerves and blood vessels by tumor cells
4. Obstruction of an organ, particularly the gastrointestinal or genitourinary tract
5. Partial or complete occlusion of blood vessels by an adjacent tumor
6. Infiltration and swelling of tissue within fascia, periosteum, or other pain-sensitive structures

7. Necrosis, infection, and inflammation of tissues sensitive to pain produced by nearby tumors of a neoplastic disease

GENERAL PRINCIPLES OF PAIN TREATMENT

The approach to treatment should include the following steps:
1. Determine the underlying cause of pain
2. Treat the underlying cause (i.e., antibiotics, chemotherapy, radiation)
3. Initiate analgesic therapy only when palliative treatment is required and treatment of the cause no longer controls the pain

Many patients with intractable or recurrent pain can be controlled on oral analgesics. Only a few need to receive high-dose parenteral medications. The following describes the basic approach to the selection of the appropriate analgesic for a patient and the use of each table.

1. The analgesic of choice for patients with mild pain is aspirin (or acetaminophen if the patient has compromised bone marrow or any bleeding disorder). Moderate pain is best treated with a combination of codeine and aspirin or acetaminophen. Severe pain should be treated with the most potent narcotic analgesic, usually morphine. Table 7-8 summarizes the usual approach to pain treatment in patients. The drugs and drug combinations are listed in order of potency and preference.
2. The selection of an analgesic must also take into consideration side effects, contraindications, and precautions so that the chosen therapy will meet the patient's needs. Tables 7-9 and 7-10 summarize these characteristics in order to enable drug comparisons.
3. All analgesics for chronic pain should be given on a regular basis

Table 7-8. Therapy for the management of chronic pain*

Kind of pain	Drug or drug combination	Comments
Mild	Aspirin 650 mg Acetaminophen 650 mg	Aspirin is contraindicative in patients with bleeding disorders or thrombocytopenia from cancer treatment Acetaminophen, codeine, pentazocine and propoxyphene do not alter platelet function or bleeding time; these drugs should be used in compromised patients instead of aspirin

*The drugs or drug combinations are listed in order of preference and of the most potent to the least potent analgesia drug or drug combination in each pain category.

Table 7-8. Therapy for the management of chronic pain—cont'd

Kind of pain	Drug or drug combination	Comments
Moderate	Codeine 65 mg + aspirin 650 mg Codeine 65 mg + acetaminophen 650 mg Pentazocine HCl 25 mg (Talwin) + aspirin 650 mg Pentazocine HCl 25 mg (Talwin) + acetaminophen 650 mg Oxycodone 9 mg + aspirin 650 mg (Percodan × 2) Oxycodone 9 mg + acetaminophen 650 mg (Percocet × 2) Propoxyphene napsylate 100 mg + aspirin 650 mg (Darvon-N with A.S.A. + aspirin 325 mg) Propoxyphene napsylate 100 mg + acetaminophen 650 mg (Darvocet-N 100)	Pentazocine has a higher incidence of gastrointestinal and central nervous system side effects than the other agents mentioned
Severe	*Oral morphine and methadone combinations* Brompton's Cocktail Morphine sulfate (10 mg/15 cc, then titrate) 98% alcohol 0%-40% Syrup 0%-50% qs 1,000 ml	
	Schlessinger's Solution Morphine 3% Ethyl Morphine 6% Scopalamine 0.025%	Schlessinger's Solution is measured in drops, leading to possible inaccurate dosing
	Val-Steck Solution Methadone 10 mg/5 cc Ethanol 5% Honey to taste qs 1,000 ml *Individual oral drugs* Hydromorphone (Dilaudid) Methadone (Dolophine) Levorphanol (Levodromoran)	Methadone should be given to patients with caution because of the long half-life of an active metabolite; cocaine has been omitted in Brompton's Cocktail—see text
Excruciating	*Parenteral form* Morphine Meperidine (Demerol) Hydromorphone (Dilaudid)	
Pain with anxiety	Add benzodiazepines to analgesic drug or drug combination	Narcotics potentiate the effects of benzodiazepines and antidepressants
Pain with depression	Add antidepressants to analgesic drug or drug combination	
Pain from bone metastases	Add nonsteroidal anti-inflammatory agent	Inhibits prostaglandin E_2 production

Table 7-9. Analgesic contraindications and precautions

Drug	Comments
Aspirin	*Contraindications* History of hypersensitivity *Use with caution* History of gastric ulcers History of asthma Bleeding tendencies Compromised bone marrow Hypoprothrombinemia During anticoagulant therapy
Acetaminophen	*Contraindications* History of hypersensitivity Glucose-6-phosphate dehydrogenase deficiency
Narcotic analgesics Codeine Hydromorphone Meperidine Methadone Morphine Pentazocine Propoxyphene Oxycodone Levorphanol	*Contraindications* History of hypersensitivity Head injury, intracranial lesions, preexisting elevated intracranial pressure *Use with caution* Narcotic analgesics may aggravate preexisting convulsive disorders *Dosage reduction* 1. Concurrent administration with a respiratory depressant (i.e., phenothiazines, other tranquilizers, sedative-hypnotics, tricyclic antidepressants, alcohol) 2. Patients with reduced respiratory reserve (i.e., COPD, cor pulmonale, acute asthmatic attack, preexisting respiratory depression) 3. Geriatric patients 4. Neonates and infants under 12 months 5. Impaired renal function, especially methadone and meperidine—toxic levels may result 6. Uremic patients—some extremely sensitive to depressant effects of strong analgesics 7. Liver disease *Other precaution* In patients with hypovolemia, give IV slowly and cautiously, IM route may be poorly absorbed

Table 7-10. Comparison of narcotic analgesics*

Drug	Analgesia	Sedation	Emesis	Respiratory depression	Constipation	Addiction	Duration of action oral route
Codeine	+	+	+	+	+	+	4 to 6 hours
Hydromorphone (Dilaudid)	++	+	+	++	+	++	3 to 4 hours
Levorphanol (Levo-Dromoran)	++	++	+	++	?	++	6 to 8 hours
Meperidine (Demerol)	++	+	?	++	+	++	3 hours
Methadone (Dolophine)	++	+	+	++	+	+	6 to 8 hours
Morphine	++	++	++	++	++	++	3 to 4 hours
Oxycodone (Percodan)	+	++	++	++	++	++	4 to 5 hours
Pentazocine (Talwin)	+	++ or 0	++	++	+	+	3 hours
Propoxyphene (Darvon, various)	0 or +	+	+	+	?	+	4 to 6 hours

*+, degree; 0, none; ?, unknown.

rather than only when necessary (PRN). PRN therapy results in intervals during which the anxiety and depression of the patient are heightened because of anticipation of the pain reappearing. The result is higher doses of the analgesic and less pain control.

4. Doses should be spaced at intervals according to the drug's duration of action. This should only serve as a guide, however, for not all patients respond the same.
5. Be careful not to *underdose* patients. Table 7-11 can be used as a guide in figuring out equivalent doses when switching from one drug to another and from one dosage form to another. Underdosing patients is a common occurrence. Patients should be given adequate therapy to produce a painfree state if possible.
6. When the patient has experienced a stable analgesic response for several days, begin titrating the dose of the analgesic down until the pain reappears. Then increase the dosage slightly to prevent relapse. Usually the dose can continue to be decreased to a therapeutic plateau unless a new pathologic condition necessitates a higher analgesic dose.
7. Do not fear drug addiction in terminally ill patients. Studies and the experience of those in pain hospices have shown that it is an

Table 7-11. Analgesic dose equivalents

MILD TO MODERATE ANALGESICS

Drug	Oral dose equivalent
Aspirin (various)	650 mg
Acetaminophen (Tylenol, various)	650 mg
Codeine	32 mg
Meperidine (Demerol)	50 mg
Propoxyphene HCl (Darvon, various)	65 mg
Propoxyphene napsylate (Darvon-N)	100 mg
Pentazocine (Talwin)	30 mg

OPIUM ALKALOIDS AND DERIVATIVES

Drug	Parenteral dose equivalent	Parenteral-oral efficacy ratio	Oral dose equivalent
Morphine	10 mg	1/6-1/2	20-60 mg
Hydromorphone (Dilaudid)	1.5 mg	1/6 low	9 mg
Meperidine (Demerol)	75-100 mg	1/4-1/3	225-400 mg
Levorphanol (Levo-Dromoran)	2-3 mg	1/2 high	4-6 mg
Methadone (Dolophine)	7.5-10 mg	1/2 high	15-20 mg
Codeine	120 mg	1/2-2/3 high	180-240 mg
Oxycodone (Percodan)* (Percocet)	10 mg†	1/2 high	20 mg
Pentazocine (Talwin)	45-60 mg	1/3	135-180 mg
Propoxyphene HCl (Darvon)			130-240 mg
Propoxyphene napsylate (Darvon-N)			360 mg

*Combination drug of oxycodone HCl, 4.5 mg; oxycodone terephthalate, 0.38 mg; aspirin, 224 mg; phenacetin, 160 mg; and caffeine, 32 mg.
†Not available in the United States.

unlikely occurrence. This issue should not be paramount in the minds of a health professional working with terminal patients.

8. Since constipation is the most frequent side effect of pain therapy, the patient should be counseled accordingly to prevent bowel impaction.
9. Nausea and vomiting of ambulatory patients who are receiving narcotics can be controlled with cyclizine. (See section on Analgesic-induced Vomiting.)
10. Finally, in renal and hepatic failure narcotics should be used with caution, especially those with long half-lives such as methadone, meperidine, and propoxyphene HCl.

ANALGESIC AGENTS FOR MILD TO MODERATE PAIN

Less potent analgesics include the nonsteroidal antipyretic–anti-inflammatory agents and "weak" narcotics; they have the advantages of producing few side effects, having low addiction liability, and relieving pain by mechanisms other than central neural pathways. The nonsteroidal antipyretic–anti-inflammatory agents used in pain management include primarily aspirin, acetaminophen, indomethacin, phenylbutazone, ibuprofen, and naproxen.

When combined with weak narcotics such as codeine or oxycodone, aspirin or acetaminophen has an additive analgesic effect. When patients are receiving concurrent cytotoxic chemotherapy, acetaminophen is the preferred nonsteroidal agent because of its lack of platelet-inhibiting effect. In addition, acetaminophen lacks the gastrointestinal irritant effects of other nonsteroidal analgesics, such as indomethacin, phenylbutazone, ibuprofen, and naproxen.

The weak narcotics include codeine, pentazocine, and oxycodone. Codeine and oxcodone are very useful in mild to moderate pain and produce few side effects. The most notable is constipation, which can be prevented with the use of mild laxatives. While effective against mild pain, pentazocine, in contrast to codeine or oxycodone, produces more severe central nervous system side effects, such as confusion, hallucinations, and dysphoria.

In pain causally linked to prostaglandin E_2 production such as bone pain from primary or metastatic cancer, the nonsteroidal anti-inflammatory analgesics may be very effective either when used alone or in combination with narcotic analgesics. In this regard, ibuprofen and naproxen may be more effective than indomethacin or phenylbutazone because of their more potent effect on prostaglandin production. Doses of nonsteroidal analgesics should be increased to their maximum level if response is not observed at usual initial doses. For example, 800 to 1200 mg of ibuprofen may produce greater total pain relief than 400 mg.

ANALGESIC AGENTS FOR SEVERE PAIN

The most useful potent analgesic for severe pain is morphine. It sets the standard by which all other analgesia are compared. Table 7-12 lists the other commonly used narcotics and their pharmacologic characteristics. Morphine has a rapid onset of action, usually within 30 minutes after parenteral injection, and a duration of 3 to 4 hours. Sedation is common early in the course of treatment but tends to disappear within a few days after effective therapy. Hydromorphone (Dilaudid) is also effective parenterally but offers no major advantage over morphine. Meperidine (Demerol) and similar derivatives such as anileridine have the disadvantage of a shorter duration of action than morphine. In addition, meperidine is metabolized to normeperidine, which is more slowly eliminated than the parent compound and is well known to precipitate seizures. In those patients with severe pain

Text continued on p. 331.

Table 7-12. Analgesics used in chronic pain

Drug class	Form	Type of patient	Dose	Onset	Duration	Half-life
Analgesics						
Acetaminophen/OTC (Tylenol, various)	Tablet: 120 mg (chewable), 325, 500 mg Capsule: 500 mg Elixir: 24, 26, 65 mg/ml Syrup: 24 mg/ml Drops: 60 mg/0.6 ml, 120 mg/2.5 ml Suppository: 125, 130, 300, 325, 600 mg	Adult	Oral: 325-650 mg every 4-6 hours (max. 3.0 g/day) Rectal: 325-650 mg every 4-6 hours (max. 3,900 mg—6 suppositories in 24 hours)	15-30 minutes	2-3 hours	2.75-3.25 hours
		Pediatric	Oral and rectal: 3-6 months, 30 mg every 4-6 hours 6-12 months, 60 mg every 4-6 hours 1-3 years, 60-120 mg every 4-6 hours 3-6 years, 120 mg every 4-6 hours 6-12 years, 240 mg every 4-6 hours			
Aspirin/OTC (various)	Tablet: 81 mg (chewable), 200, 300, 325, 650 mg Capsule: 325, 600 mg Suppository: 65, 100, 130, 195, 325, 650, 975, 1300 mg	Adult	Oral and rectal: 325-975 mg every 4 hours (max. 4 g/day)	30 minutes	4 hours	Aspirin: 14-20 minutes Salicylate (dose dependent): 0.25 g—2.4 hours 1.0 g—5.0 hours 1.3 g—6.1 hours 10-20 g—19 hours
		Pediatric	Oral and rectal: 65 mg/kg/24 hours divided every 4-6 hours			

Codeine/C-II (various)	Tablet: 15, 30, 60 mg Hypo. tablet: 15, 30, 60 mg	Adult	Oral or SC or IM:15-60 mg every 4-6 hours	15-30 minutes	4-6 hours	
	Syrup: 10 mg/5 ml (varies—check strength) Injection: 15, 30, 60 mg/ml	Pediatric	Oral or SC: 3 mg/kg/day divided dose every 4 hours			
Hydromorphone/C-II (Dilaudid)	Tablet: 1, 2, 3, 4 mg Injection: 1, 2, 3, 4 mg/ml	Adult	Oral: 2 mg every 4-6 hours	15-30 minutes	3-4 hours	
	Suppository: 3 mg		SC or IM: 2 mg every 4-6 hours; severe pain: 3-4 mg every 6 hours; may be given by *slow* IV (3-5 minutes to administer)	15-30 minutes	4-5 hours	
			Rectal: 3 mg			
Levorphanol/C-II (Levo-Dromoran)	Tablet: 2 mg Injection: 2 mg/ml	Adult	Oral or SC; 2 mg, may increase to 3 mg	60 minutes	5-8 hours	
		Pediatric	*Has not been approved for children*			
Meperidine/C-II (Demerol)	Tablet: 50, 100 mg Elixir: 10 mg/ml Injection: 25, 50, 75, 100 mg/ml	Adult	Oral: 50-150 mg every 3-4 hours (50% absorbed); half as effective as parenteral route	20 minutes	3 hours	
			SC or IM: 50-150 mg every 3-4 hours	10 minutes	2-4 hours	2-3 hours; active metabolic normeperidine T½
			Very slow IV: 50-100 mg every 3-4 hours (preferably diluted)			14-21 hours

Continued.

Table 7-12. Analgesics used in chronic pain—cont'd

Drug class	Form	Type of patient	Dose	Onset	Duration	Half-life
Meperidine—cont'd		Pediatric	Oral, SC, IM, or IV: 6 mg/kg/24 hours in divided doses every 4 hours (max. 100 mg/dose); oral dose, 50% is absorbed—less than half as effective as parenteral			
Methadone/C-II (Dolophine)	Tablet: 5 mg Injection: 10 mg/ml	Adult	Oral: 2.5-10 mg every 3-4 hours (*Note:* oral dose is equivalent to half the parenteral dose)	30-60 minutes	6-8 hours	25 hours
			SC or IM: 2.5-10 mg every 3-4 hours (*Caution:* because of long half-life and short dosage intervals, *plasma levels should be monitored* to prevent toxic and lethal drug accumulations from occurring)	10-15 minutes	3-6 hours	
		Pediatric	*Has not been approved for use*			
Morphine/C-II	Tablet: 10, 15, 30 mg Injection: 8, 10, 15 mg/ml	Adult	Oral: 8-20 mg every 4 hours		3-4 hours	

			SC or IM: 5-15 mg every 4 hours (10 mg/70 kg optional initial dose)	15-30 minutes	Up to 7 hours	2.6 hours
			IV: 4-10 mg (dilute) given slowly over 4-5 minutes		3-4 hours	
		Pediatric	SC or IM: 0.1-0.2 mg/kg/dose every 4 hours (max. 15 mg) IV: 0.05-0.1 mg given over 4-5 minutes (max. 15 mg)			
Oxycodone/C-II (Percodan, Percodan-Demi, Percocet-5)	Tablet: Percodan oxycodone HCl 4.5 mg oxycodone terephthalate .038 mg aspirin 224 mg phenacetin 160 mg caffeine 32 mg	Adult	1-2 tablets (~4.88 mg oxycodone) every 4-6 hours	10-15 minutes	4-5 hours	
	Percodan-Demi oxycodone HCl 2.25 mg oxycodone terephthalate 0.19 mg aspirin 224 mg phenacetin 160 mg caffeine 32 mg Percocet-5 oxycodone HCl 5 mg acetaminophen 325 mg	Pediatric	12 years or older: 1 tablet (~2.44 mg oxycodone) every 4-6 hours 6-12 years: ½ tablet (~1.22 mg oxycodone) every 4-6 hours			

Continued.

Table 7-12. Analgesics used in chronic pain—cont'd

Drug class	Form	Type of patient	Dose	Onset	Duration	Half-life
Pentazocine/Rx (Talwin)	Tablet: 50 mg Injection: 30 mg/ml	Adult	Oral: 50-100 mg every 3-4 hours (max. 600 mg/day)	15-30 minutes	3+ hours	
			SC or IM: 30-60 mg every 3-4 hours (max. 360 mg/day)	15-20 minutes	2-3 hours	2.1 hours
			IV: 30 mg every 3-4 hours (max. 360 mg/day)	2-3 minutes	1 hour	
		Pediatric	*Not recommended for use in children under 12 years*			
Propoxyphene/C-IV (Darvon, various)	Capsule (HCl): 32, 65 mg Capsule (napsylate): 100 mg Suspension (napsylate): 10 mg/ml	Adult	Oral: HCl, 65 mg every 4 hours; napsylate, 100 mg every 4 hours	1 hour	4-6 hours	11.8 hours active metabolic norpropoxyphene 36.6 hours
		Pediatric	*Not recommended for children*			
Analgesic oral preparations						
Brompton's Cocktail/C-II	See Table 7-8	Adult and pediatric	Oral: see Morphine: titrate to pain relief, 15 ml (1 tbsp) every 4 hours with or without phenothiazine		4 hours	2.6 hours
Schlessinger's solution/C-II	See Table 7-8	Adult	Oral: 0.3-1 ml every 4 hours in liquid; 1 ml = 60 mg morphine SO_4		4 hours	2.6 hours
Val-Steck Solution/C-II	See Table 7-8	Adult and pediatric	Oral: See Methadone; 5 ml (1 tsp) every 5-6 hours		3-5 hours	25 hours

and CNS metastases, regular meperidine usage is especially hazardous and thus is not recommended in treatment of chronic cancer pain.

Once pain is adequately controlled, the patient can be switched to an oral potent narcotic. Useful oral agents appear to be those with a high parenteral-oral ratio (Table 7-11). It is generally believed that oral morphine has a low parenteral-oral ratio (about 0.15). However, we find many patients have apparent ratios of about 0.5, especially when morphine is administered as a solution. Other agents with high ratios are methadone and levorphanol. The advantages of methadone, good oral absorption and a longer duration of effect, are overridden by cumulative toxicity of the drug. Levorphanol also has the advantages of good absorption, a duration of 5 to 8 hours, and potency greater than morphine, but experience with this agent has generally been limited and it is relatively expensive. We have had success substituting levorphanol for other agents in patients with narcotic-associated nausea or vomiting. Hydromorphone has a parenteral-oral ratio of only 0.2, but it has the advantages of higher potency and apparent less sedative effect in our experience. Thus patients who are controlled on IM morphine 10 mg every 4 hours can be given oral hydromorphone 8 mg every 4 hours with continued control.

A new analgesic, butorphanol (Stadol), has analgesic activity equivalent to morphine and similar side effects. A few long-term clinical studies suggest that it may have a lower physical dependency than morphine. However, its current use is limited because of its high cost in parenteral dosage form and the fact that addiction is not a major concern in the management of the patient with chronic pain.

An investigational parenteral analgesic of interest is buprenorphine, an opiate-like partial agonist-antagonist. It is a potent analgesic with 0.3 mg equivalent to the analgesia produced by 10 mg of morphine. One of its appealing features is the fact that its duration of action is at least twice that of morphine. It may prove to be a useful addition to this class of analgesics.

ANALGESIC "COCKTAILS"

Due to the successful experience of hospices in England, oral liquid analgesics have become a popular dosage form in the treatment of chronic and intractable pain. Table 7-12 lists the most popular one at present: Brompton's Cocktail, Schlessinger's Solution, and Val-Steck Solution, which substitutes methadone for morphine. The United States requires no special clearance to prescribe these solutions to patients. Their advantages are that doses are easily titratable to analgesia in patients. They are easy to swallow and allow the patient greater independence and mobility.

Brompton's Cocktail was perhaps the first oral narcotic solution of wide use and interest. Its original formula contained an opiate, cocaine, alcohol, chloroform water, and other agents such as phenothiazines. Twycross recently investigated whether the cocaine in Brompton's Cocktail had any beneficial effect in chronic cancer pain and showed that it only produced a greater incidence of CNS side effects. The high concentration of alcohol in the original cocktail appeared to be pharmacologically inappropriate, since its depressant properties on respiration and central nervous system can add to those of the opiate.

A phenothiazine in the cocktail was included to decrease anxiety and narcotic-induced nausea and vomiting. However, it was found that frequent administration of this fixed-dose cocktail could lead to an overdose of phenothiazine with subsequent parkinsonian adverse reactions. Lastly, the FDA banned chloroform water from the market because of its carcinogenic properties. We believe that if a morphine liquid is desired, a solution of morphine in syrup or syrup with a small percentage of alcohol (to preserve the preparation) is all that is necessary.

ADJUNCTIVE AGENTS IN THE TREATMENT OF CHRONIC PAIN

As stated earlier, the patient's psychological status can play an important role in the evaluation of agonizing pain. Several authors have described a pain-anxiety-depression cycle that frequently occurs in chronic cancer pain. In order to effectively treat such pain, the cycle must be broken. Thus, it may be beneficial to add psychotropic drugs such as antidepressants, tranquilizers, and CNS stimulants. Table 7-13 summarizes those used in pain therapy.

In addition to their effect on reducing anxiety and depression, the phenothiazines and tricyclic antidepressants appear to have pharmacologic properties for relief of pain. Apparently, concentrations of 5-hydroxytryptamine (5HT) or dopamine (DA) are increased and decreased, respectively, in patients with chronic pain. Both 5HT and DA appear to act as neuromodulators on pain stimuli by lowering the pain threshold. Since phenothiazines decrease 5HT levels, they may be effective in some patients whose pain might be modulated by these substances. Similarly, since tricyclic antidepressants, especially the tertiary agents, amitriptyline and imipramine, increase DA levels, they may be effective in patients with severe pain and associated depression. Halpern and Budd have reported that psychotropic agents are effective and should be considered in the management of selected patients with chronic pain.

CNS stimulants, such as dextroamphetamine or methylphenidate, also have analgesic properties as well. Some investigators claim that these agents can be substituted for potent narcotics. However, no mention is made of

Table 7-13. Psychotropic drugs useful in the management of chronic pain

Drug	Action
Phenothiazines	
Chlorpromazine, perphenazine, levopromazine	Decrease 5-hydroxytryptamine levels Antipsychotic Sedation Analgesic
Antidepressants	
Amitriptyline, imipramine, doxepin	Increase dopamine Elevate mood Analgesic Sedation
Sedatives	
Diazepam, oxazepam, diphenhydramine, hydroxyzine	Antianxiety Sedation Mild analgesic
Sympathomimetics	
Dextroamphetamine, methylphenidate	Antidepressant Respiratory stimulant Analgesic
Cannabis derivatives	
Marijuana, delta-9-tetrahydrocannabinol (THC)	Antianxiety Antidepressant

long-term usage of these agents. Tolerance is expected and usually occurs within 10 to 14 days. This characteristic would appear to preclude the use of amphetamines and similar drugs from prolonged therapy. Also their dysphoric CNS side effects are disturbing to patients with chronic pain.

MANAGEMENT OF ANTICANCER DRUG TOXICITIES

Nausea and vomiting[50-77b]

Nausea and vomiting of cancer patients are symptoms caused by any of the numerous pathologic changes associated with the disease or its therapy. Such pathologic changes as increased cranial pressure owing to brain metastasis, infection, or pressure effects of tumors may lead to potent stimulation of the vomiting center. Both radiation and chemotherapy when initially implemented often cause massive cell death, which is thought to liberate chemicals that stimulate the vomiting center indirectly through the chemoreceptor trigger zone. Other common causes of vomiting in cancer patients are psychogenic vomiting, postsurgical vomiting, vomiting as a result of pain, pain therapy (narcotics), hormone therapy, water intoxication, adrenal failure, electrolyte abnormalities, uremia, hypotension, and labyrinthine disturbances.

Nausea and vomiting is a complex reflex mediated by the vomiting center located in the medullary reticular formation. The vomiting center receives impulses from three sources: (1) the chemoreceptor trigger zone (CTZ), (2) the periphery, and (3) higher central nervous system structures such as the vestibular apparatus of the ear or cerebral cortex. Two model systems have been established to distinguish two major pathways for impulses that cause vomiting—one from the chemoreceptor trigger zone and the other from the periphery. The apomorphine model is one in which IV apomorphine (a blood-borne emetic substance) directly stimulates the chemoreceptor trigger zone, an area located in the floor of the fourth ventricle that is sensitive to vomiting stimuli. The impulse then is transmitted to the vomiting center to cause the act of vomiting. The vomiting center itself is insensitive to apomorphine. Apomorphine acts both as a choline esterase inhibitor and a dopamine agonist in addition to having other effects. The second model system traces a major pathway from the periphery. Copper sulfate is given by mouth or IV, producing irritation of the gastric mucosa to produce the vagal impulses. These impulses run directly to the vomiting center. Such peripheral emetic action can be eliminated by a vagotomy.

The complications of nausea and vomiting can be acute or chronic in nature. Protracted vomiting can cause life-threatening fluid and electrolyte imbalance, especially in the elderly and the pediatric patient. Such electrolyte imbalances are likely to perpetuate the vomiting in the patient. Forceful vomiting accompanied by strain and retching can result in the Mallory-Weiss syndrome. Patients with medical histories of sliding hiatus hernias are particularly susceptible. A more common complication is anorexia, which can be severe. It has been observed that as the patient becomes more debilitated, the side effects of the disease and treatment, including nausea and vomiting, become more severe and frequent.

Uncontrolled nausea and vomiting compromise the quality and quantity of therapy. Treatment should be aimed at removal of the cause. Symptomatic therapy is indicated only after the primary disease process has been adequately diagnosed and therapeutic steps are initiated. Antiemetic therapy is used when no alternative exists and the benefit outweighs the risk of adverse effects.

MINIMIZING NAUSEA AND VOMITING

Several methods have been used to minimize nausea and vomiting in cancer patients. They are as follows:

1. The treatment area should be a calm, reassuring environment. Ideally the patient should be alone and away from sight or smell of food.
2. Keeping the patient quiet and nonambulatory often helps to mini-

mize vomiting. Motion increases the sensitivity of the labyrinth apparatus of the inner ear, which may induce motion sickness. This is particularly true with patients who have received opiates.

3. Timing of therapy can be important. Some patients benefit by receiving chemotherapy early in the morning with a small amount of food in their stomach. Others tolerate therapy better at nighttime when given in combination with a sedative. Vomiting can occur in a sedated patient; the chances of aspiration increase, and this must be kept in mind when using this approach.
4. Gastritis frequently accompanies the nausea and vomiting from chemotherapy or radiation therapy and can produce further nausea and vomiting of the patient. It is caused by the local effects of the oral agents or radiation or the selective toxicity of oral agents on the rapidly dividing cells of the gastrointestinal tract. Precede treatments with antacids or small amounts of cold food (ice cream) to buffer the gut. This may help to decrease the gastritis in these patients.
5. Frequent small meals that would not be anorexigenic or nauseating to the patient are desirable rather than large meals during or after receiving therapy.
6. Finally, patients with severe anorexia and malnutrition often benefit from hyperalimentation. It has been observed that these patients may have fewer side effects (that is, nausea and vomiting) when receiving hyperalimentation with therapy.

ANTIEMETIC THERAPY

There are several well known groups of antiemetic agents. Table 7-14 lists them and gives their sites of action and comparative antiemetic effects and toxicity. They include the phenothiazines, antihistamines, butyrophenones, anticholinergic agents, cannabinoids, sedatives, hypnotics, and a miscellaneous group that consists of trimethobenzamide, benzquinamide, diphenidol, metoclopramide, and pyridoxine. Antiemetics prevent nausea and vomiting by their action on one or more of the following sites: (1) chemoreceptor trigger zone, (2) vomiting center, (3) aural vestibular apparatus in the labyrinth, and (4) cerebral cortex.

The phenothiazines, because of their primary action on the chemoreceptor trigger zone, have been found to be the most effective group of antiemetics in the treatment of cancer chemotherapy-induced vomiting. They are also the most effective agents in treating narcotic-induced vomiting in postoperative patients and in the treatment of pain. Next to the butyrophenones, they have been found to be quite effective in the treatment of radiation sickness.

Table 7-14. Antiemetic comparative mechanisms of action, toxicities, and therapeutic effects

Drug	Site	Sedative effects	Extra pyramidal effects	Hypotensive effects	Other	Antiemetic potency
Phenothiazines						
Piperazine compounds						
Prochlorperazine (Compazine)	CTZ (VC)*	Moderate	High	Low		High
Thiethylperazine (Torecan)	CTZ (VC)	Low	Moderate	Moderate		High
Perphenazine (Trilafon)	CTZ (VC)	Moderate	High	Low		High
Aliphatic compounds						
Chlorpromazine (Thorazine)	CTZ (VC)	High	Moderate	High		Moderate
Triflupromazine (Vesprin)	CTZ (VC)	Moderate	High	Moderate		High
Promazine (Sparine)	CTZ (VC)	Moderate	Moderate	High		Moderate
Promethazine (Phenergan)	Labyrinth + CTZ	Moderate	Low	Low		Low
Antihistamines						
Cyclizine (Marezine)	Labyrinth, ?CTZ (VC)	Moderate	None	None	Dryness of mouth Blurred vision Urinary retention	Low
Meclizine (Antivert, Bonine)	Labyrinth, ?CTZ (VC)	Moderate	None	None	Dryness of mouth Blurred vision Urinary retention	Low
Butyrophenones						
Haloperidol (Haldol)	CTZ (VC)	Low	High	Moderate		High
Droperidol (Inapsine)	CTZ	Low	High	Moderate		Moderate

Anticholinergic agent						
†TTS Scopolamine	CNS depressant Labyrinth Vestibular-cerebellar CTZ	Moderate	None	None	Dryness of mouth Blurred vision	High
Miscellaneous						
Trimethobenzamide (Tigan)	CTZ	Low	Low	None		Low/moderate
Benzquinamide (EmeteCon)	CTZ (VC)	Moderate	None	Low/none		High/none
Diphenidol (Vontrol)	Vestibular-cerebellar	Moderate	None	Low	Hallucinations Disorientation Confusion	High
†Delta-9-tetrahydrocannabinol (THC)	Not known	Low	None	Low	Dysphoria Tachycardia	High
†Nabilone	Not known	Moderate	None	Low	Hallucinations Dizziness Transient psychosis Animal studies: seizures, death	Very high
Pyridoxine (Vitamin B_6)	Not known	None	None	None		Low/high
†Metoclopramide (Reglan)	CTZ (VC) Normalizes aberrant gut motility	Low	Low	Low		High

*CTZ, chemoreceptor trigger zone; VC, vomiting center.
†Investigational.

The antihistamines, which include cyclizine (Marezine), dimenhydrinate (Dramamine), diphenhydramine (Benadryl), hydroxyzine (Atarax, Vistaril), meclizine (Antivert, Bonine) and buclizine (Bucladin-S) are the agents of choice in the treatment of motion sickness. Motion sickness is caused by stimulation of the labyrinth of the inner ear. Cyclizine (Marezine) and meclizine (Antivert, Bonine) have shown some effectiveness in the treatment of nausea and vomiting caused by radiation therapy. All antihistamines, because of their primary action on the labyrinth of the inner ear, are *not effective in the treatment of nausea and vomiting caused by cancer chemotherapeutic agents.*

The butyrophenones, particularly haloperidol (Haldol), are considered the most effective agents in the treatment of radiation-induced vomiting except in pediatric patients. Their high incidences of extrapyramidal effects prevent their use in these patients. They are also effective in the treatment of cancer chemotherapy-induced vomiting but are seldom used in this capacity owing to their side effects.

The anticholinergic drug scopolamine is considered the most effective drug in the prevention of motion sickness. Recently it has been shown investigationally that it has some activity in the prevention of cancer chemotherapy-induced vomiting in pediatric patients.

The cannabinoids are investigational agents of delta-9-tetrahydrocannabinol (THC) and its derivative nabilone. They have been found effective in treating nausea and vomiting in cancer patients refractory to standard antiemetic therapy. Their mechanisms of action are unknown.

Sedatives and hypnotics primarily act by the depression of the central nervous system and are used in the control of psychogenic vomiting. They in themselves have no antiemetic effects.

The agents of the miscellaneous group will be discussed individually in the following sections. Their sites of actions are also summarized in Table 7-14.

The most common causes of vomiting that require antiemetic therapy in cancer patients are (1) cancer chemotherapy, (2) radiation therapy, (3) hormone therapy, (4) psychogenic factors, and (5) the effects of narcotics. In the selection of the appropriate antiemetic, not only the etiology of the nausea and vomiting must be taken into consideration but also the site of action of the antiemetic and its toxicity.

Table 7-15 presents each etiology and lists the antiemetic agents in order of preference in their use. A patient may have one or more of these etiologies. For example, he may have both psychogenic vomiting and radiation-induced vomiting. In these cases more than one drug may be required in the treatment. Table 7-15 is merely a guide presenting the most common sys-

Table 7-15. Therapy for the management of nausea and vomiting*

Etiology	Adult	Pediatric
Radiation therapy	1. Haloperidol (Haldol) 2. Prochlorperazine (Compazine) Chlorpromazine (Thorazine) 3. Cyclizine (Marezine) Meclizine (Atarax, Bonine) †4. Ibuprofen (Motrin) 5. Pyridoxine (Vitamin B_6)	1. Promethazine (Phenergan) Chlorpromazine (Thorazine) †2. Domperidone 3. Cyclizine (Merezine) 4. Pyridoxine (Vitamin B_6)
Chemotherapy	1. Prochlorperazine (Compazine) Thiethylperazine (Torecan) Perphenazine (Trilafon) 2. Chlorpromazine (Thorazine) Triflupromazine (Vesprin) Promazine (Sparine) 3. Haloperidol (Haldol) 4. Trimethobenzamide (Tigan) 5. Benzquinamide (Emete-Con) †6. Dexamethasone (Decadron) 7. Diphenidol (Vontrol) †8. Nabilone (not available)	1. Promethazine (Phenergan) 2. Chlorpromazine (Thorazine) †3. TTS scopolamine (ALZA)
Refractory vomiting	†1. Delta-9-tetrahydrocannabinol (THC)	
Cisplatin (vomiting refractory to standard antiemetics)	†1. Metoclopramide (Reglan) †2. Droperidol (Inapsine)	
Therapy for breast cancer	1. Trimethobenzamide (Tigan)	
Hormone therapy	1. Promethazine (Phenergan)	
Psychogenic vomiting (anxiety, sight, smell, taste, etc.)	1. Diazepam (Valium) 2. Chlordiazepoxide (Librium) 3. Phenobarbital (various)	†1. Chloral hydrate (Noctec, Somnos, various) Hydroxyzine (Vistaril) 2. Chloral hydrate (Noctec, Somnos, various) 3. Phenobarbital (various)
Analgesic therapy (opiates)		
Nonambulatory vomiting	1. Benzquinamide (Emete-Con) 2. Prochlorperazine (Compazine) Thiethylperazine (Torecan) †3. Metoclopramide (Reglan)	
Ambulatory vomiting	1. Promethazine (Phenergan) Cyclizine (Marezine) Meclizine (Antivert, Bonine)	

*Drugs are listed in order of preference.
†Investigational.

tematic approach to treating nausea and vomiting in cancer patients. Patient variability in their response to various antiemetic agents must be taken into consideration in its use. The clinician may have to resort to trial and error. An antiemetic such as trimethobenzamide (Tigan), considered in general not to be that effective in preventing nausea and vomiting in cancer patients, has been observed clinically to be quite effective in some patients.

Oral dosage forms of antiemetics are normally used for *prophylactic therapy* of nausea and vomiting in cancer patients. This route is also the one most preferred by the patient. Parenteral and suppository dosage forms are used in the *treatment* of nausea and vomiting. The use of the parenteral form should be reserved for the hospital setting.

DOSING ANTIEMETICS

Unsuccessful antiemetic therapy often reflects less than optimal use of the agents themselves by the clinician. Effective use of these drugs depends on the understanding of their dose response characteristics and the etiology of the nausea and vomiting. The primary goal of antiemetic therapy should be to utilize the least amount of antiemetic drug and at the same time maximize the control of the nausea and vomiting with minimal side effects in the cancer patient. One of the most common errors in dosing antiemetics is the failure to keep constant therapeutic blood levels of the antiemetic during the time the vomiting center is being stimulated. Table 7-16 presents the common agents used in antiemetic therapy, giving the dose intervals based on the pharmacokinetics of the drug rather than the intervals recommended by the manufacturer.

In accomplishing the goal of using the least amount of drug while providing maximal antiemetic therapy with minimal side effects, the following factors must be kept in mind:

1. It is more effective to use prophylactic therapy to prevent nausea and vomiting than to treat it after it has begun.
2. The action of the antiemetic should match the determined etiology or etiologies of nausea and vomiting in the cancer patient.
3. Patterns of sickness should be determined. Onset and duration of nausea and vomiting should be documented. Most cancer chemotherapy agents do not produce sickness longer than 48 hours. In Table 6-17 commonly known nausea and vomiting patterns for individual oncolytic agents are presented to assist the clinician in tailoring the antiemetic therapy to meet the needs of the patient receiving these drugs.
4. Antiemetic therapy should be started prior to the anticipated nausea and vomiting at a time interval in which the clinician is certain a therapeutic blood level of the antiemetic will be present when vomiting

Text continued on p. 348.

Table 7-16. Antiemetics

Drug	Form	Type of patient	Dose	Onset	Duration	Cautions
Phenothiazines						
Prochlorperazine (Compazine)	Tablets: 5, 10, 25 mg Syrup: 5 mg/5 ml Injection: 5 mg/ml Suppository: 2½ mg (young child) 5 mg (older child) 25 mg (adult)	Adult	Oral: 5-10 mg every 3-4 hours IM: 5-10 mg every 3-4 hours (max. 40 mg) PR: 25 mg every 3-4 hours	30-40 minutes 10-20 minutes 60 minutes	3-4 hours 3-4 hours 3-4 hours	Give lower range doses in geriatric patients
		Pediatric	Oral: 0.4 mg/kg/day divided every 6-8 hours IM: 0.2 mg/kg/day divided every 6-8 hours PR: 0.4 mg/kg/day divided every 6-8 hours			Extrapyramidal symptoms more likely in children than adults, especially with high doses; *do not* give to children under 9 kg or 2 years
Thiethylperazine (Torecan)	Tablets: 10 mg Injection: 5 mg/ml Suppository: 10 mg	Adult	Oral: 10-30 mg every 4 hours IM: 10 mg every 4 hours Suppository: 10 mg every 4 hours	30 minutes	4 hours	
		Pediatric	Has not been determined; >12 years, use lowest limit of adult dose			
Perphenazine (Trilafon)	Tablets: 2, 4, 8, 16 mg Repetabs: 8 mg Injection: 5 mg/ml	Adult	Oral: 2-4 mg every 6 hours 1 Repetab every 12 hours (24 mg may be necessary)			Injection is more potent than oral; equal or higher oral doses should be given when transferring from injection to oral

Continued.

Table 7-16. Antiemetics—cont'd

Drug	Form	Type of patient	Dose	Onset	Duration	Cautions
			IM: 5 mg every 6 hours (max. 15 mg ambulatory patients; 30 mg hospitalized patients)	10 minutes (max. 1-2 hours)	6 hours (occasionally 12-24 hours)	
		Pediatric	Has not been determined; > 12 years, use lowest limit of adult dose			
Chlorpromazine (Thorazine)	Tablets: 10, 25, 50, 100 mg	Adult	Oral: 10-25 mg every 4-6 hours	30-60 minutes	4-6 hours	
	Syrup: 10 mg/5 ml Injection: 25 mg/ml		IM: 25-50 mg every 3-4 hours	30 minutes	3-4 hours	
	Suppository: 25, 100 mg		PR: 50-100 mg every 3-4 hours	60 minutes	3-4 hours	
		Pediatric	Oral: 2 mg/kg/day in divided doses of 6 hours IM: 2 mg/kg/day in divided doses of 6 hours Max. dose per day: 40 mg, child less than 5 yrs (50 lbs); 75 mg, child 5-12 yrs (50-100 lbs) PR: 1.1 mg/kg every 6-8 hours			Thorazine should not be given to children less than 6 months of age
Triflupromazine (Vesprin)	Tablets: 10, 25, 50 mg Suspension: 50 mg/5 ml	Geriatric	IM: 2.5 mg every 4 hours (up to 15 mg/day)			
	Injection: 10, 20 mg/Liter	Adult	Oral: 5-15 mg every 4 hours (up to 60 mg/day)			

			IV: 1 mg (up to 3 mg/day)			
		Pediatric	Oral: 0.2 mg/kg/day divided into 3 doses (up to 10 mg/day) IM: 0.2-0.25 mg/kg/day (up to 10 mg/day) IV: not recommended			Not used in children less than 2½ years of age
Promazine (Sparine)	Tablets: 10, 25, 50, 100 200 mg Syrup: 10 mg/5 ml Injection: 25, 50 mg/ml	Adult	Oral: 25-50 mg every 4-6 hours IM: 50 mg			
		Pediatric	Doses have not been established			
Promethazine (Phenergan)	Tablets: 12.5, 25, 50 mg Syrup: 6.25, 25 mg/5 ml Injection: 25, 50 mg/ml Suppository: 25, 50 mg	Adult	Oral, IM, IV, PR: 25 mg, then 12.5-25 mg every 4-6 hours	30-60 minutes	4-6 hours	High incidences of drowsiness
		Pediatric	Oral, IM, PR: 0.25-0.5 mg/kg/dose every 4-6 hours			
Butyrophenones						
Haloperidol (Haldol)	Tablets: 1, 2, 5 mg Injection: 5 mg/ml	Adult	Oral: 0.5-2.0 mg every 4-8 hours		Peaks 2-6 hours	
			IM: 2-5 mg every 4-8 hours	10 minutes	T ½ 13-35 hours	
		Pediatric	Doses have not been established			
Droperidol (Inapsine)	Injection 2.5 mg/ml	Adult	IM or IV: 2.5-10 mg in 1 dose	3-10 minutes	6-8 hours	
		Pediatric	IM or IV: 2-12 yrs, 1.0-1.5 mg/20-25 lbs in 1 dose			Safety in children less than 2 years has not been established

Continued.

Table 7-16. Antiemetics—cont'd

Drug	Form	Type of patient	Dose	Onset	Duration	Cautions
Antihistamines						
Hydroxyzine (Atarax, Vistaril)	Tablets: 10, 25, 50, 100 mg Capsules: 25, 50, 100 mg Suspension: 25 mg/5 ml Syrup: 10 mg/5 ml Injection: 25, 50 mg/ml	Adult	Oral: 25-100 mg 3-4 times daily IM: 25-100 mg	15-30 minutes	Unknown	Drowsiness
		Pediatric	Oral: 2 mg/kg/day divided every 6-8 hours IM: 0.5 mg/lb			
Cyclizine (Marezine)	Tablets: 50 mg Injection: 50 mg/ml Suppository: 50, 100 mg	Adult	Oral: 50 mg every 4-6 hours IM: 50 mg every 4-6 hours PR: 100 mg every 4-6 hours	4-6 hours		
		Pediatric	Oral: 3 mg/kg/divided into 3 doscs IM: 3 mg/kg/day divided into 3 doses PR: 9 mg/kg/day divided into 3 doses			
Meclizine (Antivert, Bonine)	Tablets: 25 mg (chewable), 12.5, 25 mg	Adult	Oral: 25-100 mg/day in divided doses		24-48 hours	
		Pediatric	Skin patch behind ear maintains level of hyoscine equivalent to an oral dose of 0.2 mg for 60 hours (transdermal administration)		60 hours	

Miscellaneous						
Trimethobenzamide (Tigan)	Capsules: 100, 250 mg Injection: 100 mg/ml Suppository: 200 mg	Adult	Oral: 400 mg every 3-4 hours	10-40 minutes	3-4 hours	
			IM: 200 mg every 2-3 hours	15-30 minutes	2-3 hours	
			PR: lacking substantial evidence of effectiveness			
		Pediatric	Oral: (13-40 kg) 100-200 mg every 3-4 hours			
			IM: not recommended in children			
			PR: lacking substantial evidence of effectiveness			
Benzquinamide (Emete-Con)	Injection: 50 mg vial	Adult	*Oral: 100 mg every 3-4 hours			
			IM: 50 mg (0.5 mg-1.0 mg/kg initially; may repeat in 1 hour, then give every 3-4 hours	15 minutes	3-4 hours	
			IV: 25 mg (0.2-0.4 mg/kg); give slowly (25 mg/½-1 minute)	15 minutes	3-4 hours	IV route has been associated with sudden increase in BP and cardiac arrhythmias; IM is preferred route
			*PR: 100-200 mg every 3-4 hours			
			*Note: Oral and PR routes are not available commercially but these doses have been given effectively in chemotherapy			
		Pediatric	Doses have not been established			

Continued.

Table 7-16. Antiemetics—cont'd

Drug	Form	Type of patient	Dose	Onset	Duration	Cautions
Diphenidol (Vontrol)	Tablets: 25 mg Suspension: 20 mg/5 ml Injection: 20 mg/ml Suppository: 25, 50 mg	Adult	Oral: 25-50 mg every 3-6 hours	30-45 minutes	3-6 hours	Use only in hospitalized or closely supervised patients; hallucinations, disorientation, and confusion may result; onset 2 days; subsides 24-48 hours after discontinuation; use IV only twice, then switch to IM; do not use SC
			IM, IV: 20-40 mg initially; may repeat 1 hour later, then give every 3-6 hours (max. 300 mg/day)	15 minutes	3-6 hours	
		Pediatric	Oral and PR: 0.88 mg/kg/24 hours given in divided doses every 4 hours (max. dose daily 5.5 mg/kg) IM: 0.44 mg/kg/24 hours given in divided doses every 4 hours (max. dose daily 3.3 mg/kg)			IV or SC is not used in children at any age; note recommended for use in infants under 6 months or 25 pounds
Pyridoxine (Vitamin B_6)	Tablets: 5, 10, 25, 50 mg Injection: 50, 100 mg/ml	Adult and pediatric	Oral, IM, IV: 25-100 mg/day (up to 200 mg/day)			
Sedative, hypnotics, tranquilizers						
Diazepam (Valium)	Tablets: 2, 5, 10 mg Injection: 5 mg/ml	Adult	Oral: 2-10 mg every 4-6 hours	30 minutes-1 hour	Peak 2-3 hours T ½ 7-8 hours	
			IM: 2-20 mg, may repeat in 1-4 hours	15-30 minutes		
			IV: Same as IM	More rapid than IM	3 hours	

		Pediatric	Oral: >6 mo. of age 1 mg-2.5 mg 3-4 times daily IV: >30 days of age 0.25 mg/kg in 1 dose given *slowly* over 3minutes; may repeat in 15-30 minutes			
Chlordiazepoxide (Librium)	Capsules: 5, 10, 25 mg Tablets: 5, 10, 25 mg Injection: 100 mg	Adult	Oral: 5-10 mg every 6 hours IM: 50-100 mg IV: 50-100 mg	30 minutes-1 hour 15-30 minutes 3-30 minutes	Peaks 2-4 hours T ½ 20-24 hours	
		Pediatric	Oral: <6 years of age not recommended; 5 mg 2-4 times daily (may be increased in some children to 10 mg, 2-3 times daily) IM and IV: >12 years of age do not exceed 25-50 mg			
Phenobarbital (various)	Tablets: 8, 16, 32, 65, 100 mg Elixir: 20 mg/5 ml, 40 mg/5 ml Injection: 65, 130, 162 mg/ml Powder for injection: 65, 130, 200 mg	Adult	Oral or deep IM: 15-30 mg every 6-10 hours	30 minutes-1 hour	6-10 hours T ½ 2-5 days	
		Pediatric	Oral, IM, or PR: 2-3 mg/kg/day in 3-4 divided doses		T ½ 1.6 to 2.9 days	Children may become paradoxically excited and hyperactive; IV administration may cause respiratory arrest or hypotension
Chloral hydrate (Noctec, Somnos, various)	Capsules: 250, 500 mg Elixir: 250 mg/5 ml, 500 mg/5 ml Syrup: 250 mg/5 ml, 267 mg/5 ml, 500 mg/5 ml Suppository: 324, 500, 650, 975 mg, 1.3 g	Adult	Oral and PR: 250 mg every 4-8 hours after meals (max. 2 g/day)	30 minutes-1 hour	4-8 hours T ½ 8-11 hours	
		Pediatric	Oral and PR: 20-40 mg/kg/day (may be divided in 3-4 doses)			Wide margin of safety in children

is anticipated. The best time of administration may not be immediately prior to the injection of chemotherapy or other forms of therapy. The patient may have a characteristic pattern of not getting sick until 24 hours after therapy has been initiated. The best time of initiation will vary according to the patient. The clinician may find that the patient has erratic vomiting that cannot be anticipated. In these cases, antiemetic therapy with constant therapeutic blood levels over 48 hours during the anticipated vomiting period is often found effective.

5. To insure constant therapeutic blood levels of an antiemetic in patients, dosage times of administration should be *written on a sheet of paper or patient medication calendar* to encourage the compliance of the patient.
6. Antiemetic therapy should be given through the entire anticipated duration of the nausea and vomiting, then discontinued.
7. *Antiemetic agents given on a PRN basis should be avoided.* Abuse of the drug is likely, since cancer patients do not have the knowledge of the drug to properly dose themselves. Most patients when left to themselves in this manner wait until they are too sick for drug administration. The patient often cannot keep his medication down in order to stop his sickness or he may take more than the amount of antiemetic required.

RADIATION-INDUCED VOMITING

The cause of radiation-induced vomiting has not been clearly determined. It has been thought to be caused by damage of the intestinal mucosa, choline poisoning, vitamin B_6 deficiency, histamine release, shock, chloride depletion, or stimulation of the CTZ by circulating factors from cellular breakdown. Irradiation of the abdomen, especially the epigastric area, is associated with a higher incidence of vomiting than that of the chest or extremities. Symptoms are relieved by potent blockers of the CTZ such as the butyrophenones and phenothiazines. When these agents are not effective, pyridoxine (vitamin B_6) has been found at times to be effective in these circumstances. Its mechanism of action is not clearly understood and its effectiveness is not always clinically consistent in alleviating or minimizing nausea and vomiting in radiation patients. Some even question whether it is useful and attribute the clinical effectiveness to a placebo response in these patients. Severe avitaminosis of B_6 with high concentrations of urinary xanthurenic acid often follows in patients who have received radiation therapy. Because of this pathologic condition, some feel that it may be associated with the radiation sickness patients experience after therapy and may explain why pyridoxine is effective in its treatment. Cyclizine (Marezine) and meclizine (Atarax, Bonine) have shown activity in minimizing nausea and vomiting caused by radiation in cancer patients. They are usually considered the second drugs of choice in the treatment of radiation-induced vomiting. Since pediatric patients cannot receive the butyrophenones or the most effective phenothiazines because of the high incidence of extrapyramidal effects, phenothiazines that have shown minimal side effects in pediatric patients are used. Promethazine (Phenergan) has become the drug of choice. Chlorpromazine (Thorazine) is more effective than promethazine, but it has greater sedative properties that prevent its frequent use.

Two new investigational drugs have been used recently in the treatment of nausea and vomiting of radiation therapy. Stryker reported that 35 patients who were to begin pelvic irradiation randomly received prophylactically ibuprofen (Motrin) 400 mg four times daily with other standard antiemetic therapy. None of the patients who received Motrin experienced nausea or vomiting, whereas 27% of the control group reported vomiting.

Domperidone, a new antiemetic, has also been found effective in the treatment of radiation-induced vomiting. It is a dopamine-blocker that, in contrast to antipsychotic neuroleptics, does not induce psychotropic or neurotropic effects at therapeutic doses. It has been found to be safe in both adults and children for nausea and vomiting, producing minimal to no side effects. Reyntjins found that 30 adult patients (80%) when given domperidone 10 mg three times daily experienced a marked decrease or complete disappearance of nausea and vomiting following radiation therapy.

CHEMOTHERAPY-INDUCED VOMITING

Chemotherapy-induced vomiting is thought to be caused primarily by the direct stimulation of chemotherapeutic agents on the chemoreceptor trigger zone. Some agents, such as nitrogen mustard, also have peripheral effects. Other possible causes are the local irritant effects of oral agents on the gastrointestinal mucosa or the selective toxicity of several agents on the rapidly dividing tissues of the lining of the gastrointestinal tract. When cancer chemotherapy is first initiated, the massive cell lysing of normal and neoplastic cells is thought to release chemical substances that stimulate the chemoreceptor trigger zone to cause vomiting.

The group of drugs found to be the most effective in the treatment of chemotherapy-induced vomiting is the phenothiazines. They act primarily to block the stimulation of the chemoreceptor trigger zone and to a lesser extent, the vomiting center. They are all good inhibitors of the apomorphine response, and some of them are inhibitors of the copper sulfate response, which is representative of vomiting caused by peripheral stimulation.

There are two pharmacologic groups of phenothiazines used in the treatment of nausea and vomiting, the piperazine compounds and the aliphatic compounds.

Piperazine compounds, with the halogenated side chain, have the greatest antiemetic effect and the least sedation and hypotension when compared with the aliphatic compounds. However, their characteristic structure causes them to have an increased incidence of extrapyramidal side effects owing to their interference with dopaminergic transmission. It has been found that the incidences of extrapyramidal side effects increase as the milligram potency of these compounds increases. Because of this side effect, these compounds are recommended for short-term use only. They should be avoided in pediatric patients and given with caution in the elderly since extrapyramidal side effects occur more frequently in these age groups than in adults.

The piperazine compounds most frequently used in nausea and vomiting are prochlorperazine (Compazine), thiethylperazine (Torecan), and perphenazine (Trilafon). Both perphenazine and thiethylperazine raise the oral copper sulfate threshold as well as act as good inhibitors of the apomorphine response. Prochlorperazine is the most widely used but thiethylperazine appears to have fewer side effects (less sedation). Its second antiemetic action may be playing a role in its increasing popularity. Both can be given by the oral, parenteral, and rectal routes. Perphenazine has no advantage over either prochlorperazine or thiethylperazine.

The aliphatic compounds, except for triflupromazine (Vesprin), have low incidences of extrapyramidal side effects. Therefore they are used primarily in children. When used in adults, they are given for chronic use or for their sedative effects that help minimize the anxiety of the patient. They are also considered the alternative to the piperazine compound failures. The aliphatic compounds consist of chlorpromazine (Thorazine) triflupromazine (Vesprin), promazine (Sparine) and promethazine (Phenergan). Chlorpromazine and promethazine are the most frequently used of this group. Promethazine is rather unique in that it has antihistaminic properties that can be used in motion sickness as well as in blocking the apomorphine response in patients. It has the weakest antiemetic effects of the four compounds. Both promazine and chlorpromazine have moderate antiemetic effects. Even though promazine is comparable to chlorpromazine with less sedation, it is not as versatile. Chlorpromazine can be given to both pediatric and adult patients, and like promethazine, it also can be given by the rectal route. Chlorpromazine produces the greatest sedation and hypotension of the four compounds. Triflupromazine is comparable antiemetically to prochlorperazine except for its greater tendency for hypotension and fewer dosage forms. It should be avoided in children.

The extrapyramidal side effects, even though rarely seen, manifest themselves with the phenothiazines in a variety of specific symptoms. The most common are the dystonic reactions and dyskinesias characterized by torticollis, opisthotonos, tics, grimacing dysarthria, and various involuntary muscle movements such as oculogyric crisis. These are most often seen after the administration of prochlorperazine and perphenazine. A higher incidence occurs in children and the elderly. These symptoms are rapidly reversed with diazepam 10 mg IV or diphenhydramine 50 mg IV.

The Parkinson symptoms characterized by tremor, rigidity, and akinesia are more prevalent with chlorpromazine after several weeks of high-dose therapy. They are very unlikely to appear at the doses and duration of common antiemetic therapy.

Phenothiazines should be used with caution in patients who have brain metastasis with a history of seizures. They lower the seizure threshold in patients and have been known to precipitate seizures in cancer patients.

Phenothiazines at antiemetic doses also cause the release of prolactin by suppression of the prolactin inhibitory factor. The role of prolactin in increasing the progression of breast cancer is highly controversial. Because of this unsettled question, phenothiazines are given in very short courses in breast cancer patients, or an antiemetic that does not cause prolactin release is given, such as trimethobenzamide (Tigan).

There is much controversy concerning the effectiveness of trimethobenzamide as an antiemetic. Recently bioavailability studies revealed that the blood levels of the 250 mg capsule and the 200 mg suppository are 60% and 32% respectively of a 200 mg IM blood level. The Tigan suppository has been reclassified as lacking substantial evidence of effectiveness by the U.S. Food and Drug Administration. Twice the oral dosage form (400 mg) has been found to be equivalent to a 200 mg injection of trimethobenzamide. Its use has been approved for gastroenteritis and for postoperative conditions. Results of studies currently taking place will resolve the question of its effectiveness for other indications. Trimethobenzamide has a structure similar to reserpine and antihistamines. It is thought to have a blocking effect on the apomorphine response as its mechanism of action.

The butyrophenones, which include haloperidol and droperidol, are considered as effective as the phenothiazines in the treatment of chemotherapy-induced vomiting. Because of their higher incidences of side effects, they are usually not chosen over the phenothiazines as first-line therapy. A recent study revealed that droperidol was successful in treating vomiting refractory to standard antiemetic therapy during cisplatin therapy. The antiemetic effects of butyrophenones are similar to the phenothiazines.

Benzquinamide is a nonphenothiazine antiemetic that is effective against apomorphine-induced vomiting. Its use in the treatment of cancer chemotherapy-induced vomiting has been limited. One reason for its limited use is that it exists in parenteral form only. An early study also revealed that it was ineffective in the treatment of nausea and vomiting from 5-fluorouracil.

Diphenidol is an antiemetic as effective as prochlorperazine, but its use is limited because of its high incidence of side effects. Side effects characteristic of this drug are hallucination, dizziness, disorientation, and confusion; they can be so severe that the manufacturer recommends that all patients who receive this drug be hospitalized or be closely supervised.

Investigational antiemetics (Table 7-17). Antiemetics of investigational interest for some time are the cannabinoids. Their mode of action is yet to be determined but both delta-9-tetrahydrocannabinol (THC) and its derivative nabilone have been proven to be more effective than a placebo. Delta-9-tetrahydrocannabinol has been observed clinically to be effective in stopping or minimizing refractory nausea and vomiting. Its side effects are primarily a "high" and in some patients dysphoria and tachycardia.

In a recent study nabilone, when compared with prochlorperazine, proved to be superior in its antiemetic action. Research with this agent has diminished because of animal studies that revealed that nabilone has the potential of causing seizures and death. However, most patients who receive the drug experience primarily somnolence and dizziness. Some note incoordination and spacial disorientation. A few patients may require medical intervention for transient psychosis and hallucinations.

Metoclopramide recently became available commercially with approved indications to facilitate small bowel intubation in adults and children after standard procedures have been taken and to stimulate gastric emptying and intestinal transit of barium in delayed emptying of the stomach and small intestines that is interfering with radiologic exams. Its use in the treatment of cancer chemotherapy-induced vomiting is yet to be determined.

In an early investigational study in which metoclopramide was given orally, it was found ineffective in the treatment of nausea and vomiting produced by 5-fluorouracil. In a recent study, however, it has shown significant activity in stopping or minimizing the nausea and vomiting produced by cisplatin refractory to standard emetic therapy. It is considered to be equipotent parenterally to prochlorperazine and perphenazine. In animals it is a potent antagonist of vomiting induced by both apomorphine and copper sulfate. Thus it has both central and peripheral action. Metoclopramide also tightens the distal esophageal sphincter and enhances gastric emptying. It has some cardiovascular sedative and antihistaminic side effects. Recently there have been reports of dystonic reactions in patients

Table 7-17. Investigational antiemetic agents

Drug	Form	Use	Dose	Side effects
Delta-9-tetrahydro-cannabinol (THC)[70,71]	Capsules Cigarette or smoking apparatus	Cancer chemotherapy and refractory vomiting in cancer chemotherapy	Oral: 10 mg/m every 4 hours in 3 doses Smoking: Patient titrates to desired effect plasma levels >5.0 mg/ml	"High" 2% disphoric reactions
Nabilone[67,68]	Tablet: 2 mg Capsule: 1 mg	Cancer chemotherapy (not currently available in U.S.)	Oral: Tablet, 2 mg every 12 hours in 3-5 doses Capsule, 2 mg every 8 hours or 2 mg every 6 hours	Drowsiness, dizziness, dry mouth, hallucinations and/or dysphoria, incoordination, disorientation, transient psychosis, severe hypotension; animal studies: seizures and death
Metopimazine (Vogalene)[77b] France	Oral liquid preparation	Cancer chemotherapy	Oral: 45 mg/day for 2 days given in divided doses (10 ml [2 tsp] 1 hour before each meal with the first dose prior to chemotherapy)	Mild drowsiness, dry mouth
Droperidol (Inapsine)[74]	Injection: 2.5 mg/ml	Refractory cisplatin vomiting	Adult IM or IV: 0.5 mg 1 hour before cisplatin, then 0.5 mg every 4 hours when necessary Note: After repeated courses, may require dose increase to 0.75-1.5 mg to achieve antiemetic effect; type of tolerence builds in patients; recovery is complete in 6-12 hours after use	Mild somnolence

Continued.

Table 7-17. Investigational antiemetic agents—cont'd

Drug	Form	Use	Dose	Side effects
Metoclopramide (Reglan)[64,65,66]	Injection: 10 mg/ml	Refractory cisplatin vomiting	Adult IM, IV, oral: 20 mg every 3-4 hours before and after cisplatin administration	Sedation
Domperidone[75,76,77]	Drops: 1% solutior Tablets: 10 mg IM, IV: 10 mg Suppository: 1.3 rr kg	Pediatric: Chronic vomiting and nausea Postoperative vomiting Radiation-induced vomiting	Pediatric oral: 0.3 mg/kg 3 times daily before meals Postoperative vomiting: 10 mg every 6 hours	Minimal to none
Ibuprofen (Motrin)[73]	Tablets: 400 mg	Radiation-induced vomiting and nausea	Adult oral: 400 mg 4 times daily during radiotherapy	None reported
Dexamethasone (Decadron)[69]	Injection: 4 mg/ml	Cancer chemotherapy	Adult IM: 10 mg in 1 dose	None reported
TTS Scopolamine (ALZA)[60,72,77a]	Skin patch	Cancer chemotherapy	Maintains hyosine level equivalent to 0.2 mg oral dose	Minimal to none; dry mouth

with advanced renal failure and in people from Sardinia. It is thought that the latter is caused by genetic differences in the sensitivity of dopamine receptors.

A surprising discovery of a new way to use an old drug, dexamethazone, was reported by Baker and co-workers in treating nausea and vomiting associated with various chemotherapy regimens, including such drugs as semustine, cyclophosphamide, doxorubicin, nitrogen mustard, and mitomycin C. Seventy per cent of patients had marked to moderate relief of nausea and vomiting. A further study has been initiated to compare its efficacy with prochlorperazine.

In treating cancer chemotherapy-induced vomiting in pediatric patients, a unique investigational drug, TTS scopolamine, has appeared and received great interest. It utilizes the transdermal therapeutic system (TTS), a new drug delivery system that allows a controlled continuous delivery of scopolamine through intact skin into the blood stream. During 1980 it will be made commercially available for the treatment of motion sickness. It provides effective antiemetic action for a duration of 60 to 72 hours. In preliminary studies it has also shown promise in the treatment of cancer chemotherapy-induced vomiting in children. Sawicka and co-workers found it effective in a pilot study of 12 children receiving high-dose methotrexate. Minimal or no side effects were observed in the children. Scopolamine is a centrally acting cholinergic that has been found effective in preventing emesis caused by oral copper sulfate. It is also thought to have some action on the chemoreceptor trigger zone, the vestibular apparatus, and the cerebral cortex of the brain.

Another investigational drug of interest is domperidone. Even though there are no known reported clinical trials of its use in cancer chemotherapy-induced vomiting, it is similar to metoclopramide in its mechanism of action as a potent dopamine blocker, which suggests that it may have promise. It has already been demonstrated as being effective and safe in treating chronic pediatric vomiting with minimal side effects.

PSYCHOGENIC VOMITING

Psychogenic vomiting is an ingrained conditioned reflex that results from the patient experiencing sounds, sights, smells, tastes, or thoughts associated with a previous act of vomiting, perhaps caused by direct or indirect stimulation of the vomiting center by blood-borne emetic substances, motion, or a vagal stimulation from the periphery simply because of the intense anxiety of the patient. Psychogenic vomiting is a common occurrence in cancer patients. It often creates problems in the patient receiving radiation therapy or chemotherapy.

Psychogenic vomiting has not been studied extensively and is usually treated empirically. Whether responses can be attributed to a placebo effect or the effect of the agents used in treating it one cannot say. It has been observed clinically that antianxiety agents, the benzodiazepines, and the antihistamine hydroxyzine, and sedative-hypnotics used alone or in combination are more effective than standard emetics used in treating nausea and vomiting.

In adult patients diazepam or chlordiazepoxide have been found to miniimize or stop psychogenic-vomiting in cancer patients. Phenobarbital has been given successfully to adults prior to bedtime before administration of chemotherapy.

Psychogenic vomiting may occur concurrently with the nausea and vomiting from other etiologies such as chemotherapy or radiation therapy. If this is determined or suspected and the nausea and vomiting is out of control, the combination of diazepam and prochlorperazine has been found to be successful in some adult patients. Basically the clinician has to use his good judgment and knowledge of these drugs and the possible etiologies of the vomiting. From this information he can determine combinations by trial and error until he meets the needs of his patients.

In pediatric patients, a recent clinically observed successful combination for psychogenic vomiting is hydroxyzine (Vistaril) and chloral hydrate (Noctec, Somnos). Chloral hydrate or phenobarbital given alone has also been successful in some patients.

ANALGESIC-INDUCED VOMITING

Morphine and its derivatives, which are commonly used postoperatively or for chronic pain in terminal cancer patients, often produce nausea and vomiting by their direct stimulation of the chemoreceptor trigger zone. Nausea and vomiting is quite common with the first administration. It is unusual, however, after therapeutic blood levels are achieved that vomiting continues, owing to morphine's depressant effect on the chemoreceptor trigger zone unless it is given on a PRN basis, in which case vomiting may follow after each dose. Narcotic antagonists and some phenothiazines, especially those with dopamine blocking action such as prochlorperazine and thiethylperazine, are quite effective in its treatment. Benzquinamide is the drug of choice since, unlike the phenothiazines, it does not potentiate narcotic-induced hypotension or respiratory depression. It is limited in its use, however, because it is only available in parenteral form. Investigationally, it has been used successfully when given orally and rectally. Metoclopramide and domperidone have also been found effective.

Nausea and vomiting that occurs after subsequent doses is usually caused by a different mechanism of action and requires a different approach to treatment. Morphine and its derivatives also increase the sensitivity of the vestibular apparatus of the inner ear to motion. As a result, nausea and vomiting occurs more commonly in ambulatory patients than recumbent patients. Drugs used to treat motion sickness, such as promethazine, cyclizine or meclizine, are found to be the most effective agents in controlling this type of morphine-induced vomiting in cancer patients.

Hyperuricemia[78-85]

Hyperuricemia in cancer patients is usually the result of increased nucleic acid turnover from the mass of abnormal neoplastic cells in the cancer patient or from nucleic acids that are released by the rapid lysis of tumor cells from radiation or chemotherapy received by the patient. Purines of the nucleic acids released are metabolized to hypoxanthine, then to xanthine (both water soluble metabolites), then to uric acid, which is excreted into the urine (Fig. 7).

The normal serum uric acid level is 7 mg/100 ml. In both acute myelogenous leukemia and acute lymphocytic leukemia, uric acid levels may be as high as 20 mg/100 ml prior to therapy, sometimes resulting in acute renal failure. At least half of the patients with chronic myelogenous leukemia experience hyperuricemia, but it is rarely seen in patients with chronic lymphocytic leukemia. Myeloma is the only other neoplastic disease in which hyperuricemia may be seen before therapy is initiated. Of course, any form of malignancy that undergoes rapid destruction and release of nucleic acid constituents after treatment with radiation or chemotherapy may produce hyperuricemia, which is easily treated in the cancer patient. However, it is more common to prevent hyperuricemia in cancer patients than to treat it. Thus, prophylactic therapy should consider avoidance of exacerbating factors such as dehydration, a low urinary pH, renal disease, and obstructive uropathy. Concurrent diuretic therapy may increase the risk of urate nephropathy by inducing dehydration, producing secondary renal dysfunction, and inhibiting urate excretion.

Clinical signs and symptoms of hyperuricemia are usually related to renal insufficiency owing to the precipitation of uric acid into the renal tubules, collecting ducts, and parenchyma of the kidneys. These symptoms are lethargy, nausea, vomiting, hematuria, renal colic, oliguria, or anuria.

Purines ⟶ Hypoxanthine ⟶ (Xanthine oxidase) Xanthine ⟶ (Xanthine oxidase) Uric acid

Fig. 7. Metabolism of nucleic acids.

Gouty symptoms from hyperuricemia are rarely seen in cancer patients, but they may occur in patients with chronic leukemia or solid tumors. Acute leukemia patients lack the polymorphonuclear cells to mediate the inflammatory joint changes characteristic of gout.

The major goal of therapy of hyperuricemia in cancer patients is to prevent urate nephropathy. When uric acid levels are 15 mg/100 ml or greater, urate nephropathy is a definite danger to the patient with tumors that are rapidly responsive to therapy. Thus prophylactic therapy is given to patients prior to radiation or chemotherapy with the objective of keeping serum uric acid levels less than 6 mg/100 ml and urine in an optimum urate solubilizing state.

MANAGEMENT OF HYPERURICEMIA

The reduction of serum uric acid levels in hyperuricemia consists of three approaches:

1. To decrease uric acid production
2. To increase uric acid solubility in the urine
3. To reduce the uric acid concentration in the urine

Uric acid production is decreased by allopurinol, which acts as a competitive inhibitor of the enzyme xanthine oxidase, which catalyzes the final steps in the degradation of purines to uric acid (see Fig. 7). It also diminishes excessive rates of purine synthesis in patients. Allopurinol has a half-life of 2 to 3 hours, and its major active metabolite, oxypurinol, has a half-life of 18 to 30 hours. Because of oxypurinol's long half-life, it has been found that single doses of allopurinol are as effective as divided doses. However, when doses are greater than 300 mg, divided doses are usually given.

Allopurinol comes in 100 mg and 300 mg tablets commercially. Its onset of action is 1 to 2 days with its maximum effects occurring 7 to 10 days after initiation of therapy. The response of uric acid levels to the dose is directly proportionate. The higher the dose used, the greater the fall in serum uric acid levels. Mild hyperuricemia is usually treated with 200-300 mg/day, and moderate to severe with 400-600 mg/day. Up to 1,800 mg/day has been given.

The second approach is to increase the uric acid solubility in the urine by raising the pH of the urine. A urinary pH of 5 or less causes uric acid to crystalize when present in high concentrations. Since normal urine pH ranges from 5.5 to 6.0, producing an alkaline urine will have to be achieved by the use of exogenous agents such as sodium bicarbonate or acetazolamide.

In the third approach the uric acid concentration in the urine is reduced by hydration of the patient. The average uric acid concentration and daily excretion rate in normal patients is 60 mg/100 ml and 600 mg, respectively.

In hyperuricemia, this concentration is much greater and larger amounts of uric acid are excreted each day. Along with increasing the uric acid solubility with an alkaline pH, vigorous hydration with fluids can prevent a supersaturated solution of uric acid from forming.

The following is an outline format of the prophylactic therapy and treatment of hyperuricemia. Each clinical situation is presented and followed by the treatment that would be given under those conditions.

A. High-risk patients with no prior hyperuricemia about to receive radiation or chemotherapy
   1. Premedicate 48 hours prior to therapy with:
      Allopurinol 300 mg twice daily
      Thereafter:
      Allopurinol 300 mg/day
      Normal uric acid levels (6-7 mg/100 ml) will appear in 1-3 weeks; allopurinol is usually discontinued after uric acid is normalized
   2. Establish adequate hydration orally or IV (if necessary) by giving 3 liters of fluid per day with a daily output of 2 liters or greater (100 ml/m^2/hour)

B. High-risk patients with no prior hyperuricemia about to receive radiation or chemotherapy who have had a *prior drug reaction to allopurinol*
   1. Vigorously hydrate the patient 48 hours prior to therapy with:
      3000 ml/m^2/day to produce urine output of ≥100 ml/m^2/hour
   2. Alkalinization of the urine to maintain a pH of 7.0-7.5 with:
      6-8 g/day of $NaHCO_3$ continuous IV drip (or 3 g orally three or four times daily) and in some cases acetazolamide (Diamox) 250 mg orally once or twice daily may be added
   3. *Do not give* allopurinol since a more severe hypersensitivity reaction such as vasculitis and toxic epidermal necrolysis can occur which may lead to death. The most frequent side effect of allopurinol seen is a maculopapular skin rash, but exfoliative, urticarial, purpuric, and erythema multiform lesions may also occur; occasionally, reversible hepatotoxicity, nausea, vomiting and abdominal pain may appear

C. An *adult* patient with preexisting hyperuricemia with no renal failure about to receive chemotherapy or radiation therapy
   1. Premedicate 48 hours prior to therapy with:
      Allopurinol 300 mg twice daily
      Thereafter:
      Allopurinol 300 mg/day

Discontinue allopurinol after normal uric acid levels have been established

2. Adequate hydration orally or IV (if necessary)
   3000 ml/m^2 daily of fluid to produce urine output of 100 ml/m^2/hour
3. Alkalinization of the urine to maintain a pH of 7-7.5
   3 g $NaHCO_3$ orally three or four times daily *or* 6-8 g/day $NaHCO_3$ continuous IV drip. Acetazolamide (Diamox) may be added or given in place of $NaHCO_3$ in doses of 250 mg orally once, twice, or four times daily

   Plus: 40-80 mEq KCl should be given

D. *Pediatric* patient with preexisting hyperuricemia with no renal failure about to receive chemotherapy or radiation therapy; *Note:* a child should be hospitalized with uric acid levels greater than 10 mg/100 ml, WBC >75,000/mm^3, or massive organomegaly
   1. Premedicate 48 hours prior to therapy with:
      Allopurinol 100 mg orally three times daily (for children >6 years)
      Allopurinol 50 mg orally three times daily (for children <6 years)

      Discontinue allopurinol after normal uric acid levels have stabilized
   2. Adequate hydration with:
      3,000 ml/m^2 of D5, 0.25 normal saline to produce urine output of ≥100 ml/m^2/hour
   3. Alkalinization of the urine to maintain a pH of 7.0-7.5
      $NaHCO_3$ 35-90 mEq/m^2/daily

      Note: If the urine is not alkaline in 6 hours, give acetazolamide (Diamox) 200 mg/m^2/day; once the serum uric acid levels fall below 6.0 mg/100 ml, discontinue the $NaHCO_3$ and Diamox

E. Alternatives for *pediatric or adult* patients who cannot receive allopurinol orally because of nausea and vomiting
   1. Crush allopurinol tablet and administer through a nasal gastric tube
   2. Investigational IV allopurinol for injection (NSC-1390) is available in a 300 mg vial; it has been found effective

      Reconstitute: 5-10 ml D_5W or NS

      Stable: 7 days

      Administration: IV push or IV infusion in 100 ml D_5W or normal saline over 30-60 minutes

      Incompatible with: 6-mercaptopurine sodium and methotrexate in D_5W

3. Allopurinol suppository: A crushed 300 mg tablet in cocoa butter base has been found effective
4. Vigorously hydrate the patient with:
   3,000 ml/m^2/day to produce urine output of $\geq$100 ml/m^2/hour
5. Alkalinization of the urine to maintain a pH of 7.0-7.5:
   Adult: $NaHCO_3$ 6-8 g/day continuous IV drip (or 3 g orally three or four times daily)
   Pediatric: 35-90 mEq/m^2/day $NaHCO_3$
   May add:
   Adult: Acetazolamide (Diamox) 250 mg orally once or twice daily
   Pediatric: Acetazolamide (Diamox) 200 mg/m^2/day once or twice daily

F. Emergency therapy for severe hyperuricemia or azotemia secondary to uric acid nephropathy
1. Allopurinol 200 mg four times daily

Note: If creatinine clearance is:	then give dose:
10-20 ml/min	200 mg/day
<10 ml/min	$\leq$100 mg/day
<3 ml/min	Lengthen dose interval

2. Hydration with 3 to 4 liters of fluid per day
3. Alkalinization of urine to maintain a pH of 7.0-7.5 with:
   $NaHCO_3$ 6-8 g/day continuous IV drip (or 3 g $NaHCO_3$ orally three or four times daily
   May add:
   Acetazolamide (Diamox) 250 mg orally once, twice, or four times daily

G. Anuric or oliguric patients
1. Allopurinol, $NaHCO_3$, and hydration may aggravate the nephropathy and be dangerous unless excess fluid is removed
2. Perform osmotic diuresis:
   Mannitol (12.5-25 g/m^2 IV over 10-15 minutes) following insertion of ureteral catheter; *if successful:* alkalinize the urine as presented in section E; *if unsuccessful:* treat as acute renal failure by appropriate fluid, protein restriction, and removal of uric acid by peritoneal dialysis or hemodialysis
3. In severe cases, with serum urate levels above 25-30 mg/100 ml, emergency hemodialysis or peritoneal dialysis should be done immediately

Leucovorin rescue (LR)[86-88]

High-dose methotrexate with leucovorin rescue (HDMTX-LR) is being used for several human malignancies (Table 7-18), even though its superi-

Table 7-18. HDMTX-LR in various malignancies

Cancer	Response rate
Osteogenic sarcoma	42%
Non-Hodgkin's lymphoma	77%
Head and neck	70%
Breast	26%
Melanoma	36%
Pancreas	27%

ority over conventional doses of the drug has not been clearly demonstrated. There are several ongoing clinical trials at the present time with various methods for MTX infusion and several dose schedules for leucovorin administration. This discussion will consider the rationale and current recommendations for using leucovorin rescue.

The toxicity of methotrexate is dependent upon both concentration and duration of exposure to the drug effect. The early toxic effect of the drug is related to its action on cellular renewal systems of the bone marrow and gastrointestinal tract (normal cells with a high growth fraction). After more than 40 hours of effective drug exposure, stem cells of bone marrow and gastrointestinal mucosa are more extensively damaged. MTX continues to be cytotoxic as long as serum concentrations are above 0.1 μM (1×10^{-7} M). Thus, high-dose MTX protocols (>0.5 g/m^2) produce greater clinical toxicity unless leucovorin is used to limit or prevent toxic effects to normal tissue.

Leucovorin is transported into the cell by the same active transport system as MTX, and it is at the cell membrane where leucovorin competes with MTX for entry into the cell. Once inside the cell, leucovorin counteracts the effects of MTX in several ways: (1) it bypasses the MTX block of dihydrofolate reductase, (2) it enhances the efflux of MTX from the cell, and (3) it restores DNA, RNA, and protein synthesis. The critical factors in "rescue" therapy are to administer leucovorin *within 40 hours* of MTX infusion and to administer doses of leucovorin that will *effectively compete* with MTX for entry into the cell. Leucovorin is effective only when it is equal to or exceeds MTX serum concentration by tenfold. These considerations suggest that when high serum concentrations ($\geq$10 μM) of MTX exist after short-term infusion (6 hours), early administration of small doses of leucovorin (10 mg/m^2) will not provide effective rescue, while later administration (12 to 24 hours post-MTX) will provide a greater competitive inhibition because MTX levels will be much lower. Doses of leucovorin commonly used are 10 to 15 mg/m^2, which give serum concentrations of 1 to 5 μM.

Factors which decrease the effectiveness of leucovorin rescue are listed

Table 7-19. Factors decreasing the effect of leucovorin rescue

Renal dysfunction
"Third" space
Pleural effusion
Ascites
Severe edema
High concentrations of MTX (>10 μM)

in Table 7-19. Of note is the presence or development of renal dysfunction, which can substantially decrease the body clearance of MTX and subsequently increase blood levels. High serum MTX concentrations are associated with a greater incidence of bone marrow and gastrointestinal toxicity. This increased risk of toxicity from delayed MTX clearance can be minimized by increasing the dosage of leucovorin from 10 mg/m^2 to 50 mg/m^2. In either dosage, the duration of leucovorin rescue should be continued until serum MTX levels fall to less than 0.1 μM (1×10^{-7} M).

Extravasation[89-91]

Vesicant reactions after extravasation of some cancer chemotherapeutics account for 2% to 5% of their adverse effects. Table 7-20 provides the specific clinical findings for those anticancer drugs commonly associated with severe tissue necrosis.

The factors associated with an increased risk of extravasation are listed in Table 7-21. The risk of extravasation can be minimized by using a systematic technique of drug administration. Table 7-22 provides guidelines for the intravenous administration of chemotherapy.

Controlled studies have been initiated to determine the best method for treatment of extravasation. Table 7-23 is our recommendation for managing an extravasation that has recently occurred. Some anticancer drugs have antidotes that are recommended by the manufacturer and others do not. Most of the empirical antidotes, although having theoretical rationale, have not been well documented in humans or animals to prevent local tissue necrosis. Both types of antidotes are listed in Table 7-24.

If patients continue to complain of inflammation and pain at the site of extravasation after 2 to 3 weeks, a plastic surgeon should be consulted for consideration of debridement and engraftment.

Oral mucositis[92-95]

Stomatitis occasionally leads to severe nutritional complications in patients treated with anticancer drugs. The mechanism of toxicity to the oral

Table 7-20. Vesicant anticancer drugs and their clinical manifestations

Drug	Type of reaction	Onset of inflammation	Symptoms	Duration of reaction	Mechanism
Carmustine	Vein phlebitis	10-14 days	Pain	7 days	Endothelial alkylation
Dactinomycin	Vesicant, recall	1-2 weeks	Pain	Several weeks	Inhibition of DNA-directed RNA synthesis
Daunorubicin	Vesicant	1-2 weeks	Pain	Several weeks	Tissue DNA intercalation superoxide formation
Doxorubicin	Vesicant, recall	1-2 weeks	Pain	Several weeks	Tissue DNA intercalation superoxide formation
Fluorouracil	Discoloration	1 week	No pain	1 week	Unknown
Mechlorethamine	Vesicant	12-24 hours	Pain	4-6 weeks	Tissue alkylation
	Vein discoloration	2 weeks	No pain	3-4 weeks	Endothelial alkylation
Mithramycin	Vesicant	1 week	Pain	Several weeks	Tissue alkylation
Mitomycin C	Vesicant	1 week	Pain	Several weeks	Tissue alkylation superoxide formation
Vinblastine	Vesicant	12-24 hours	Pain	Several weeks	Mitotic inhibition
Vincristine	Vesicant	12-24 hours	Pain	Several weeks	Mitotic inhibition

Table 7-21. Factors associated with increased risk of extravasation

Sclerotic vascular disease
Venous obstruction in the arm of patients with axillary lymph node dissection
Prior local irradiation near the site of drug injection
High drug concentration
Site of injection
Multiple venipunctures
Iatrogenic disease

Table 7-22. Guidelines for administering chemotherapy

1. Dilute the drug in the appropriate amount of diluent to avoid high concentrations.
2. Select an infusion site in the following order of preference: forearm > dorsum of hand > wrist > antecubital fossa.
3. Insert a 20 or 21 gauge "butterfly" needle (one venipuncture only) into the vein.
4. Lightly tape the tubing of the "butterfly" distal to the needle. Do not obscure the injection site by covering it with tape.
5. Administer 5 ml of normal saline solution (NS) and withdraw a small amount of blood to test vein integrity and flow. Observe for extravasation.
6. If extravasation of NS is obvious, select another site (the other arm, or lateral or proximal to the initial site in that arm). Avoid a distal point on the same vein because of the potential for extravasation "upstream."
7. Administer the drug over at least 3 minutes or approximately 5 ml per minute. (See Section 5 for administration rate of specific agents). Withdraw blood once for each 1 to 2 ml of solution administered to assure proper needle placement. Repeatedly ask the patient if he feels any pain or burning.
8. Follow the drug injection with 5 to 10 ml or more of a saline infusion to flush tubing and needle of all drug.
9. If multiple drugs are prescribed, inject the nonvesicant agents first. If all drugs are vesicants, inject the one with the least amount of diluent first. Separate each administered drug with 3 to 5 ml of saline.

Table 7-23. Management of chemotherapy extravasation

1. Stop injection immediately, leaving needle in place.
2. Withdraw 3 to 5 ml of blood and solution (if possible).
3. Administer 25 mg hydrocortisone into the needle (optional) and remove needle.
4. With a 27-gauge TB syringe, aspirate any extravasated solution not removed by procedure (2).
5. Purposely administer the antidote subcutaneously in a "pin-cushion" manner in the extravasated area (use 4 to 5 injections).
6. Apply cold compresses for 1 hour to allow time for the antidote to interact with the vesicant.
7. Apply warm compresses at the extravasated site for 1 hour.*
8. Follow-up should be obtained weekly (or earlier if mechlorethamine), observing for signs of inflammation and necrosis.
9. Surgical excision should be considered at the first sign of tissue breakdown or ulceration.

*It is well known that drug absorption from subcutaneous or intramuscular injections is enhanced in the presence of heat and decreased by cold. Some clinicians prefer cold over heat in the setting of extravasation. In our opinion, we think that a combination of initial cold compresses followed by heat may be more rational than either method alone.

Table 7-24. Antidotes for vesicant cancer drugs

Drug	Antidote	Dose
Manufacturer-recommended antidote		
Mechlorethamine	Sodium thiosulfate 10%	4 ml
Vincristine	Heat + hyaluronidase (150 μ/ml)	150 units
Theoretical antidote		
Actinomycin C	Sodium thiosulfate 10%	4 ml
	or	
	Ascorbic acid injection (50 mg/ml)	1 ml
Carmustine	Sodium bicarbonate 8.4%	5 ml
Daunorubicin	Sodium bicarbonate 8.4% plus dexamethasone 4 mg/ml	5 ml 1 ml
Doxorubicin	Sodium bicarbonate 8.4% plus dexamethasone 4 mg/ml	5 ml 1 ml
Mithramycin	EDTA 150 mg/ml	1 ml
Mitomycin C	Sodium thiosulfate 10%	4 ml
	or	
	Ascorbic acid 50 mg/ml	1 ml
	or	
	Pyridoxine HCl 50 mg/ml	1 ml
Vinblastine	Sodium bicarbonate 8.4%	5 ml
	or	
	Heat + hyaluronidase (150 μ/ml)	150 units

mucosa appears to be related to the effect of these agents on the continual cell renewal process of this rapidly dividing tissue. The onset of oral stomatitis can occur as early as 4 days to as late as 14 days after chemotherapy.[40]

Not all anticancer drugs produce stomatitis. Remarkably, the alkylating agents rarely produce the problem. Table 7-25 lists those anticancer drugs that have induced documented oral ulceration. Most of these agents are antitumor antibiotics and antimetabolites, and therefore, certain patients may be more likely to develop stomatitis.

Leukemic patients commonly receive combination chemotherapy with antitumor antibiotics (daunorubicin or doxorubicin) and antimetabolites (cytarabine or mercaptopurine) in very high doses. Thus the chance that patients treated for acute myeloblastic leukemia with these agents will develop stomatitis is very high (probably greater than 80% at University of California at San Francisco). Acute physical stress, certainly common in the leukemic patient, is also a known risk factor in the development of stomatitis.[41,42]

There are few studies addressing the issue of symptomatic or preventive care for stomatitis. Some nursing units employ a systematic protocol for

Table 7-25. Anticancer drugs toxic to the oral mucosa

Drug	Incidence	Comment
Doxorubicin	75% at 90 mg/m² or 30 mg/m² for 3 days 15%-20% at 45-60 mg/m² for 1 day	Dose-related
Acridinyl anisidide	75% at 200 mg/m² for 5 days 50% at 120 mg/m² for 5 days 5% at 120 mg/m² for 1 day	Dose-related
Azacitidine	5%-10% at 150-200 mg/m² for 5 days	
Bleomycin	16%-40%	Dose-related; more common with doses 10 mg/m² given twice weekly
Cytarabine	10%-30%	Dose-related; more common with doses of 100 mg/m² for 5 days by continuous infusion
Dactinomycin	20%	Dose-related
Daunorubicin	11%	Dose- and schedule-related; 20 mg/day for 3 days produces 30%-40% incidence
Fluorouracil	50%-75% at 1 g/m² for 5 days 4%-8% at 1 g/m² weekly	
Hydroxyurea	10%-20% at high doses (4 g/day)	
Mercaptopurine	5%	
Methotrexate	25% at conventional doses 90% in high doses with low-dose leucovorin rescue in children; 6%-21% in high doses with leucovorin rescue	Low-dose leucovorin (3 mg per dose) is associated with a higher incidence of mucositis
Mithramycin	2% at 0.010 mg/kg for 5 days 20% at 0.015 mg/kg for 5 days	Dose-related

oral care.[43] Such programs improve the oral status of patients and decrease the number of infections arising from the oral mucosa.[43] Dental programs stressing oral hygiene prior to aggressive antileukemia therapy also have been shown to decrease morbidity to the oral mucosa.

A frequent infection that complicates mucositis is oral candidiasis. Many institutions utilize prophylactic nystatin locally to prevent *Candida* infections. There are several dosage forms for this agent in present use. Our patients prefer nystatin diluted to make popsicles (formula by M. D. Anderson). The usual dose of nystatin is 500,000 units 3 to 4 times daily. Nystatin lozenges are also very useful in providing 15 minutes of drug exposure per dose, even though they are somewhat unpalatable. Nystatin suspension, which provides a short duration of local effect, may be used but is not preferred.

If stomatitis is caused by chemotherapy alone, local therapy with topical anesthetics may be necessary for adequate pain control. Many oncologists have used mixtures of diphenhydramine elixir, Maalox, and 1% viscous xylocaine, but no systematic studies have been reported. Others have used viscous xylocaine or Kenalog or Orabase ointment. In our experience these preparations are very unpalatable and unacceptable to patients. We have used 2% lidocaine solution in an atomizer with significantly greater success. This solution can be easily sprayed onto oral lesions any time the patients require local pain control. Oral absorption of lidocaine is poor, and thus toxicity is a minimal risk.

In patients refractory to local therapy, systemic analgesics with narcotics may be necessary (see section on Pain Management).

SELECTED REFERENCES

Malignant effusions

1. Friedman, M. A., and Slater, E.: Malignant pleural effusions, Cancer Treat. Rev. **5**:49-66, 1978.
2. Leff, A., et al.: Pleural effusion from malignancy, Ann. Intern. Med. **88**:532-537, 1978.
3. Chernow, B., et al.: Carcinomatosis involvement of the pleura: an analysis of 96 patients, Am. J. Med. **63**:695-702, 1977.
4. Dollinger, M. R.: Management of recurrent malignant effusions, CA **22**:138, 1972.
5. Light, L. W., et al.: Cells in pleural fluid, Arch. Intern. Med. **132**:854, 1973.
6. Wallach, H. W.: Intrapleural tetracycline for malignant pleural effusion, Chest **68**:510, 1975.
7. Paladine, W., et al.: Intracavitary bleomycin in the management of malignant effusions, Cancer **38**:1903, 1976.
8. Davis, S., et al.: Intrapericardial tetracycline for tamponade secondary to malignant effusions, N. Engl. J. Med. **299**:1113-1114, 1978.
9. Lokich, J. J.: The management of malignant pericardial effusions, J.A.M.A. **224**:1401-1404, 1973.

Electrolyte abnormalities

SIADH and hyponatremia

10. Cadman, E.: Toxicity of chemotherapeutic agents, In Becker, F. F., editor: Cancer, vol. 5, New York, 1977, Plenum Press, section 11.
11. DeFronzo, R. A., et al.: Water intoxication in man after cyclophosphamide therapy: time course and relation to drug activation, Ann. Intern. Med. **78**:861-869, 1973.
12. Weiss, H. D., et al.: Neurotoxicity of commonly used antineoplastic agents, N. Engl. J. Med. **291**:75-81, 127-133, 1974.
13. Robertson, G. L., et al.: Vincristine neurotoxicity and abnormal secretion of antidiuretic hormone, Arch. Intern. Med. **132**:717, 1973.
14. Forrest, J. N., et al.: Superiority of demedocycline over lithium in the treatment of chronic SIADH, N. Engl. J. Med. **298**:173-177, 1978.

15. Bayssas, M., et al.: Phase 2—trial with dimdesin for regression induction in patients with leukemia, Cancer Chemother. Pharmacol. **2**:247-255, 1979.

Hypokalemia

16. O'Regan, S., et al.: Electrolyte and acid-base disturbances in the management of leukemia, Blood **49**:345-353, 1977.
17. Mir, M. A.: Hypokalemia in acute myeloid leukemia, Ann. Intern. Med. **82**:54-57, 1975.
18. Bar, R. S., et al.: Hypomagnesemia, hypocalcemia, secondary to renal magnesium wasting: a possible consequence of high dose gentamicin therapy, Ann. Intern. Med. **82**:646-649, 1975.
19. Klostersky, J., et al.: Carbenicillin and hypokalemia, Ann. Intern. Med. **78**:774-775, 1973.

Hyperkalemia

20. Morse, B. M., et al.: Metabolic complications of aggressive therapy of chronic lymphocytic leukemia, Am. J. Med. Sci. **267**:311-314, 1974.
21. Arseneau, J. C., et al.: Hyperkalemia, a sequel to chemotherapy of Burkitt's lymphoma, Lancet **1**:10, 1973.
22. Fennelly, J. J., et al.: Extreme hyperkalemia due to rapid cell lysis of leukemia cells, Lancet **1**:27, 1974.

Hyperphosphatemia and hypocalcemia

23. Cadman, E. C., et al.: Hyperphosphatemia and hypocalcemia accompanying rapid cell lesions in a patient with Burkitt's lymphoma, Burkitt's cell leukemia, Am. J. Med. **62**:283-290, 1977.
24. Zuzman, J.: Hyperphosphatemia, hyperphosphaturia, and hypocalcemia in acute lymphoblastic leukemia, N. Engl. J. Med. **289**:1335, 1973.

Hypercalcemia

25. Gordon, G. F., et al.: Clinical endocrinology of parathyroid hormone excess, Recent Prog. Horm. Res. **18**:297-336, 1962.
26. Mazzaferri, E. L., et al.: Treatment of hypercalcemia associated with malignancy, Semin. Oncol. **5**:141-151, 1978.
27. Muggia, F. M., et al.: Hypercalcemia associated with neoplastic disease, Ann. Intern. Med. **73**:281-290, 1970.
28. Besarab, A., et al.: Mechanisms of hypercalcemia in malignancy, Cancer **41**: 2276-2285, 1978.

Therapy of CNS metastases

29. Pochedly, C.: Neurotoxicity due to CNS therapy for leukemia, Med. Pediatr. Oncol. **3**:101-115, 1977.
30. Bleyer, W. A.: Clinical pharmacology of intrathecal methotrexate. I. Pharmacokinetics in nontoxic patient after lumbar injection, Cancer Treat. Rep. **61**:703-708, 1977.
31. Bleyer, W. A., et al.: Clinical pharmacology of intrathecal methotrexate. II. An improved dosage regimen derived from age-related pharmacokinetics, Cancer Treat. Rep. **61**:1419-1425, 1977.

32. Bleyer, W. A., et al.: Neurotoxicity and elevated cerebrospinal fluid methotrexate concentration in meningeal leukemia, N. Engl. J. Med. **289:**770-773, 1973.
33. Shapiro, W. R., et al.: Distribution in cerebrospinal fluid and intravenous, intraventricular and lumbar injections, N. Engl. J. Med. **293:**161-166, 1975.

Pain management

34. Goodman, L. S., and Gilman, A.: The pharmacological basis of therapeutics, ed. 5, New York, 1975, Macmillan Publishing Co.
35. Lipman, A. G.: Drug therapy in chronic pain, J. Continuing Educ. Hosp. Clin. Pharm., Feb., 1979.
36. Catalano, R. B.: The medical approach to management of pain caused by cancer, Semin. Oncol. **2:**379-392, 1975.
37. Lewis, B. J.: The use of opiate analgesics in cancer patients, Cancer Treat. Rep. **63:**341-342, 1979.
38. The Brompton Cocktail, Lancet (June 9):1220-1221, 1979.
39. Heel, R. C., et al.: Buprenorphine: a review of its pharmacological properties and therapeutic efficacy, Drugs **17:**81-110, 1979.
40. Dorr, R. T., et al.: Cancer Chemotherapy Manual, New York, 1977, American Elsevier Publishing Co., pp. 64-72.
41. Postoperative Pain, Br. Med. J. **6136:**517-518, 1978.
42. Beaver, W. T.: The pharmacologic basis for the choice of an analgesic, I. Potent analgesics, Pharmacol. Physicians **4:**1-7, 1970.
43. Szeto, H. H., et al.: Accumulation of normeperidine, an active metabolite of meperidine, in patients with renal failure or cancer, Ann. Intern. Med. **86:**738-741, 1977.
44. Effinger, D. S., et al.: Important clinical pharmacologic considerations in the use of methadone in cancer patients, Cancer Treat. Rep. **63:**457-459, 1979.
45. Marks, R. M., et al.: Undertreatment of medical inpatients with narcotic analgesics, Ann. Intern. Med. **78:**173-181, 1973.
46. Mount, B. M., et al.: Use of the Brompton mixture in treating the chronic pain of malignant disease, Can. Med. Assoc. J. **115:**122-124, 1976.
47. Lipman, A. G.: Drug therapy in terminally ill patients, Am. J. Hosp. Pharm. **32:**270-276, 1975.
48. Drug Evaluation: Morphine, Drug Information Analysis Service/Rocky Mountain Drug Consultation Center, University of California, San Francisco, Denver General Hospital, 1979, pp. 1-4.
49. Drug consult Schlessinger's Solution therapy of cancer pain, Drug Information Analysis Service/Drug Consultation Center, University of California, San Francisco, Denver General Hospital, 1979, pp. 1-2.
49a. Halpern, L. M.: Psychotropic, ataractic, and related drugs. In Bonica, J., editor: Advances in Pain Research and Therapy, vol. 2, New York, 1977, Raven Press, pp. 276-283.
49b. Budd, K.: Psychotropic drugs in the treatment of chronic pain, Anaesthesia **33**(6):531-534, 1978.
49c. Seyverth, H. W., et al.: Prostaglandins as mediators of hypercalcemia associated with certain types of cancer, N. Engl. J. Med. **293:**1278, 1975.

Nausea and vomiting

50. Harris, J. G.: Nausea, vomiting and cancer treatment, CA **28**:194-201, 1978.
51. Dorr, et al.: Cancer Chemotherapy Manual, American Elsevier Publishing Co., New York, 1977, pp. 50-57.
52. Israel, L., et al.: Treatment of nausea and vomiting related to anti-cancerous multiple combination chemotherapy: results of two controlled studies, J. Int. Med. Res. **6**:235-240, 1978.
53. Dudrick, S. J.: Summary of the informal discussion of nutritional management, Cancer Res. **37**:2462-2468, 1977.
54. Holland, J., et al.: Psychological aspects of anorexia in cancer patients, Cancer Res. **37**:2425-2428, 1977.
55. Gibbs, D.: Diseases of the alimentary system—nausea and vomiting, Br. Med. J. **2**:1489-1492, 1976.
56. Moertel, C. G., et al.: A controlled clinical evaluation of antiemetic drugs, J.A.M.A. **186**:116-118, 1963.
57. Moertel, C. G., et al.: Controlled clinical studies of orally administered antiemetic drugs, Gastroenterol. **57**:262-268, 1969.
58. Mellencamp, E., et al.: The patient with nausea. III. Cancer pregnancy or surgery, Drug Therapy, June, 1977, pp. 102-112.
59. Mellencamp, E., et al.: The patient with nausea. I. Cancer, Drug Therapy, April, 1977, pp. 28-32.
60. Wood, C. D.: Antimotion sickness and antiemetic drugs, Drugs **17**:471-479, 1979.
61. Crout, J. R.: Trimethobenzamide hydrochloride suppositories, Fed. Register **44**:2021-2022, 1979.
62. Crout, J. R.: Trimethobenzamide hydrochloride injection and capsules, Fed. Register **44**:2017-2071, 1979.
63. Kahn, T., et al.: A single dose of metoclopramide in the control of vomiting from cis-dichlorodiammine-platinum (II) in man, Cancer Treat. Rep. **62**:1106-1107, 1978.
64. Caralps, A.: Metoclopramide and renal failure, Lancet **1**(8115):554, March 10, 1979.
65. Corsini, G. U., et al.: Metoclopramide and dystonic reactions in sardinians, Lancet **1**(8130):1344, June 23, 1979.
66. Pinder, R. M., et al.: Metoclopramide: a review of its pharmacological properties and clinical use, Drugs **12**:81-131, 1976.
67. Herman, T. S., et al.: Superiority of nabilone over prochlorperazine as an antiemetic in patients receiving cancer chemotherapy, N. Engl. J. Med. **300**:1295-1297, 1979.
68. Steele, N., et al.: Double-blind comparison of the antiemetic effects of nabilone and prochlorperazine on chemotherapy-induced emesis, Proc. Am. Soc. Clin. Oncol. **20**:337, 1979.
69. Baker, J. J., et al.: Nabilone as an antiemetic, N. Engl. J. Med. **301**:728, 1979.
70. Sallan, S. E., et al.: Antiemetic effect of delta-9-tetrahydrocannabinol in patients receiving cancer chemotherapy, N. Engl. J. Med. **293**:795-797, 1975.
71. Chang, A. E., et al.: A prospective randomized trial of delta-9-tetrahydrocannabinol (THC) as an antiemetic in patients receiving high dose methotrexate (MTX), Proc. Am. Soc. Clin. Oncol. **20**:377, 1979.

72. TTS scopolamine communication with the manufacturer, Alza, Palo Alto, Calif.
73. Stryker, J. A., et al.: Ibuprofen (Motrin) prophylaxis during pelvic irradiation, Proc. Am. Soc. Clin. Oncol. **20:**294, 1979.
74. Grossman, B., et al.: Droperidol prevents nausea and vomiting from cis-platinum, N. Engl. J. Med. **301:**47, 1979.
75. Reyntieus, A.: Domperidone as an antiemetic; summary of research reports, Postgrad. Med. J. **55**(1):50-54, 1979.
76. Clara, R., et al.: A multicenter pilot study of parenteral and rectal administration of domperidone in the treatment of severe vomiting in children, Postgrad. Med. J. **55**(1):43-44, 1979.
77. Boulanger, M., et al.: Domperidone in the prevention of post-operative nausea and vomiting, Postgrad. Med. J. **55**(1):45-47, 1979.
77a. Sawicka, J., et al.: Transdermal therapeutic system scopolamine: prevention of vomiting associated with cancer chemotherapy, Proc. Am. Soc. Clin. Oncol. **18:**302, 1977.
77b. Israel, L., and Rodary, C.: Treatment of nausea and vomiting related to anticancerous multiple combination chemotherapy, J. Int. Med. Res. **6:**235-240, 1978.

Hyperuricemia

78. Perry, M. C., et al.: Uric acid nephropathy, J.A.M.A. **236:**961-962, 1976.
79. Boss, G. R., et al.: Hyperuricemia and gout, N. Engl. J. Med. **300:**1459-1468, 1979.
80. DeConti, R. C., et al.: Use of allopurinol for preventing and control of hyperuricemia in patients with neoplastic disease, N. Engl. J. Med. **274:**481-486, 1966.
81. Krakoff, I. H.: Use of allopurinol in preventing hyperuricemia in leukemia and lymphoma, Cancer **19:**1489-1496, 1966.
82. Simkin, P. A.: Management of gout, Ann. Intern. Med. **90:**812-816, 1979.
83. Ignoffo, R. J.: Cancer chemotherapy. In Koda-Kimble, M. A., et al., editors: Applied therapeutics for clinical pharmacists, San Francisco, 1978, Applied Therapeutics, Inc.
84. Knoben, J. E., et al.: Handbook of clinical drug data, ed. 4, Hamilton, Ill., 1978, Drug Intelligence Publications, Inc.
85. Dorr, R. T., et al.: Cancer chemotherapy manual, New York, 1977, American Elsevier Publishing Co.

Leucovorin rescue

86. Bertino, J. R.: Rescue techniques in cancer chemotherapy: use of leucovorin and other rescue agents after methotrexate treatment, Semin. Oncol. **4:**203-216, 1977.
87. Tattersall, M., et al.: The pharmacology of methotrexate rescue studies. In Pharmacologic Basis of Cancer Chemotherapy, The Williams & Wilkins Co., Baltimore, 1975, pp. 105-107.
88. Von Hoff, D. D.: "Single" agent activity of high-dose methotrexate with citrovorum factor rescue, Cancer Treat. Rep. **62:**233-235, 1978.
88a. Phase I trial of high-dose methotrexate with modified citrovorum factor rescue, Cancer Treat. Rep. **62:**397-399, 1978.

Extravasations

89. Ignoffo, R. J., et al.: Treatment of local toxicities from cancer chemotherapeutic agents, Cancer Treat. Rev., March, 1980.
90. Rudolph, R., et al.: Skin ulcers due to adriamycin, Cancer **38**:1087-1094, 1976.
91. Reilly, J. J.: Clinical course and management of accidental adriamycin extravasation, Cancer **40**:2053-2056, 1977.

Oral mucositis

92. Dreizen, S.: Somatotoxic manifestations of cancer chemotherapy, J. Prosthet. Dent. **40**:650-655, 1978.
93. Bottomley, W. K., et al.: Antineoplastic agents and their oral manifestations, Oral Surg. **44**:527-533, 1977.
94. Segelman, A. E., et al.: Treatment of oral complications of leukemia, J. Oral Surg. **35**:469-477, 1977.
95. Beck, S.: Impact of a systemic oral care protocol on stomatitis after chemotherapy, Cancer Nurs. **2**:185-199, June, 1979.

Section 8

INFECTIONS IN CANCER PATIENTS: MANAGEMENT AND PREVENTION

Infection is the most frequent serious complication as well as the most frequent cause of death in patients with cancer.[1] Nearly 90% of the deaths are caused by bacteria. Seven major defects in host defenses are responsible for this high incidence (Table 8-1). The first defect, immunosuppression, may be caused by the malignant disease process itself or induced by radiation or chemotherapy. Several diseases are associated with defective cellular immunity, which is responsible for poor antigenic recognition, impaired mobilization of leucocytes, macrophages, and interferon and transfer factor release. These diseases include acute leukemia, lymphoma, multiple myeloma, and primary immunodeficiency states.[5] Humoral immunity, which is related to neutrophil function, is impaired not only by the diseases above but also by the aggressive chemotherapy used as treatment. Splenectomy, occasionally performed in lymphoma or leukemia patients, results in a large decrease in reticuloendothelial phagocytosis. Malnutrition, a frequent sequela in the cachexia of malignancy, results in impaired cellular and humoral immunity. Surgical manipulations, instrumentation, and cancer chemotherapy disrupt mucociliary defenses, resulting in a portal of entry for infectious organisms.

INFECTIONS IN PATIENTS WITH LEUKEMIA

The most frequent types of infection in patients with leukemia are bacteremias, disseminated infection, pneumonia, and soft tissue infections.[1] The most common causes of bacteremia and fungemia in this population are *Escherichia coli, Pseudomonas aeruginosa, Klebsiella* species, and *Candida* species.[6] Disseminated fungal infections are caused primarily by *Aspergillus* and *Candida* species.[3] Pneumonia in these patients is frequently caused by gram-negative bacilli and fungi, particularly *Aspergillus.*[1,2,3,7,8] Soft tissue infections such as cellulitis are predominantly bacterial.

Table 8-1. Predisposing factors to infection in patients with malignancies[2-4]

Immunosuppression
Humoral immunity (immunoglobulins, complement)
Cellular immunity (lymphocyte function)
Neutropenia
Malnutrition
Splenectomy
Surgery
Foreign bodies (catheters, shunts)
Adverse drug reactions

Viral infections are uncommon in patients with leukemia, but can be fatal if dissemination occurs. Of particular importance to this discussion are infections caused by herpesviruses, since effective therapy may be available. Herpesviruses (simplex and zoster) may cause localized or disseminated infection in leukemic patients.[4] Herpes simplex causes oral or genital lesions in the normal host, which may also occur in the compromised host. However, disseminated infection is quite serious and frequently fatal. Herpes zoster (varicella zoster), the cause of chickenpox and "shingles," may cause severe disseminated disease in the immunosuppressed host.

INFECTIONS IN PATIENTS WITH LYMPHOMA

Patients with Hodgkin's disease and non-Hodgkin's lymphomas become susceptible to infection by chemotherapeutic destruction of bone marrow leading to bacterial infection with *Staphylococcus aureus* and gram-negative bacilli.[9] Additionally, localized or disseminated varicella zoster infection is not uncommon in patients with lymphoma.[10] Finally, because of the depressed cellular immunity in such patients, dissemination of tuberculosis and infection with intracellular parasites such as *Listeria monocytogenes* may be anticipated. Splenectomy in these patients may predispose them to severe pneumococcal infection, but this would probably occur only during staging laparotomy for Hodgkin's disease.

INFECTIONS IN PATIENTS WITH SOLID TUMORS

Patients with solid tumors such as adenocarcinomas of the breast, liver, or bowel become susceptible to infection in basically two ways. First, the space-occupying effects of the tumor lead to destruction of normal tissue and obstruction of lumenal organs such as in bowel, biliary, or uteral obstruction where retrograde infection and sepsis is common. Bacterial infections predominate in this situation. Second, the treatment of solid tumors with chemotherapy and radiation not uncommonly produces immunosuppression and neutropenia, and thus any type of infection may occur.

MANAGEMENT OF THE FEBRILE PATIENT WITH CANCER

It is estimated that fever greater than 38.5 C (101 F) that is not drug or blood-product induced is a sign that implies severe infection in approximately 80% of patients with malignancies and neutropenia (<1,000 PMN/mm^3).[1,2] Other common signs of infection usually present in the normal host, such as erythema, tenderness, and pus, may be diminished or absent in these patients due to a suppressed inflammatory response or lack of neutrophils.

Elevated temperature may be due to either infection, underlying malignancy, or an allergic reaction to drugs or blood products. Fever during granulocytopenia appears to be due to infection in 64% to 78% of cases.[1,12] The duration of fever appears to be directly proportional to the degree of granulocytopenia, being more prolonged with severe neutropenia of less than 100/mm^3.[1,12] This suggests that infection is a cause of fever even though it cannot be documented. Evidence for this notion is supported by the fact that many patients with fever of undetermined origin will respond to empiric antimicrobial therapy.

Possible etiologies

Bacterial and fungal infections are the most frequent cause of fever in the neutropenic cancer patient (Table 8-2).[1-3,6-12] The most common bacteria are gram-negative bacilli, predominantly *Klebsiella pneumoniae, E. coli,* and *Pseudomonas aeruginosa.* Infection with a gram-positive organism is less frequent and is usually from *Staphylococcus aureus.* Fungi most frequently identified as pathogens in these patients are *Candida* species and *Aspergillus.* Occasionally, phycomycetes such as the Mucoraceae may be responsible for infection but this is unusual. Fungal infection accounts for very few, if any, of the episodes of *acute* infection in the neutropenic patient. However, *prolonged* undiagnosed fever in the patient with leukemia, lymphoma, or solid tumor may well be due to fungi such as *Candida, Aspergillus,* or *Histoplasma.*[3,13] Unfortunately, most of these infections are documented postmortem. Moreover, infections caused by *Nocardia* species, *Pneumocystis carinii,* herpes simplex, and varicella zoster, although uncommon in the neutropenic patient, should be considered in patients who do not respond to empiric antimicrobial therapy directed at bacteria, and in whom the clinical setting suggests such a diagnosis. The management of these infections is discussed below.

Table 8-2. Infectious etiologies in patients with malignancies

Disease	Organisms
Myeloproliferative disorders (acute leukemia, myeloma)	Gram-negative bacilli Gram-positive cocci Fungi (leukemia) Viruses
Chronic lymphocytic leukemia, lymphomas	Tuberculosis *Salmonella* *Listeria* Viruses
Neutropenia	Gram-negative bacilli Fungi?

Table 8-3. Sites and etiology of infection in neutropenic cancer patients

Infection	Organism
Pharyngitis, esophagitis	*Candida albicans* Gram-negative bacilli *Klebsiella* *Pseudomonas* *E. coli* Herpes simplex
Respiratory tract	Gram-negative bacilli *Staphylococcus aureus* Fungi
Skin, soft tissues	*Staphylococcus aureus* Gram-negative bacilli
Perianal area	Gram-negative bacilli *Bacteroides fragilis* Other anaerobes
Septicemia	Gram-negative bacilli *Staphylococcus aureus*

Diagnostic considerations

Infection can occur in almost any site and can be caused by any organism. However, certain sites of infection are more common than others and are listed in Table 8-3 along with the most common pathogens.

It should be noted that common pathogens in the normal host such as streptococci and *Hemophilus* species are very uncommon in these patients. Also, it is unusual for the neutropenic patient to become acutely infected with an organism that would normally be contained by the cellular immune system (varicella zoster, cryptococcosis, pneumocystosis, toxoplasmosis, salmonellosis, listeriosis, and tuberculosis).[14]

Attempts to arrive at a diagnosis are frustrated by several factors. A poor inflammatory response prevents the development of the usual signs and symptoms of infection. This is especially true in patients who have profound neutropenia (≤100 granulocytes per ml),[14] as noted above. Finally, concurrent and sequential infections with different organisms are not uncommon. For example, patients being treated for a pneumonia may develop a new pulmonary infiltrate with persistent fever.[3] In this difficult situation, the diagnosis may have to be obtained by invasive techniques (biopsy, pneumocentesis).

Empiric therapy

After appropriate cultures of blood, urine, sputum, and other tissues have been obtained, empiric antibiotic therapy is instituted promptly in the febrile neutropenic patient (Table 8-4). The antibiotics should be bacteriocidal and active against the most likely offending organisms, namely gram-negative bacilli. It is probably best to administer these antibiotics by the intravenous route because (1) oral absorption may be erratic in patients who are very ill, and (2) neutropenic patients are often thrombocytopenic, which precludes intramuscular administration. Also, patients who are in septic shock have compromised peripheral blood flow, which would decrease the absorption of drug from oral and intramuscular sites.

SINGLE-DRUG VERSUS COMBINATION THERAPY[15,16]

In planning empiric therapy, single antibiotics with a broad spectrum are desirable but not yet widely available, so current therapy should be initiated with two antibiotics. The most frequently used combinations have included a cephalosporin, an aminoglycoside, an expanded spectrum penicillin, or most recently trimethoprim/sulfamethoxazole (co-trimoxazole).

Both two-drug and three-drug combinations are of equal efficacy, about a 70% to 75% response rate in documented infections. However, two drugs appear to be as effective as three drugs[15,22] when the combination is synergistic against all possible organisms.[23-26] There are some differences in toxicity among the combinations studied. When an aminoglycoside is combined with cephalothin, a greater incidence of nephrotoxicity is observed. When cephalothin is replaced by a newer cephalosporin such as cefazolin,

Table 8-4. Empiric antibiotic regimens

Agent	Dosage	Comments
Gentamicin or Tobramycin	5-6 mg/kg/day	Equally effective against sensitive organisms but tobramycin appears to have less potential for nephrotoxicity
or		
Amikacin	15-20 mg/kg/day	Should either be reserved for documented infection resistant to gentamicin or tobramycin or employed as empiric therapy in those institutions where primary resistance to gentamicin or tobramycin is high (≥10%-15%)
plus		
Carbenicillin	400-500 mg/kg/day	Equally effective against sensitive organism
or		
Ticarcillin	300 mg/kg/day	Since lower dosages of ticarcillin are used, it should be reserved for those patients who cannot tolerate the sodium content of carbenicillin
or		
Cefazolin	50-75 mg/kg/day	Cefazolin combined with an aminoglycoside has not been demonstrated to be more nephrotoxic
or		
Cefamandole	100-150 mg/kg/day	Untested in clinical trials in this setting but should be efficacious; nephrotoxic potential is unknown
or		
Cefoxitin	100-150 mg/kg/day	Less active against *S. aureus*

cefamandole, or cefoxitin, the incidence of nephrotoxicity is not increased over the aminoglycoside alone.[29]

Single agents currently are not recommended for empiric therapy for several reasons. Even when an aminoglycoside is active against a gram-negative organism such as *Pseudomonas* or *Klebsiella* in vitro, it is often nonbactericidal in vivo.[19,21] Carbenicillin or ticarcillin used alone or as the only active agent in a combination remains bactericidal in the neutropenic patient.[18,20,22]

The question of whether the various possible combinations in Table 8-4 would adequately control staphylococci has been posed by several investigators. Despite the absence of penicillinase-resistant penicillin in the various empiric regimens tested, the response of staphylococcal infection to aminoglycosides plus antipseudomonal penicillins is equivalent to those regimens that include a cephalosporin.[18,20] This is not unexpected since nearly all staphylococci are susceptible to clinically achievable levels of carbenicillin or ticarcillin and are uniformly susceptible to the aminoglycoside. Moreover, combinations of aminoglycosides plus carbenicillin or ticarcillin are synergistic in vitro against *S. aureus*.[27]

The appropriate duration of antibiotic therapy when no infectious source can be identified is unknown. Rodriguez and co-workers[36] studied the effects of continuing or discontinuing antibiotic therapy after 4 days in a small number of neutropenic patients with presumed infection who had responded to empiric therapy. Several patients died of infection in the group randomized to discontinue antibiotics on the fourth day. The ability to diagnose infection was the same regardless of continuation of therapy. This suggests that antibiotic therapy should be continued for a longer period of time in those neutropenic patients who respond to empiric therapy. Regarding the length of therapy, Pizzo and co-workers[37] have recently reported the results of a large-scale clinical trial in which antibiotics were either continued or discontinued in persistently neutropenic patients after 7 days of therapy to which the patients had become afebrile. The patients who continued to receive therapy (range 8 to 25 days) until their neutrophil counts were more than 500/mm^3 had no infectious sequelae. However, 40% of the patients randomized to discontinue therapy had infectious sequelae within 2 days. These data suggest that antibiotic therapy should be continued in those patients who respond to therapy even if cultures are negative. It must be emphasized that the search for the infectious etiology should be continued during continued antibiotic therapy.

EFFECT OF NEUTROPHIL COUNT AND EFFICACY OF NEUTROPHIL TRANSFUSIONS

It is well established that the return of bone marrow function during or shortly after the onset of gram-negative infection is associated with a relatively good prognosis. It has also been noted that a rise in neutrophil counts *during therapy* is correlated with a good prognosis; and conversely, a fall in neutrophils during therapy is correlated with a decreased response to treatment. However, the possibility of inadequate antibiotic dosage or suboptimal choice of antibiotics may have contributed to this poor response. Many of these studies do not provide these details.

The role of neutrophil transfusions is unclear. Strauss[35a] has summarized the literature to date and made the following points: (1) Those patients randomized to receive either transfusions or placebo in most cases had failed 48 to 72 hours of appropriate antibiotic therapy and the result was to select patients who were unlikely to have been cured by antibiotics alone. Therefore, the efficacy of transfusions versus placebo in *all* neutropenic patients is unknown. (2) The infections treated were heterogeneous and may not respond uniformly. Conversely, results of treating one type of infection may not apply to all. (3) The antibiotic therapy prior to and during transfusions may not have been optimal. Very little data is provided and the results of the studies published to date cannot be compared in this regard. The conclusions are that certain neutropenic patients with proven infection will benefit from neutrophil transfusions and that this may justify exposing both recipients and donors to the risks and expenses of neutrophil transfusions. However, this therapy should not be indiscriminately given to all neutropenic patients with suspected infection.

PROTECTED ENVIRONMENTS AND PROPHYLACTIC ANTIBIOTICS

A desirable approach to the problem of infection in the cancer patient is to protect them from exogenous and endogenous sources of infection. The total protected environment (protected environment of laminar air flow room or reverse isolation) plus prophylactic antibiotics (usually gentamicin, vancomycin, nystatin) has been shown to decrease the number of days and incidence of severe infection.[58] However, these protective regimens are unpalatable, cumbersome, and expensive as well as psychologically demanding because of isolation. In addition, even with the decrease in the number of days of infection, benefits in terms of remission rate and duration or long-term survival in acute leukemias have not been increased.[58-60]

Nearly all studies utilizing protected environments in leukemia have demonstrated a significant reduction in the incidence of severe infection in adult leukemia patients undergoing remission-induction chemotherapy.[58] Protected patients have 5% to 25% fewer severe infections than control patients. The role of isolation *alone* has not been adequately studied. However, since most infections in the compromised host are secondary to endogenous flora, it would be surprising if isolation and air filtration would have a major impact. The role of prophylactic antibiotics without isolation has been extensively studied, and in prospective controlled trials little benefit has been noted from their use.[58,59] Moreover, it has been noted that the presence of antibiotic-resistant organisms was greater in those patients who received prophylactic antibiotics.

The role of total protected environments in patients with solid tumors, including lymphomas, seems to be similar to that role in acute leukemias. Dosage escalations of chemotherapeutic agents, potentially resulting in improved response rates, were accomplished more often among protected patients. However, no significant differences in response rates or duration of remission were seen as a result of the protected environment with prophylactic antibiotics, despite significant reductions in the incidence of infection.[58,61]

Adverse reactions from nonabsorbable antibiotics are frequent and include nausea, anorexia, and diarrhea, leading to poor compliance. In this regard, Bender and co-workers[63] not only improved the palatability of the preparation by removing the vancomycin component, but decreased the incidence of microbiologically documented, severe gram-negative bacillary infection. Nutritional malabsorption has been reported secondary to the use of oral aminoglycosides.[62] Also, antibiotic therapy appears to decrease absorption of oral methotrexate.

Placebo and trimethoprim/sulfamethoxazole (TMP/SMX) (320 mg/1600 mg) daily have been compared randomly in neutropenic patients with various malignancies.[64] The results indicated that the incidence of bacteremias and urinary tract infections was significantly less in the treated group and that patients were not colonized with *S. aureus, P. aeruginosa,* or *Candida.* No significant side effects were noted other than skin rash in a few patients. Compared to most oral nonabsorbable regimens, TMP/SMX proved palatable and inexpensive. Its efficacy must be confirmed in other large-scale clinical trials.

In summary, the most efficacious and least toxic combination of antimicrobials for empiric therapy in the febrile neutropenic patient appears to be an aminoglycoside, such as gentamicin, tobramycin, or if resistance is a problem, amikacin, plus a semisynthetic penicillin that has antipseudomonal activity, such as carbenicillin or ticarcillin. The value of prophylactic antibiotics, including TMP/SMX, must be examined more carefully before their use can be generally recommended.

Specific therapy in the neutropenic patient

BACTERIAL INFECTION

An important question, however, has yet to be answered. Once an organism has been identified, must combination therapy be continued or can the treatment be tailored to utilize a single bactericidal antibiotic?

Although synergistic combination therapy is the standard of practice, recent studies have utilized single-agent therapy with sisomicin[31] or amikacin[32] given by continuous infusion and both have produced results similar to other trials using combination therapy. It is claimed that failure of single-agent gentamicin in early trials was due to inadequate dosage with subtherapeutic serum concentrations.[32] Some evidence exists for the potential use of single agents rather than combinations. Bodey[33] and the EORTC group[20] reported a response rate for carbenicillin and a cephalosporin alone was equivalent to combinations, even in infections resistant to the cephalosporin. Issel and co-workers,[34] using continuous infusion tobramycin with carbenicillin, demonstrated that results were no different if the organism treated was sensitive to one or both drugs, indicating the importance of adequate aminoglycoside serum concentrations. Therefore, it does not seem unreasonable to suggest that antibiotic therapy may be tailored to a single agent once an etiologic organism has been identified. However, large-scale trials are needed to confirm these impressions.

Specific antibiotic therapy (Table 8-5) may differ among institutions because sensitivity patterns differ; but gentamicin, tobramycin, or amikacin should provide the broadest spectrum of gram-negative coverage.

Antibiotics. Gentamicin and tobramycin should be used in doses of at least 5 to 6 mg/kg/day and perhaps higher. Amikacin dosage should be 15 to 20 mg/kg/day. Continuous infusions to maintain serum levels of these drugs in the "therapeutic" range necessitate larger daily dosages, and comparative toxicity studies have not been done to determine any difference in ototoxicity or nephrotoxicity of aminoglycoside given by rapid or continuous infusion. We recommend the rapid infusion technique because it avoids logistic problems in drug administration.

Carbenicillin or ticarcillin used in daily dosages of 450 to 500 mg/kg and 300 mg/kg respectively should provide adequate therapy for most gram-negative rods with the exception of *Klebsiella*. The emergence of resistance during therapy reported in early trials was probably related to inadequate dosage.

Table 8-5. Specific antibiotic therapy

Type of organisms	Antibiotic(s)	Daily dosage	Comments
Gram-positive organisms			
Staphylococcus aureus	Nafcillin	100-150 mg/kg	Less toxic than methicillin, bactericidal
	or		
	Cefazolin	50-75 mg/kg	Bactericidal
	or		
	Vancomycin	20 mg/kg	Bactericidal
Streptococcus faecalis	Penicillin G	200,000 U/kg	Bactericidal only with combination
	or		
	Ampicillin	100-150 mg/kg	Unusual infection in neutropenic patients
	or		
	Vancomycin	20 mg/kg	Neutropenia
	plus		
	Gentamicin or tobramycin	4-5 mg/kg	Urinary tract infection will respond to a penicillin alone
Listeria monocytogenes	Ampicillin	100-150 mg/kg	A penicillin alone may be only bacteriostatic
	plus		
	Gentamicin or tobramycin	5-6 mg/kg	
	or		
	Chloramphenicol	30-50 mg/kg	

Continued.

Table 8-5. Specific antibiotic therapy—cont'd

Type of organisms	Antibiotic(s)	Daily dosage	Comments
Gram-negative organisms			
Escherichia coli *Proteus mirabilis*	Ampicillin or Cefazolin or Cefamandole or cefoxitin	100-150 mg/kg 50-75 mg/kg 100-150 mg/kg	Little evidence that combination of antibiotics is more effective; all choices are bactericidal
Klebsiella pneumoniae	Cefazolin or Cefamandole or cefoxitin *plus* Gentamicin or tobramycin or Amikacin	50-75 mg/kg 100-150 mg/kg 5-6 mg/kg 15-20 mg/kg	Synergistic combination may be more effective, but strong evidence is lacking; may be nephrotoxic
Pseudomonas aeruginosa	Gentamicin or tobramicin or Amikacin *plus* Carbenicillin or Ticarcillin	5-6 mg/kg 15-20 mg/kg 400-500 mg/kg 300 mg/kg	Synergistic combination probably more effective; choice of agents depends upon susceptibility of isolate
Proteus (indole positive) *(P. vulgaris, P. morgani, P. rettgiri)*	Gentamicin or tobramycin or Amikacin or Cefamandale or cefoxitin	5-6 mg/kg 15-20 mg/kg 100-150 mg/kg	Little evidence that synergistic combinations are more effective; all choices are bactericidal
Enterobacteriaceae species	Gentamicin or tobramycin or Amikacin or Cefamandole	5-6 mg/kg 15-20 mg/kg 100-150 mg/kg	Same
Bacteroides fragilis	Carbenicillin or ticarcillin or Metronidazole or Clindamycin	400-500 mg/kg 25-30 mg/kg 30-40 mg/kg	Metronidazole is investigational parenterally; clindamycin may be only bacteriostatic

The cephalosporins, cephalothin, cephapirin, or cefazolin, provide adequate treatment for infections caused by *E. coli, Proteus mirabilis,* and some strains of *Klebsiella.* The newer cephalosporins, cefamandole and cefoxitin, have a wider spectrum of activity and are effective in the above infections plus those caused by indole-positive *Proteus* species, Enterobacter, and some strains of *Serratia marcescens.* These new drugs are also bactericidal as single agents.

In contrast, chloramphenicol and tetracycline are not appropriate agents for the treatment of aerobic gram-negative bacillary infection because they are not bactericidal or synergistic with other antibiotics. Response rates, especially for septicemia, are lower than those for "synergistic" combinations.[34a]

Finally, trimethoprim/sulfamethoxazole as a fixed combination has been utilized in the infected neutropenic patients and has been found to be efficacious in serious gram-negative infection.[35] Adequate dosage would be trimethoprim 10 mg/kg with sulfamethoxazole 50 mg/kg given in 2 to 3 divided doses daily.

FUNGAL INFECTIONS

As mentioned above, the most frequently encountered fungal infections in this setting are due to *Candida albicans, Cryptococcus neoformans, Aspergillus* species, and the phycomycetes. There are two reliable criteria for the diagnosis of invasive fungal infection: (1) the demonstration of the fungus in otherwise viable tissue and (2) positive culture from cerebral spinal fluid or other body fluid (excluding blood and urine) where the fungus is never normally present.[3,6,7] The specific treatment for the fungal infection depends upon the severity of the illness, the organism involved, and the site of the infection. This will range from topical nystatin for mucocutaneous candidiasis to intravenous amphotericin B for invasive fungal disease.

General principles of amphotericin B therapy. Amphotericin B should be dissolved in *sterile water only* and then further diluted in 250 to 500 ml of 5% dextrose solution and infused over 4 to 6 hours each day. In critically ill patients the dosage of amphotericin B may be escalated to 0.25 mg/kg within the first 24 to 36 hours after administration of a test dose of 1 mg. Thereafter, dosage may be increased to 0.5 to 0.75 mg/kg over the next several days as tolerated. This gradual increase in dosage may help to minimize the acute constitutional side effects such as headache, fever, chills, nausea, and vomiting as well as to decrease the incidence and severity of nephrotoxicity due to the drug. Management of side effects is discussed below. Fungal infection in the central nervous system generally requires intrathecal or intraventricular amphotericin B (0.1 to 0.5 mg/day). Daily intravenous dosage of 0.5 to 0.75 mg/kg is continued until the patient has improved, then long-term thrice-weekly dosage is instituted until the dosage or duration has been reached.

Candidiasis. Oropharyngeal candidiasis is one of the most common fungal infections in cancer patients and frequently prevents the patient from taking adequate nutrition because of discomfort. Local infection will usually respond to topically applied antifungal agents such as nystatin, miconazale, or clotrimazole.[38] These agents are generally applied 3 to 6 times daily. Nystatin suspension used as mouthwash in dosage of 500,000 to 1,000,000 U swished in the mouth every 3 to 6 hours may be effective. Perhaps more effective are nystatin troches (vaginal tablets), which are allowed to dissolve in the mouth (1 or 2 every 3 to 6 hours). These provide more prolonged contact time than a suspension. Alternatively, a more palatable preparation might be nystatin "popsicles," which are frozen flavored dilutions of nystatin suspension with 500,000 U in 30 ml.

Invasive local candidiasis can occur in one or many organs after hematogenous dissemination. Deeper oropharyngeal tissue involvement and esophageal candidiasis may require intravenous amphotericin B in low dosage as described by Medoff and co-workers.[39] Dosages of intravenous amphotericin B as low as 10 to 15 mg/day for 10 to 14 days have been used in several patients with esophageal candidiasis refractory to topical therapy. The results have been most promising, with minimal to no toxicity.

Systemic candidiasis is frequently suspected but often undiagnosed in patients with cancer. The treatment requires intravenous amphotericin B alone or in combination with flucytosine. *Candida* is especially susceptible to amphotericin B and high daily dosages are generally not necessary. Doses of amphotericin B of 0.5 mg/kg/day should be adequate to treat most cases of disseminated infection.[40] The duration of therapy or total dosage for the treatment of disseminated candidiasis is unknown.

The value of the addition of flucytosine to this therapy is unknown. It should not be used alone. Flucytosine may be of benefit in candidal urinary tract infection because of its high renal clearance. In sepsis, however, the in vitro synergy between amphotericin B and flucytosine is not uniform and the bone marrow toxicity of flucytosine may be a relative contraindication in the cancer patient.

Intravenous miconazole is also available for the treatment of fungal infection.[41] However, the experience with this agent in the treatment of serious candidal infection has been less than promising and cannot be recommended unless therapy with amphotericin B is impossible.

Cryptococcosis. Disseminated cryptococcal infection may occur in normal as well as immunosuppressed hosts. Cancer patients who are prone to develop this disease are those with lymphoma or chronic lymphocytic leukemia.[37] Especially feared is the development of cryptococcal meningitis, which is cured in only 50% to 60% of the cases by amphotericin B. Therapy should consist of intravenous amphotericin B (intrathecal administration is generally not necessary in this disease) plus flucytosine 150 mg/kg/day. This infection responds more rapidly to the combination, and the duration of treatment may be shortened. In a recent clinical trial the combination proved to be somewhat more effective in achieving cure as well as in preventing relapse.[46]

Aspergillosis. Significant infections due to *Aspergillus* species are generally disseminated and usually involve the respiratory tract. The clinical presentation of aspergillosis is frequently evasive. The infection may manifest as bronchopneumonia, lung abscess, or empyema.[42] Invasive procedures such as bronchial or open lung biopsy are necessary for diagnosis since sputum culture and serologies are of questionable diagnostic value.[42]

Again, intravenous amphotericin B is standard therapy for invasive infection. However, the organism is relatively resistant in vitro and response rates are only 20% to 30%.[42-44] Flucytosine and miconazole are of little value. Early diagnosis, utilizing transtracheal aspiration or transbronchial biopsy, and early treatment appear to improve the general prognosis of disseminated aspergillosis which is nearly uniformly fatal.[43]

In the leukemic patient nasal cultures that grow *Aspergillus* species should alert the clinician to carefully follow the patient and consider invasive procedures for the definitive diagnosis of aspergillosis.[44] The duration of amphotericin B therapy is unknown, but total dosage should be 1.5 to 2.0 grams.

Mucormycosis (phycomycosis). This infection, which primarily involves the head and neck and extends from the sinuses, is increasing in frequency in the immunosuppressed patient, especially with diabetes mellitus.[42] Clinical signs of mucormycosis are similar to those of aspergillosis. As with aspergillosis the treatment of this disease is difficult because the organisms are relatively insensitive to amphotericin B and are completely resistant to flucytosine. Miconazole has not been tested in this disease. Surgical intervention to excise infected tissue is nearly always necessary to produce clinical improvement.

Histoplasmosis. It should be emphasized that histoplasmosis is a regional illness usually confined to residents of Southeastern United States, the Mississippi Valley, and the Ohio River Valley. Permanent residents west of the Rocky Mountains generally do not acquire histoplasmosis.

Disseminated histoplasmosis occurs in immunocompromised hosts, predominantly in patients with Hodgkin's disease and acute and chronic lymphocytic leukemias.[45] The lungs and reticuloendothelial organs are primarily involved. The response to amphotericin B therapy is good if early diagnosis is made and a full course of treatment (>1 gram total dose) can be administered. Flucytosine has little or no activity, and miconazole has not been tested.

MISCELLANEOUS INFECTIONS

Nocardiosis. Infection with this microorganism, which is neither a bacterium nor a fungus, has been associated with intrinsic immunologic disorders and steroid therapy.[47] The primary sites of infection are the lungs, brain, and skin in all of which the organism tends to form abscesses. Diagnosis is made by culture of the organism from appropriate tissues or fluids, or by morphologic identification in stained tissue sections. The mycelia of *Nocardia asteroides* are acid fast and appear as gram-positive branching, filamentous forms. Over the years, early treatment with sulfonamides has been very effective therapy. The dosage of sulfisoxazole or sulfadiazine is 100 to 150 mg/kg/day given orally or intravenously. Therapy is continued for prolonged durations, generally 6 to 9 months or more. Other agents that may be useful include ampicillin, erythromycin, cycloserine, rifampin, and amikacin. These are generally used in combinations of two agents. In vitro evidence suggests that the trimethoprim/sulfamethoxazole combination may be effective, and limited clinical trials have borne this out.[48] However, the dosage for the combination is unclear, and the optimal ratio of each component is unknown. Generally, trimethoprim 10 mg/kg/day and sulfamethoxazole 50 mg/kg/day are recommended.

Pneumocystis carinii infections. A number of protozoan or helminth infections have been described in the immunosuppressed host. The most prevalent and serious is *Pneumocystis carinii* interstitial pneumonitis which occurs predominantly in patients who have received chronic corticosteroid therapy or who suffer from lymphoproliferative disorders.[49] Clinical manifestations are tachypnea, cyanosis, and bilateral diffuse pneumonitis on chest x ray. Complement-fixing antibody tests of serum have been tested in diagnosis, but the results are not helpful since many children and adults without the disease will have high titers of antibody.[49]

The disease is only diagnosed by obtaining samples of lung tissue by pneumocentesis, bronchoscopy, or open biopsy and by staining techniques.

If left untreated, pneumocystosis is uniformly fatal. Pentamidine isethionate has been the mainstay of therapy for many years. Significant toxicity to kidneys, bone marrow, and liver as well as severe local reactions, have prompted the search for a less toxic alternative. Dosages of trimethoprim/sulfamethoxazole (TMP/SMX) 20/100 mg/kg/day given by mouth or intravenously has been compared to pentamidine.[50,51] The results indicate that TMP/SMX is as effective as pentamidine (70% cure rate) and significantly less toxic. In the animal model the combination of TMP/SMX and pentamidine has been found to be no more effective than TMP/SMX alone.[52]

Because *Pneumocytis* has been a prevalent infecting organism in childhood leukemia, prophylactic therapy with low doses of TMP/SMX (320/1600 mg daily) has been studied and reported to substantially decrease its occurrence.[53]

Herpes zoster infection (varicella zoster). Cancer patients with Hodgkin's disease and other lymphomas are particularly susceptible to viral infections.[54] Characteristic manifestations of primary infection with varicella zoster virus are those of chicken pox. A maculopapular eruption on the trunk spreads centrifugally. Papules progress to vesicles, which crust, then scab, and go on to heal. Shingles occurs exclusively in patients who have had previous varicella zoster virus infection. This is manifested as localized pain for a variable period of time before the development of the classic eruption in a dermatomal distribution. In the immunosuppressed host dissemination may occur in as many as 25% of patients, producing lesions in the gastrointestinal tract, myocardium, lungs, and brain. Predisposing factors appear to be local irradiation, local tumor, and advanced stages of malignancy.[54] Mortality is low (≤5%) even with disseminated disease but morbidity is not infrequent. Postherpetic neuralgia may be more frequent in the immunosuppressed.

Varicella zoster infection may be prevented in patients exposed to the disease if zoster immune globulin[54] or zoster immune plasma[55] are administered with 72 hours of exposure. This passive immunity is of no value in the treatment of established infection.[55] Adenine arabinoside (vidarabine) has been tested in localized or disseminated zoster and was shown to accelerate clearing of virus from vesicles and cessation of new vesicle formation.[56] Toxicity was minimal. It is most effective when administered within the first week of infection. The dosage is 10 mg/kg/day given as a single intravenous infusion.

Finally, human leukocyte interferon appears to be highly effective in preventing dissemination of zoster and in reducing pain and the incidence of visceral complications and postherpetic neuralgia.[57] Unfortunately, this treatment is extremely expensive and not widely available.

DOSAGE REGIMENS IN RENAL INSUFFICIENCY

The following are brief descriptions of the pharmacology and pertinent pharmacokinetics of those antibiotics commonly used in the cancer patient. Several drugs require dosage adjustment in the presence of renal or hepatic

Table 8-6. Antimicrobial agents that do not require dosage adjustment in renal and hepatic failure

Amphotericin B	Erythromycin	Oxacillin
Chloramphenical	Isoniazid	Pentamidine
Clindamycin	Miconazole	Rifampin
Cloxacillin	Nafcillin	Vidarabine

insufficiency. Table 8-6 lists those antimicrobial agents for which no dosage adjustment is necessary.

Dosage adjustment is usually based upon the best measure of renal function, creatinine clearance. Actual measurement of endogenous creatinine clearance (Ccr) is preferable to estimates. However, if renal function is stable and an estimate of Ccr is needed, one may use the following equation:

$$\text{Ccr male} = \frac{140 - \text{age}}{\text{Crs}} \qquad \text{Ccr female} = 0.85 \text{ Ccr male}$$

In patients with severe renal failure or if renal function is changing, serum levels of aminoglycosides, vancomycin, and flucytosine should be obtained to assist in designing dosage regimens.

It should also be emphasized that loading doses of antibiotic need not be changed. It is only the subsequent maintenance dosages that need to be reduced.

Penicillins

Penicillin G. Although the penicillins are generally nontoxic, excessive accumulation in renal failure may lead to CNS irritation and convulsions. A useful method for adjusting dosage of penicillin G has been described by Bryan and Stone[65]: Maximum daily dosage (million units) = 3.2 + Ccr/7. Patients who are anuric with concomitant hepatic failure should receive 500,000 every 8 hours.

Ampicillin. The considerations for ampicillin are similar to penicillin G. The following guidelines are suggested for dosage:

Ccr	Fraction of normal dose
>50 ml/min	1.0
25-50 ml/min	0.75
10-25 ml/min	0.5
<10 ml/min	0.25

Carbenicillin. Excessive dosages of carbenicillin or ticarcillin may lead not only to CNS irritation but to severe hypokalemia and bleeding diatheses. The following guidelines have been adapted from Hoffman and co-workers[66]:

Ccr	Fraction of normal dose
>30 ml/min	0.8-1.0
20-30 ml/min	0.4-0.75
10-20 ml/min	0.20-0.40
<10 ml/min	0.15
<10 ml/min plus hepatic failure	0.075

Cephalosporins

Cephapirin and cephalothin. Cephalosporins are relatively nontoxic. Both of these agents are partially metabolized to biologically active desacetyl metabolites. The dosage schedule for ampicillin may be used.

Cefazolin, cefamandole, and cefoxitin. Although these three agents are essentially devoid of dose-related toxicities, excessive accumulation may occur in severe renal insufficiency, possibly leading to central nervous system toxicity. Moreover, excessive serum levels are not known to be more efficacious than those usually achieved. Although the pharmacology of these agents is somewhat different, their dosage modification is the same.

Ccr	Fraction of normal dose
>50 ml/min	1.0
25-50 ml/min	0.5
15-25 ml/min	0.25
≤10-15 ml/min	0.125

Aminoglycosides

Gentamicin, tobramycin, kanamycin, and amikacin. These agents all have similar pharmacology. They possess dose-related toxicity, and significant adjustments for renal insufficiency should be made. The most useful guide for modifying aminoglycoside dosage has been published by Sarubbi and Hull[67] (Table 8-7).

Tetracyclines

Tetracyclines, with the exception of doxycycline, should probably not be used since accumulation in renal insufficiency occurs and subsequent antianabolic effects may lead to worsening of renal function. Doxycycline dosage need not be adjusted for renal failure.

Sulfonamides

Sulfonamides/trimethoprim (co-trimoxazole). Most sulfonamides are primarily metabolized. More soluble agents such as sulfisoxazole and sulfamethoxazole are excreted approximately 50% unchanged. Thus, dosage adjustment, 50% of a normal dose, is required only when Ccr <10 ml/min. Similarly, trimethoprim is partially metabolized but may accumulate in

Table 8-7. Aminoglycoside dosing*

1. Select loading dose in mg/kg (ideal weight) to provide peak serum levels in range listed below for desired aminoglycoside.

Aminoglycoside	Usual loading doses	Expected peak serum levels
Tobramycin, Gentamicin	1.5 to 2.0 mg/kg	4 to 10 μg/ml
Amikacin, Kanamycin	5.0 to 7.5 mg/kg	15 to 30 μg/ml

2. Select maintenance dose (as percentage of chosen loading dose) to continue peak serum levels indicated above according to desired dosing interval and the patient's corrected creatinine clearance†

PERCENTAGE OF LOADING DOSE REQUIRED FOR DOSAGE INTERVAL SELECTED

C(c)cr (ml/min)	Half life‡ (hrs)	8 hrs	12 hrs	24 hrs
90	3.1	84%	—	—
80	3.4	80	91%	—
70	3.9	76	88	—
60	4.5	71	84	—
50	5.3	65	79	—
40	6.5	57	72	92%
30	8.4	48	63	86
25	9.9	43	57	81
20	11.9	37	50	75
17	13.6	33	46	70
15	15.1	31	42	67
12	17.9	27	37	61
10§	20.4	24	34	56
7	25.9	19	28	47
5	31.5	16	23	41
2	46.8	11	16	30
0	69.3	8	11	21

*From Sarubbi, F. A., and Hull, J. H.: Ann. Intern. Med. **89**:617, 1978.

†Calculate corrected creatinine clearance, C(c)cr, as:

C(c)cr male = 140 − age/serum creatinine

C(c)cr female = 0.85 × C(c)cr male

‡Alternatively, one half of the chosen loading dose may be given at an interval approximately equal to the estimated half life.

§Dosing for patients with C(c)cr ≤10 ml/min should be assisted by measured serum levels.

renal failure, potentially producing bone marrow suppression if given in high dosage. The dosage of co-trimoxazole for urinary tract infection or bacterial gastroenteritis need not be reduced. However, when higher doses of TMP/SMX are used to treat gram-negative infection (10/50 mg/kg/day) or pneumocystosis (20/100 mg/kg/day), doses may be adjusted according to the following guidelines:

Ccr	Fraction of normal dose
≥40 ml/min	0.75-1.0
20-40 ml/min	0.65
10-20 ml/min	0.50
<10 ml/min	0.25

Miscellaneous

Flucytosine. This agent is nearly entirely excreted unchanged and accumulates significantly in renal insufficiency leading to bone marrow suppression. Schonebeck and co-workers[68] designed a useful regimen for dosage adjustment, but serum levels should be followed whenever possible.

Ccr	Fraction of normal dose
≥40 ml/min	0.75-1.0
20-40 ml/min	0.5
10-20 ml/min	0.25
5-10 ml/min	0.125
<5 ml/min	0.06

Vancomycin. This antibiotic accumulates to the greatest extent. The half-life in anuria may be as long as 7 days or more. No dosage nomograms have been developed, and serum levels should always be done to avoid accumulation, which may lead to ototoxicity. The easiest regimen to follow would be to estimate the half-life of the drug by taking two or more serum levels and plotting the points on a concentration-time graph. After administration of a loading dose (10 mg/kg), one-half of the loading dose (5 mg/kg) may be given at an interval equal to one half-life.

ANTIBIOTIC-INDUCED PROBLEMS IN CANCER PATIENTS

Adverse reactions to antibiotics are relatively uncommon and can generally be broken down into two categories (1) those induced directly by the antibiotic and (2) those produced by the combined effect of the antibiotic and another drug.

However, it is difficult to distinguish the direct toxic effects of antimicrobials. For example, hypovolemia and shock secondary to sepsis have as much to do with the development of acute tubular necrosis as to concomitant aminoglycosides.[69] Preexistent renal dysfunction or prior aminoglycoside use is felt to predispose to vestibular and auditory toxicity induced by aminoglycosides.[70] The potential for development of respiratory compromise because of aminoglycoside (neuromuscular blockade) is probably only important if the drugs are given intraperitoneally in the presence of renal failure, during surgical procedures, while the patient is paralyzed with a neuromuscular blocking agent. Finally, the development of bone marrow

Table 8-8. Common antibiotic adverse reactions and interactions in cancer patients

Drug	Reaction	Interaction	Comments
Aminoglycosides	Nephrotoxicity	Cephalothin Cisplatin Diuretics?	Has not been shown with cefazolin plus amikacin
	Ototoxicity	Furosemide Ethacrynic acid	Probably related to total dose of drug; diuretic may simply produce volume contraction → ↑ serum levels
Carbenicillin, ticarcillin	Hypokalemia	Aminoglycosides	May induce tubular defect with potassium and calcium wasting; as much as 300 mEq of K^+ lost/day
	Bleeding diatheses		Inhibition of platelet aggregation; clinical significance is unclear
Cephalosporins	Nephrotoxicity	Gentamicin, tobramycin	Cephalothin

suppression from the administration of trimethoprim is generally only seen in patients who are folate depleted at the outset.[71]

Table 8-8 lists common adverse reactions to antimicrobial agents that might be anticipated in the patient with cancer. The list is organized by organ system and attempts to list the most common agents causing the reaction as well as an estimated incidence. Additionally, comments regarding predisposing factors or the role of other drugs in the development of the reaction are included in Table 8-9.

DRUG INTERACTIONS (Table 8-10)

Penicillins plus aminoglycosides—penicillin G, carbenicillin, ticarcillin, and ampicillin—have all been shown to produce significant inactivation of gentamicin or tobramycin when mixed in solution. The mechanism is a chemical interaction of an amino group disrupting the beta-lactam ring structure, and thus inactivating both agents. This reaction is concentration and time dependent and may also occur in vivo if these agents are given in combination to patients with renal insufficiency. Another implication of this interaction is that aminoglycoside concentrations may be falsely low in patient's serum that has not been assayed within several hours but rather has been left for days. Amikacin is more resistant to this inactivation. To date, however, there is no evidence that this reaction is clinically significant.

Table 8-9. Antimicrobial adverse reactions in patients with malignancies

Reaction	Clinical manifestations	Antibiotic	Incidence	Comments
Electrolyte disturbance	Hypokalemia	Carbenicillin, ticarcillin	30%-50%	Ticarcillin may produce lower incidence due to lower dosage[72]
		Amphotericin B	>50%	Probably not dose related; consider use of $KHCO_3$ if RTA present[73]
	Hypocalcemia	Aminoglycosides		Only documented with gentamicin
	Hypomagnesemia	Aminoglycosides	<10%	Only apparent after 10-14 days of therapy[74]
		Amphotericin B	<10%	Only apparent after 10-14 days of therapy[74]
Renal dysfunction	Decreased GFR	Aminoglycosides	<10%	Probably related to total dose and duration[75]
		Aminoglycosides + cephalothin	10%-20%	Synergistic toxicity questionable[69,70,76]
		Amphotericin B	>50%	Dose and duration related; irreversible toxicity only after 4-5 grams total dose[73,77]
		Polymyxin B, colistin	≥50%	Not recommended due to lack of clinical correlations with toxicity
	Interstitial nephritis	Methicillin	10%-15%	Much less frequent with oxacillin or nafcillin[78]
	Renal tubular acidosis	Amphotericin B	10%-30%	Probably related to total dose and duration of therapy[73,77]
Hepatic dysfunction	Hepatocellular damage	Oxacillin	<1%	
		Flucytosine	<1%	Probably idiosyncratic
		Isoniazid	1%-3%	Age related[79,80]
	Cholestasis	Rifampin	≤1%	Transient in most cases[80]

Continued.

Table 8-9. Antimicrobial adverse reactions in patients with malignancies—cont'd

Reaction	Clinical manifestations	Antibiotic	Incidence	Comments
Neurological dysfunction	Altered mental status, seizures	Penicillins	NA	Common if very high doses are used in presence of renal insufficiency
	Peripheral neuropathies	Isoniazid	<1%	Infrequent at daily doses <5 mg/kg; incidence may reach 10%-20% at higher doses
		Metronidazole	?	Dose and duration related
	Neuromuscular blockade	Aminoglycosides	?	Important only if antibiotics are given by peritoneal lavage, especially in presence of renal failure[75]
	Auditory damage	Aminoglycosides		Dose and duration related
	Vestibular damage	Vancomycin		
Hematologic dysfunction	Leukopenia	Nafcillin	10%-20%	Doses of 8-12 g/day for duration of 10-14 days or more[81]
		Trimethoprim	?	
	Agranulocytosis	Flucytosine	?	Probably related to excessive dose in renal insufficiency[82]
	Thrombocytopenia	Sulfonamides	?	
	Bleeding diathesis	Carbenicillin, ticarcillin	?	Possibly related to effect of inhibition of platelet aggregation[83]
	Anemia	Amphotericin B	30%-50%	Probably related to suppression of erythropoietin[84]
Gastrointestinal dysfunction	Pseudomembranous colitis	Clindamycin, penicillins	1%	Associated with overgrowth of *Clostridium* species producing enterotoxin[85]

Table 8-10. Antimicrobial drug interactions

Antibiotics	Interaction	Significance
Penicillins plus aminoglycosides	Chemical binding of two molecules and inactivation of aminoglycoside	Has not been demonstrated to be clinically significant; important in interpreting serum levels of aminoglycoside in patients with renal failure
Ampicillin plus allopurinal	Increased incidence of rash	Mechanism unknown; probably enhanced hypersensitivity
Trimethoprim plus methotrexate	Enhanced bone marrow suppression	Not proven clinically; but exercise caution nonetheless
Chloramphenicol, isoniazid plus phenytoin, warfarin	Inhibition of phenytoin metabolism	Phenytoin toxicity due to accumulation

Ampicillin plus allopurinol

The administration of these two agents simultaneously has been reported to increase the incidence of dermatologic reaction three-fold. Perhaps this is because allopurinol potentiates drug allergy.[86]

Combinations of folate inhibitors

The administration of trimethoprim or pyrimethamine to patients who are also receiving methotrexate may produce severe folate-deficient bone marrow suppression and pancytopenia. There is little clinical evidence to support this supposition, but this might be significant in patients given moderate doses of methotrexate *without* concurrent citrovorum factor "rescue."

Inhibition of phenytoin or warfarin metabolism

Antimicrobials such as isoniazid or chloramphenicol are metabolic inhibitors via blockage of protein synthesis. The result of this is decreased metabolism of drugs that are highly dependent upon inactivation or degradation for elimination. Enhanced serum concentrations of phenytoin and excessive anticoagulant effects may occur and must be carefully monitored during concomitant therapy.[87]

REFERENCES

1. Ketchel, S. J., and Rodriquez, V.: Acute infections in cancer patients, Sem. Oncol. **5**:167-179, June, 1978.
2. Valdivieso, M.: Bacterial infection in haematological diseases, Clin. Haematol. **5**:229-248, June, 1976.

3. Krick, J. A., and Remington, J. S.: Opportunistic invasive fungal infections in patients with leukemia and lymphoma, Clin. Haematol. **5**:249-310, June, 1976.
4. Feldman, S., and Cox, F.: Viral infections and haematological malignancies, Clin. Haematol. **5**:311-328, June, 1976.
5. Neu, H. C.: The role of cellular and humoral factors in infections, Clin. Haematol. **5**:449-466, June, 1976.
6. Singer, C., et al.: Bacteremia and fungemia complicating neoplastic disease: a study of 364 cases, Am. J. Med. **62**:731-742, May, 1977.
7. Hart, P. D., et al.: The compromised host and infection. II. Deep fungal infection, J. Infect. Dis. **120**:169-191, August, 1969.
8. Williams, D. M., et al.: Pulmonary infection in the compromised host. I and II, Am. Rev. Respir. Dis. **114**:359-394, 593-627, August-September, 1976.
9. Feld, R., and Bodey, G. P.: Infections in patients with malignant lymphoma treated with combination chemotherapy, Cancer **39**:1018-1025, March, 1977.
10. Schimpff, S. C., et al.: Infections in 92 splenectomized patients with Hodgkin's disease, Am. J. Med. **59**:695-701, November, 1975.
11. Weitzman, S., and Aisenberg, A. C.: Fulminant sepsis after the successful treatment of Hodgkin's disease, Am. J. Med. **62**:47-50, January, 1977.
12. Gurwith, M. J., et al.: Granulocytopenia in hospitalized patients: prognostic factors and etiology of fever, Am. J. Med. **64**:121-126, January, 1978.
13. Luft, F. C., et al.: Infections or neoplasm as causes of prolonged fever in cancer patients, Am. J. Med. Sci. **272**:65-74, July-August, 1976.
14. Schimpff, S. C.: Infection in patients with granulocytopenia, Med. Clin. North Am. **61**:1101-1118, September, 1977.
15. Schimpff, S. C., and Aisner, J.: Empiric antibiotic therapy, Cancer Treat. Rep. **62**:673-679, May, 1978.
16. Hopefl, A. W.: Empiric therapy of febrile granulocytopenic patients, Am. J. Hosp. Pharm. **36**:178-187, February, 1979.
17. Bodey, G. P., et al.: Infections in cancer patients: results with gentamicin sulfate therapy, Cancer **29**:1697-1701, 1972.
18. Klastersky, J., et al.: Empiric therapy for cancer patients: comparative study of ticarcillin-tobramycin, ticarcillin-cephalothin, and cephalothin-tobramycin, Antimicrob. Agents Chemother. **7**:640-645, May, 1975.
19. Klastersky, J., et al.: Therapy with carbenicillin and gentamicin for patients with cancer and severe infections caused by gram-negative rods, Cancer **31**: 331-336, February, 1973.
20. EORTC International Antimicrobial Therapy Project Group: Three antibiotic regimens in the treatment of infection in febrile granulocytopenic patients with cancer, J. Infect. Dis. **137**:14-29, January, 1978.
21. Murillo, J., et al.: Comparison of serum bactericidal activity among three antimicrobial combinations, Antimicrob. Agents Chemother. **13**:992-996, June, 1978.
22. Klastersky, J., et al.: Gram-negative infections in cancer: study of empiric therapy comparing carbenicillin-cephalothin with and without gentamicin, J.A.M.A. **227**:45-48, January, 1974.
23. Klastersky, J., et al.: Comparative effectiveness of combinations of amikacin with penicillin G and amikacin with carbenicillin in gram negative septicemia: double blind clinical trial, J. Infect. Dis. **134**(suppl.):5433-5440, November, 1976.

24. Lau, W. K., et al.: Comparative efficacy and toxicity of amikacin and carbenicillin versus gentamicin and carbenicillin in leukopenic patients, Am. J. Med. **62**:212-219, June, 1977.
25. Young, L. S.: Review of clinical significance of synergy in gram-negative infections at the UCLA hospital, Infection **6**(suppl.):547-551, 1978.
26. Love, L. J.: Randomized trial of empiric antibiotic therapy with ticarcillin in combination with gentamicin, amikacin, or netilmicin in febrile neutropenic patients with cancer, Am. J. Med. **66**:603-610, April, 1979.
27. Watanakunakorn, C., and Glotzbecker, C.: In vitro activity of carbenicillin, ticarcillin, aminoglycosides, and combinations against Staphylococcus aureus, J. Antimicrob. Chemother. **5**:151-158, 1979.
28. Dellinger, P., et al.: Protective effect of cephalothin against gentamicin-induced nephrotoxicity in rats, Antimicrob. Agents Chemther. **9**:172-179, 1976.
29. Bloch, R., et al.: Protection from gentamicin nephrotoxicity by cephalothin and carbenicillin, Antimicrob. Agents Chemother. **15**:46-49, 1979.
30. Young, L. S., et al.: Gram-negative rod bacteremia: Microbiologic, immunologic, and therapeutic considerations, Ann. Intern. Med. **86**:456-471, 1977.
31. Feld, R., et al.: Comparative trial of sisomicin therapy by intermittent vs. continuous infusion, Am. J. Med. Sci. **274**:179-188, 1977.
32. Bodey, G. P., et al.: Amikacin for treatment of infections in patients with malignant diseases, J. Infect. Dis. **134**:5421-5427, 1976.
33. Bodey, G. P., et al.: Carbenicillin plus cephalothin or cefazolin as therapy for infections in neutropenic patients, Am. J. Med. Sci. **273**:309-318, May-June, 1977.
34. Issell, B. F., et al.: Continuous infusion tobramycin combined with carbenicillin for infections in cancer patients, Am. J. Med. Sci. **277**:311-318, May-June, 1979.
34a. Valdivieso, M., et al.: Therapy of infections in neutropenic patients: results with gentamicin in combination with cephalothin or chloramphenicol, Med. Pediat. Oncol. **2**:99-108, 1976.
35. Grose, W. E., et al.: Sulfamethoxazole-tremethoprim for infections in cancer patients, J. Am. Med. Assoc. **237**:352-354, January 24, 1977.
35a. Strauss, R. G.: Therapeutic neutrophil transfusions: are controlled studies no longer appropriate? Am. J. Med. **65**:1001-1006, December, 1978.
36. Rodriguez, V., et al.: Management of fever of unknown origin in patients with neoplasms and neutropenia, Cancer **32**:1007-1012, 1973.
37. Pizzo, P. A., et al.: Duration of empiric antibiotic therapy in granulocytopenic patients with cancer, Am. J. Med. **67**:194-200, 1979.
38. Yap, B. S., and Bodey, G. P.: Oropharyngeal candidiasis treated with a troche form of clotrimazole, Arch. Intern. Med. **39**:656-675, 1979.
39. Medoff, G., et al.: A new therapeutic approach to *Candida* infection, Arch. Intern. Med. **130**:241-245, 1972.
40. Edwards, J. E., et al.: Severe candidal infections: clinical perspective, immune defense mechanisms, and current concepts of therapy, Ann. Intern. Med. **89**: 91-106, 1978.
41. Stevens, D. A.: Miconazole in the treatment of systemic fungal infections, Am. Rev. Resp. Dis. **116**:801-806, 1977.
42. Codish, S. D., et al.: Systemic mycotic infections. I and II. Hosp. Med. June-July, 1978, pp. 6-19, 30-48.

43. Aisner, J., et al.: Treatment of invasive aspergillosis: relation of early diagnosis and treatment to response, Ann. Intern. Med. **86:**539-543, 1977.
44. Aisner, J., et al.: Invasive aspergillosis in acute leukemia: correlation with nose cultures and antibiotic use, Ann. Intern. Med. **90:**4-9, 1979.
45. Kauffman, C. A., et al.: Histoplasmosis in immunosuppressed patients, Am. J. Med. **64:**923-932, 1978.
46. Bennett, J. E., et al.: A comparison of amphotericin B alone and combined with flucytosine in the treatment of cryptococcal meningitis, N. Engl. J. Med. **301:** 126-131, 1979.
47. Palmer, D. L., Harvey, R. L., and Wheeler, J. K.: Diagnostic and therapeutic considerations in Nocardia asteroides infection, Medicine **53:**391-401, 1974.
48. Maderazo, E. G., and Quintiliani, R.: Treatment of nocardial infection with tremithoprim and sulfamethoxazole, Am. J. Med. **57:**671-675, 1974.
49. Hughes, W. T.: Pneumocystis carinii pneumonia, N. Engl. J. Med. **297:**1381-1383, 1977.
50. Lau, W. K., and Young, L. S.: Trimethoprim-sulfamethoxazole treatment of Pneumocystis carinii pneumonia in adults, N. Engl. J. Med. **295:**716-718, 1976.
51. Hughes, W. T., et al.: Comparison of pentamidine isethionate and trimethoprim/sulfamethoxazole in the treatment of Pneumocystis carinii pneumonia, J. Pediats. **92:**285-291, 1978.
52. Kluge, R. M., Spaulding, D. M., and Spain, A. J.: Combination of pentamidine and TMP/SMX in the therapy of Pneumocystis carinii pneumonia in rats, Antimicrob. Agents Chemother. **13:**975-987, 1978.
53. Hughes, W. T., et al.: Successful chemoprophylaxis for Pneumocystis carinii pneumonitis, N. Engl. J. Med. **297:**1419-1426, 1977.
54. Dolin, R., et al.: Herpes zoster varicella infections in immunosuppressed patients, Ann. Intern. Med. **89:**375-388, 1978.
55. Groth, K. E., et al.: Evaluation of zoster immune plasma: treatment of cutaneous disseminated zoster in immunocompromised patients, J.A.M.A. **239:**1877-1879, 1978.
56. Whitley, R. J., et al.: Adenine arabinoside therapy of herpes zoster in the immunosuppressed, N. Engl. J. Med. **294:**1193-1199, 1976.
57. Merigan, T. C., et al.: Human leukocyte interferon for the treatment of herpes zoster in patients with cancer, N. Engl. J. Med. **298:**981-987, 1978.
58. Pizzo, P. A., and Levine, A. S.: The utility of protected environment regimens for the compromised host: a critical assessment, Prog. Hematol. **10:**311-332, 1977.
59. Storring, R. A., et al.: Oral non-absorbed antibiotics prevent infection in acute non-lymphoblastic leukemia, Lancet **2:**837-840, 1977.
60. Hahn, D. M., et al.: Infection in acute leukemia patients receiving oral non-absorbable antibiotics, Antimicrob. Agents Chemother. **13:**958-964, 1978.
61. Bodey, G. P., et al.: Protected environment—prophylactic antibiotic program for malignant lymphoma, Am. J. Med. **66:**74-81, 1979.
62. Cohen, M. H., et al.: Effect of oral prophylactic broad spectrum non-absorbable antibiotics on the gastrointestinal absorption of nutrients and methotrexate in small cell bronchogenic carcinoma patients, Cancer **38:**1556-1559, 1976.
63. Bender, J. F., et al.: Role of vancomycin as a component of oral nonabsorbable antibiotics for microbial suppression in leukemic patients, Antimicrob. Agents Chemother. **15:**455-460, 1979.

64. Gurwith, J. J., et al.: A prospective controlled investigation of prophylactic trimethoprim-sulfamethoxazole in hospitalized granulocytopenic patients, Am. J. Med. **66:**248-255, 1979.
65. Bryan, C. S., and Stone, W. J.: Comparably massive penicillin G therapy in renal failure, Ann. Intern. Med. **82:**189-195, 1975.
66. Hoffman, T. A., et al.: Pharmacodynamics of carbenicillin in hepatic and renal failure, Ann. Intern. Med. **73:**173-180, 1970.
67. Sarubbi, F. A., and Hull, J. H.: Amikacin serum concentrations: prediction of levels and dosage guidelines, Ann. Intern. Med. **89**(1):612-618, 1978.
68. Schonebeck, J., et al.: Pharmacokinetic studies on the oral agent flucytosine in individuals with normal and impaired renal function, Chemotherapy **18:**321-336, 1973.
69. Reymann, M. T., et al.: Correlation of aminoglycoside dosages with serum concentrations during therapy of serious gram-negative bacillary disease, Antimicrob. Agents Chemother. **16:**353-361, 1979.
70. Appel, G. B., and Neu, H. C.: Gentamicin in 1978, Ann. Intern. Med. **9:**528-538, 1978.
71. Wormaer, G. P., and Keusch, G. T.: Trimethoprim-sulfamethoxazole in the United States, Ann. Intern. Med. **91:**420-429, 1979.
72. Klastersky, J., et al.: Carbenicillin and hypokalemia, Ann. Intern. Med. **78:**774-775, 1973.
73. Maddux, M. S., and Barriere, S. L.: Management and prevention of adverse reactions due to amphotericin B, Drug Intell. Clin. Pharm., in press.
74. Bar, R. S., Wilson, H. E., and Mazzaferri, E. L.: Hypomagnesemic hypocalcemia secondary to renal magnesium wasting: a possible consequence of high dose gentamicin therapy, Ann. Intern. Med. **82:**646-649, 1975.
75. Barza, M., and Lauermann, M.: Why monitor serum levels of gentamicin? Clin. Pharmacokinet. **3:**202-215, 1978.
76. Appel, G. B., and Neu, H. C.: The nephrotoxicity of antimicrobial agents. II. N. Engl. J. Med. **296:**722-728, 1977.
77. Appel, G. B., and Neu, H. C.: The nephrotoxicity of antimicrobial agents. III. N. Engl. J. Med. **296:**784-787, 1977.
78. Appel, G. B., and Neu, H. C.: The nephrotoxicity of antimicrobial agents. I. N. Engl. J. Med. **296:**663-670, 1977.
79. Girling, D. J.: The hepatic toxicity of antituberculosis regimens containing isoniazid, rifampicin, and pyrazinamide, Tubercle **59:**13-32, 1978.
80. Dun, A. K., Jones, L., and Stead, W. W.: Short-course chemotherapy for tuberculosis with largely twice-weekly isoniazid-rifampin, Chest **75:**441-447, 1979.
81. Homayouni, H., et al.: Leukopenia due to penicillin and cephalosporin homologues, Arch. Intern. Med. **139:**827-828, 1979.
82. Diasio, R. B., Lakings, D. E., and Bennett, J. E.: Evidence of conversion of 5-fluorocytosine to 5-fluorouracil in humans: Possible factor in 5-fluorocytosine clinical toxicity, Antimicrob. Agents Chemother. **14:**903-908, 1978.
83. Brown, C. H., et al.: Hemostatic defect produced by carbenicillin, N. Engl. J. Med. **291:**265-270, 1974.
84. MacGregor, R. R., Bennett, J. E., and Erslev, A. J.: Erythropoietin concentration in amphotericin B-induced anemia, Antimicrob. Agents Chemother. **14:**270-273, 1978.

85. Keighley, R., et al.: Randomized controlled trial of vancomycin for pseudomembranous colitis and postoperative diarrhea, Brit. Med. J. **2**:1667-1669, 1978.
86. Jick, H., et al.: Excess of ampicillin rashes associated with allopurinol or hyperuricemia, N. Engl. J. Med. **286**:505-508, 1972.
87. Christensen, L. K., and Skovsted, L.: Inhibition of drug metabolism by chloramphenicol, Lancet **2**:1397-1399, 1969.

Section 9

DRUG INTERACTIONS WITH ANTICANCER DRUGS

Interactions between drugs have been shown to alter drug response and produce unexpected adverse reactions. This occurs in a variety of drug groups such as oral anticoagulants, anticonvulsants, antidiabetics, and digitalis glycosides. Fortunately, most of the drugs used in cancer chemotherapy have not been reported to be involved frequently in adverse drug interactions. This may be due to a low interactive potential of antineoplastic agents or a failure to recognize drug interaction problems among the many other problems that develop in patients receiving such drugs. Drug interactions that cause an alteration in antineoplastic drug effect are potentially quite important. Enhanced cytotoxic activity could result in life-threatening toxic effects, while inhibition of cytotoxicity could result in treatment failure with equally disastrous results. Thus practitioners should be alert for evidence of adverse drug interactions in patients receiving antineoplastic agents, even with combinations not previously reported to result in adverse consequences.

Many drug interactions in cancer chemotherapy involve the intentional use of combinations of antineoplastic agents in order to take advantage of different mechanisms of action or different toxic effects. Such combinations are discussed elsewhere in this book and will not be discussed here.

One general caution for patients receiving antineoplastic agents concerns the use of vaccines. Generalized vaccinia has resulted from the administration of live vaccines (e.g., smallpox) to patients receiving anticancer drugs with immunosuppressant activity[46,47] (see Table 9-1). Also, impaired antibody response has been reported in patients receiving chemotherapy who were given pneumococcal vaccine.[53]

L-ASPARAGINASE (ELSPAR)

General interactive properties

Asparaginase can produce a number of serious toxic effects, some of which could alter the response to concomitantly administered drugs. Hyper-

Table 9-1. Some antineoplastic drugs with immunosuppressant activity

Chlormabucil (Leukeran)	Mercaptopurine (6-MP, Purinethol)
Corticosteroids	Methotrexate
Cyclophosphamide (Cytoxan)	Thioguanine (TG, 6-thioguanine)
Cytarabine (cytosine arabinoside, Ara-C, Cytosar)	

glycemia and frank diabetes have been reported in several studies[1-3]; thus the possibility exists that antidiabetic drug requirements could be altered. Asparaginase therapy has also been associated with depression of clotting factors with corresponding increases in the partial thromboblastin time.[4] Such effects should be considered if asparaginase is used concomitantly with anticoagulants. Another interesting action of asparaginase is a marked reduction in serum thyroxine binding globulin.[5] Such decreases should be considered when assessing the need for thyroid replacement therapy. Finally, some have proposed that asparaginase administration could impair the synthesis of drug-metabolizing enzymes. However, the clinical significance of any such effect does not seem clear at this time.

Specific drug interactions[6,54]

ASPARAGINASE PLUS METHOTREXATE

Reportedly methotrexate may interfere with the action of asparaginase in some cases,[5] but the clinical significance of this remains to be established.

CARMUSTINE (BCNU, BiCNU)

General interactive properties

The metabolism of carmustine takes place, at least in part, in hepatic microsomal enzymes.[7] However, reports dealing with the effect of enzyme-inducing and enzyme-inhibiting drugs on the response to carmustine appear to be lacking.

Specific drug interactions

CARMUSTINE PLUS CIMETIDINE (TAGAMET)

A preliminary report described several patients receiving cimetidine in addition to carmustine who developed an unexpected degree of leukopenia and thrombocytopenia.[8] Since patients receiving their first course of carmustine in the absence of cimetidine seldom develop such bone marrow depression, it is possible that cimetidine may have contributed to this response. Cimetidine had previously been suspected of causing bone marrow depression in several patients.[9-12] Although the evidence for such an effect of cimetidine is not conclusive, at least two cases involved a positive challenge and de-challenge with the drug[9,10] and one case was fatal.[11] Thus patients receiving carmustine (and possibly other cytotoxic agents) should be observed closely for enhanced bone marrow suppression if cimetidine is used concomitantly.

CISPLATIN (PLATINOL)

General interactive properties

Because nephrotoxicity may occur following the use of cisplatin,[13-15] one might expect that the concomitant use of other nephrotoxic agents would enhance the likelihood of kidney damage. For example it has been suggested that aminoglycosides could be dangerous when administered with cisplatin.[14] Furthermore, since maintenance of adequate hydration appears to be important in prevention of nephrotoxicity,[15] volume-depleting drugs should be used only if careful attention is given to hydration. Ototoxicity has also been reported with cisplatin use.[13,16] Thus concomitant use of other ototoxic agents should probably be discouraged unless necessary. Finally, serum electrolyte changes such as hypomagnesemia, hypocalcemia, and hypokalemia have been noted in patients receiving cisplatin.[17,18] Thus concomitant use of cisplatin with other drugs that can produce similar electrolyte changes might be expected to increase the likelihood of such adverse effects.

Specific drug interactions

No specific drug interactions have been reported.

CYCLOPHOSPHAMIDE (CYTOXAN)

General interactive properties

Cyclophosphamide is converted to active metabolites by hepatic microsomal enzymes.[7] Thus enzyme-inducing agents might be expected to alter the pharmacokinetics of cyclophosphamide. However, if the *total* production of active metabolites is not changed, there may be little or no change in antineoplastic activity of cyclophosphamide. (See barbiturates, below.) Enzyme-inhibiting agents such as disulfiram, chloramphenicol, and allopurinol might also be expected to affect the formation of active cyclophosphamide metabolites. However, as with enzyme induction, a change in rate of formation of alkylating metabolites with no change in amount formed may not alter the response to cyclophosphamide. (See allopurinol, below.)

Specific drug interactions

CYCLOPHOSPHAMIDE PLUS ALLOPURINOL (ZYLOPRIM)

Epidemiologic evidence indicates that allopurinol may increase the likelihood of cyclophosphamide-induced bone marrow depression.[19] Preliminary evidence also indicates that allopurinol may prolong the half-life of cyclophosphamide, but the total amount of alkylating metabolites formed may not be altered.[20] Although the evidence to support the existence of a clinically important interaction is not substantial, one should be alert for altered response to cyclophosphamide in the present of allopurinol.

CYCLOPHOSPHAMIDE PLUS BARBITURATES

The rate of conversion of cyclophosphamide to active metabolites appears to be increased in the presence of barbiturates.[20,21] However, the total amount of active metabolites formed may not be affected. Also, the rate of inactivation of alkylating metabolites may be increased, thereby tending to decrease cytotoxic activity. Thus it seems clear that the pharmacokinetics of cyclophosphamide are affected by concomitant barbiturate administration. However, the clinical effect of such changes cannot be defined with available data. Certainly one should be alert for altered cyclophosphamide response in patients receiving concomitant barbiturates.

CYCLOPHOSPHAMIDE PLUS CHLORAMPHENICOL (CHLOROMYCETIN)

Chloramphenicol has been shown to prolong the half-life of cyclophosphamide, probably because of inhibition of hepatic metabolism.[22] However, the effect of chloramphenicol on the pharmacokinetics of the active metabolites of cyclophosphamide is not known. Thus the clinical importance of this interaction is not clear, but practitioners should be alert for altered cyclophosphamide response in the presence of chloramphenicol therapy.

CYCLOPHOSPHAMIDE PLUS CORTICOSTEROIDS

It has been proposed that corticosteroids inhibit the formation of active cyclophosphamide metabolites and that reduction in corticosteroid dosage in patients also receiving cyclophosphamide may result in cyclophosphamide toxicity.[23] However, this has been refuted by others[24] and the clinical significance of any interaction remains to be proven.

CYCLOPHOSPHAMIDE PLUS SUCCINYLCHOLINE (ANECTINE, QUELICIN)

A reduction in plasma pseudocholinesterase has been noted in patients receiving cyclophosphamide.[25,26] Since succinylcholine is metabolized by pseudocholinesterase, a prolonged response to succinylcholine may occur. Prolonged apnea following succinylcholine has been reported in the presence of cyclophosphamide therapy,[24] but the incidence of such an effect is not known.

5-FLUOROURACIL
General interactive properties

5-Fluorouracil (5-FU) undergoes degradative metabolism to inactive products (e.g., dihydro-5-fluorouracil) and is also activated to cytotoxic metabolites (e.g., 2′-deoxy-5-fluorouridine 5′-monophosphate).[27] However, the effect of concomitant administration of drugs with enzyme-inducing or enzyme-inhibiting activity on the response to 5-FU is not known. Drug interactions involving the renal excretion of 5-FU do not seem likely since minimal amounts of unchanged 5-FU appear in the urine.[27]

Specific drug interactions
5-FLUOROURACIL (5-FU) PLUS METHOTREXATE

Although in vitro studies indicate that methotrexate may interfere with the antitumor effects of 5-FU,[28,29] the clinical significance of this effect is not known. Indeed, some recommended cancer chemotherapy regimens include the combination of methotrexate and 5-FU.

LOMUSTINE (CCNU, CeeNU)
General interactive properties

The metabolism of lomustine takes place, at least in part, in hepatic microsomal enzymes.[7] However, reports dealing with the effect of enzyme-inducing and enzyme-inhibiting drugs on the response to lomustine appear to be lacking.

Specific drug interactions
LOMUSTINE PLUS THEOPHYLLINE

One patient treated with lomustine developed thrombocytopenia and bleeding following one cycle of treatment during which theophylline was used for her asthma.[30] Although there are reportedly experimental data to support an enhanced cytotoxic effect of carmustine (BCNU) in the presence of theophylline, additional clinical evidence is needed to assess the importance of the use of either lomustine or carmustine concomitantly with theophylline.

MERCAPTOPURINE (6-MP, PURINETHOL)
General interactive properties

The enzyme xanthine oxidase is involved in the metabolism of mercaptopurine to inactive metabolites. Thus agents that may inhibit xanthine oxidase (see allopurinol below) may enhance the cytotoxic effect of mercaptopurine. Since very little mercaptopurine appears unchanged in the urine, renal drug interactions affecting the mercaptopurine effect do not seem likely.

Specific drug interactions

MERCAPTOPURINE PLUS ALLOPURINOL (ZYLOPRIM)

Allopurinol inhibits xanthine oxidase, which in turn is responsible for the inactivation of mercaptopurine. Thus enhanced mercaptopurine toxicity may result.[31-33] Patients receiving both drugs may require a reduction in mercaptopurine dose to 25% of the original dose.

MERCAPTOPURINE PLUS ORAL ANTICOAGULANTS

A reduced hypoprothrombinemic response to warfarin with mercaptopurine administration has been documented in one patient and confirmed in animal studies.[34,35] However, the incidence and magnitude of this effect will not be known until further clinical studies are done. Certainly one should be alert for altered response to oral anticoagulants if mercaptopurine is started or stopped.

METHOTREXATE

General interactive properties

A significant amount of orally administered methotrexate is degraded by intestinal bacteria. Thus antibiotics that reduce gastrointestinal bacteria would be expected to increase systemic availability of methotrexate. Oral kanamycin appears to do so,[36] but oral neomycin has the opposite effect (see aminoglycosides, below). Methotrexate is only about 50% bound to plasma proteins.[36] Thus even though some drugs (e.g., aspirin, para-aminobenzoic acid) appear to displace methotrexate from plasma protein binding, the clinical impact of such displacement remains to be determined. Since the primary route of excretion of methotrexate is renal (about 80%), hepatic microsomal enzyme inducers or inhibitors would not be expected to significantly alter methotrexate disposition. The renal excretion of methotrexate involves both glomerular filtration and active tubular secretion. The latter mechanism involves the organic acid transport mechanism, which can be affected by several other drugs. Thus the active renal tubular secretion of methotrexate may be inhibited, resulting in a greater than expected methotrexate effect (including toxicity). Salicylates, probenecid, para-aminobenzoic acid (PABA) and possibly phenylbutazone appear to affect methotrexate in this way (see below).

Specific drug interactions

METHOTREXATE PLUS ETHYL ALCOHOL (ETHANOL)

It has been proposed that ethanol may enhance the possibility of methotrexate-induced hepatotoxicity. In one study of five cases of methotrexate-induced cirrhosis,[37] one patient ingested 28 to 85 g/week of ethanol and two ingested more than 85 g/week. This finding is consistent with the contention of others that ethanol may enhance the liver toxicity of methotrexate[38,39] but certainly does not establish such an association. Some workers feel strongly that ethanol should be avoided in patients receiving methotrexate,[38] and the manufacturer of methotrexate also recommends the avoidance of ethanol.[39] Even though the evidence for additive hepatotoxic effects is not conclusive, alcohol restriction is probably appropriate for most patients receiving methotrexate.

METHOTREXATE PLUS AMINOGLYCOSIDES

Because methotrexate undergoes bacterial degradation in the intestine, one would expect antibiotics that inhibit such organisms to result in increased absorption of intact methotrexate. Although this may be the case for oral kanamycin, oral neomycin appears to *decrease* systemic availability of methotrexate.[36] This may be related to the known ability of neomycin to produce malabsorption of various substances. Oral paromomycin (in combination with oral polymyxin B, nystatin, and vancomycin) has also been associated with reduced gastrointestinal absorption of methotrexate.[40] Thus one should be alert for altered methotrexate response in the presence of oral administration of aminoglycosides.

METHOTREXATE PLUS FOLIC ACID

Methotrexate product information states that vitamin preparations containing folic acid may alter the response to methotrexate.[39] Although clinical reports describing inhibition of methotrexate response from folate-containing vitamins appear to be lacking, it would be prudent to avoid such vitamins in methotrexate-treated patients.

METHOTREXATE PLUS PARA-AMINOBENZOIC ACID (PABA)

PABA has been shown in vitro to displace methotrexate from plasma protein binding, thus increasing the free methotrexate concentrations. However, in the absence of clinical studies, it is impossible to determine if there is any danger in concomitant methotrexate and PABA administration. Until results of studies on man are available, it would be wise to give PABA with caution to patients receiving methotrexate or to avoid it, as the manufacturer recommends.[39] It should be noted that PABA is found in several proprietary analgesic mixtures.

METHOTREXATE PLUS PHENYLBUTAZONE (BUTAZOLIDIN)

Although it has been proposed that phenylbutazone may displace methotrexate from plasma protein binding,[41] it also seems possible that phenylbutazone could affect renal clearance of methotrexate. Two patients receiving methotrexate for psoriasis developed evidence of excessive methotrexate effects during concomitant administration of phenylbutazone.[41] Both patients developed widespread cutaneous ulcerations, and one died following bone marrow depression and septicemia. Although the adverse responses seemed to be related to the concomitant use of phenylbutazone and methotrexate, the evidence is circumstantial. Although only limited clinical evidence exists, the potential severity of the purported interaction indicates that phenylbutazone should be used only with caution in patients receiving methotrexate.

METHOTREXATE PLUS PROBENECID (BENEMID)

Probenecid has been shown to considerably enhance serum methotrexate concentrations,[42,43] probably as a result of reduced active tubular secretion of methotrexate. Although it has been proposed that this interaction could be used to reduce the cost of methotrexate therapy, the inadvertent use of this combination could result in methotrexate toxicity. Concomitant use of methotrexate and probenecid need not be avoided, but one should be alert for the necessity of reducing the dose of methotrexate in patients receiving both drugs.

METHOTREXATE PLUS SALICYLATES

Study in man has shown a decreased clearance (about 35%) of methotrexate following salicylate administration as well as a decrease in plasma protein binding of about 30%.[44] Both of these factors would tend to increase the amount of active methotrexate, and therefore, toxicity. In another study[45] two patients receiving methotrexate and salicylate rapidly developed pancytopenia and died. A subsequent retrospective review of 176 patients who had received methotrexate infusions revealed that 66 patients also received salicylate in a dose greater than 600 mg/day. Of the seven patients who rapidly developed a severe pancytopenia, six were in the group who had received salicylates. Studies in mice also indicated that salicylates can enhance methotrexate toxicity.[45] In one study a patient with psoriatic arthritis developed methotrexate hepatotoxicity while also taking moderate doses of aspirin for the arthritis.[21] Also, two elderly patients with psoriasis developed signs of excessive methotrexate effect with concomitant aspirin therapy.[22] Considering all of the above evidence, it appears that some patients on methotrexate may be adversely affected by concomitant salicylate therapy. Thus it would be wise to administer salicylates to methotrexate-treated patients with caution or not at all. The manufacturer of methotrexate recommends that salicylates be avoided in patients receiving methotrexate.[39] Patients receiving methotrexate should be reminded of the many nonprescription mixtures which contain salicylates.

METHOTREXATE PLUS SULFONAMIDES

In vitro studies have shown that certain sulfonamides are capable of displacing methotrexate from plasma protein binding, thus increasing free methotrexate concentrations. Studies in man have shown sulfisoxazole (Gantrisin) infusions to decrease plasma protein-bound methotrexate by about one fourth. Sulfisoxazole may also have a minor inhibitory effect on the renal tubular secretion of methotrexate.[44] Clinical reports of combined toxicity have not appeared. However, it is possible that sulfisoxazole could enhance methotrexate toxicity because of protein displacement. Other less highly bound sulfonamides could have a similar, but less pronounced, effect. It has also been cautioned that other types of sulfonamides (e.g., sulfonylurea hypglycemics, thiazide diuretics) could also displace methotrexate from plasma protein binding.[39] Although the clinical evidence for this interaction is scanty, one should be alert for excessive methotrexate effect if sulfonamides are given concurrently.

PROCARBAZINE (MATULANE)

General interactive properties

It is thought that procarbazine is converted to active metabolites by hepatic metabolism. Since hepatic microsomal enzymes may be involved in the disposition of procarbazine and its metabolites, enzyme induction or inhibition might be expected to alter procarbazine response. However, clinical documentation for such an effect appears lacking. Another potential interactive property of procarbazine involves a purported ability to inhibit monoamine oxidase. However, this is based primarily on a study in animals.[49] Thus the ability of procarbazine to produce monoamine oxidase inhibition under clinical conditions is not established (see also Sympathomimetics, below). It should be noted for medicolegal reasons that the product information for procarbazine warns against the concomitant use of sympathomimetics and tricyclic antidepressants.[50]

Specific drug interactions

PROCARBAZINE PLUS CENTRAL NERVOUS SYSTEM DEPRESSANTS

Procarbazine reportedly may augment the effects of central nervous system depressants such as barbiturates, narcotic analgesics, and phenothiazines.[50,51] Although clinical information on the magnitude and incidence of combined central nervous system depression appears scanty, practitioners should be alert for such effects.

PROCARBAZINE PLUS ETHYL ALCOHOL (ETHANOL)

A disulfiram-like reaction reportedly may occur following ethanol ingestion in patients receiving procarbazine.[50,51] Although information on this effect is limited, patients should probably be warned of the possibility. Additive central nervous system depression might also be expected with combined procarbazine and ethanol.

PROCARBAZINE PLUS SYMPATHOMIMETICS

Animal studies indicate that procarbazine inhibits monoamine oxidase.[49] If procarbazine inhibits monoamine oxidase in man, one would expect potentially dangerous hypertensive episodes with administration of indirect acting sympathomimetics such as amphetamines, phenylpropanolamine, or ephedrine. However, clinical evidence to support such interactions is lacking. One patient receiving procarbazine developed a manic reaction following administration of lidocaine plus epinephrine for extraction of three teeth.[52] However, it seems unlikely that the epinephrine was responsible. More study is needed to determine if procarbazine is a monoamine oxidase inhibitor in man. However, until it is determined whether the interaction occurs in humans, sympathomimetics (especially indirect acting) should be used cautiously in patients receiving procarbazine.

REFERENCES

1. Gailani, S., et al.: Diabetes in patients treated with asparaginase, Clin. Pharmacol. Ther. **21**:487-490, 1971.
2. Carpentieri, U., and Balch, M. T.: Hyperglycemia associated with the therapeutic use of L-asparaginase: possible role of insulin receptors, J. Pediatr. **93**:775-778, 1978.
3. Lavine, R. L., et al.: The effect of E. coli L-asparaginase on oral glucose tolerance and insulin release in man, Diabetologia **15**:113-116, 1978.
4. Biggs, J. C., Chesterman, C. N., and Holliday, J.: L-asparaginase—clinical experience in leukaemia, lymphoma and carcinoma, Aust. N.Z. J. Med. **1**:1-7, 1971.
5. Garnick, M. B., and Larsen, P. R.: Acute deficiency of thyroxine-binding globulin during L-asparaginase therapy, N. Engl. J. Med. **301**:252, 1979.

6. Zager, R. F., et al.: The effects of antibiotics and cancer chemotherapeutic agents on the cellular transport and antitumor activity of methotrexate in L-1210 murine leukemia, Cancer Res. **33**:1670-1676, 1973.
7. Chabner, B. A., Myers, C. E., and Oliverio, V. T.: Clinical pharmacology of anticancer drugs, Semin. Oncol. **4**:165-191, 1977.
8. Selker, R. G., Moore, P., and LoDolce, D.: Bone-marrow depression with cimetidine plus carmustine (letter), N. Engl. J. Med. **299**:834, 1978.
9. Posnett, D. N., et al.: Cimetidine-induced nutropenia: a possible dose-related phenomenon, Arch. Intern. Med. **139**:584-586, 1979.
10. Littlejohn, G. O., and Urowitz, M. B.: Cimetidine, lupus erythematosus, and granulocytopenia (letter), Ann. Intern. Med. **91**:317-318, 1979.
11. Chang, H. K., and Morrison, S. L.: Bone marrow suppression associated with cimetidine, Ann. Intern. Med. **91**:580, 1979.
12. Freston, J. W.: Cimetidine and granulocytopenia (editorial), Ann. Intern. Med. **90**:264-265, 1979.
13. Prestayko, A. W., et al.: Cisplatin (*cis*-diamminedichloroplatinum II), Cancer Treat. Rev. **6**:17-39, 1979.
14. Einhorn, L. H., and Williams, S. D.: The role of cis-platinum in solid-tumor therapy, N. Engl. J. Med. **300**:289-291, 1979.
15. Stark, J. J., and Howel, S. B.: Nephrotoxicity of cis-platinum (II) dichlorodiammine, Clin. Pharmacol. Ther. **23**:461-466, 1978.
16. Helson, L., et al.: cis-Platinum ototoxicity, Clin. Toxicol. **13**:469-478, 1978.
17. Schilsky, R. L., and Anderson, T.: Hypomagnesemia and renal magnesium wasting in patients receiving cisplatin, Ann. Intern. Med. **90**:929-931, 1979.
18. Winkler, C. F., Mahr, M. M., and DeBandi, H.: Cisplatin and renal magnesium wasting (letter), Ann. Intern. Med. **91**:502-503, 1979.
19. Boston Collaborative Drug Surveillance Program: Allopurinol and cytotoxic drugs: interaction in relation to bone marrow depression, J.A.M.A. **227**:1036, 1974.
20. Bagley, C. M., Jr., et al.: Clinical pharmacology of cyclophosphamide, Cancer Res. **33**:226, 1973.
21. Jao, J. Y., Jusko, W. J., and Cohen, J. L.: Phenobarbital effects on cyclophosphamide pharmacokinetics in man, Cancer Res. **32**:2761-2764, 1972.
22. Faber, O. K., Mouridsen, H. T., and Skovsted, L.: The effect of chloramphenicol and sulphaphenazole on the biotransformation of cyclophosphamide in man, Br. J. Clin. Pharmacol. **2**:281-285, 1975.
23. Kaplan, S. R., and Calabresi, P.: Immunosuppressive agents (first of two parts), N. Engl. J. Med. **289**:952-955, 1973.
24. Faber, O. K., and Mouridsen, H. T.: Cyclophosphamide activation and corticosteroids (letter), N. Engl. J. Med. **291**:211, 1974.
25. Mone, J. G., and Mathie, W. E.: Qualitative and quantitative defects of pseudocholinesterase activity, Anaesthesia **22**:55, 1967.
26. Walker, I. R., et al.: Cyclophosphamide, cholinesterase and anaesthesia, Aust. N.Z. J. Med. **2**:247, 1972.
27. Sadee, W., and Wong, C. G.: Pharmacokinetics of 5-fluorouracil: inter-relationship with biochemical kinetics in monitoring therapy, Clin. Pharmacokinet. **2**: 437-450, 1977.

28. Maugh, T. H.: Cancer chemotherapy: an unexpected drug interaction, Science **194:**310, 1976.
29. Jackson, R. C., and Harrap, K. R.: Computer models of anticancer drug interaction, J. Pharmacol. Ther. **4:**245-280, 1979.
30. Zeltzer, P. M., and Feig, S. A.: Theophylline-induced lomustine toxicity (letter), Lancet **2:**960-961, 1979.
31. Coffey, J. J., et al.: Effect of allopurinol on the pharmacokinetics of 6-mercaptopurine (NSC 755) in cancer patients, Can Res. **32:**1283, 1972.
32. Calabro, J. J., and Castleman, B.: Case records of the Massachusetts General Hospital (Case 4-1972), N. Engl. J. Med. **286:**205, 1972.
33. Berns, A., et al.: Hazard of combining allopurinol and thiopurine (letter), N. Engl. J. Med. **286:**730, 1972.
34. Spiers, A., and Misbashan, R. S.: Increased warfarin requirement during mercaptopurine therapy: a new drug interaction (letter), Lancet **2:**221, 1974.
35. Martini, A., and Jahnchen, E.: Studies in rats on the mechanisms by which 6-percaptopurine inhibits the anticoagulant effect of warfarin, J. Pharmacol. Exp. Ther. **201:**547, 1977.
36. Shen, D. D., and Azarnoff, D. L.: Clinical pharmacokinetics of methotrexate, Clin. Pharmacokinet. **3:**1-13, 1978.
37. Tobias, H., and Auerbach, R.: Hepatotoxicity of long-term methotrexate therapy for psoriasis, Arch. Intern. Med. **132:**391, 1973.
38. Pai, S. H., et al.: Severe liver damage caused by treatment of psoriasis with methotrexate, N.Y. State J. Med. **73:**2585, 1973.
39. Methotrexate product information, Lederle Laboratories, Pearl River, N.Y., 1979.
40. Cohen, M. H., et al.: Effect of oral prophylactic broad spectrum nonabsorbable antibiotics on the gastrointestinal absorption of nutrients and methotrexate in small cell bronchogenic carcinoma patients, Cancer **38:**1556-1559, 1976.
41. Adams, J. D., and Hunter, G. A.: Drug interactions in psoriasis, Aust. J. Dermatol. **17:**39, 1976.
42. Aherne, G. W., et al.: Prolongation and enhancement of serum methotrexate concentrations by probenecid, Br. Med. J. **1:**1097, 1978.
43. Ramu, A., et al.: Probenecid inhibition of methotrexate excretion from cerebrospinal fluid in dogs, J. Pharmacokinet. Biopharm. **6:**389-397, 1978.
44. Liegler, D. G., et al.: The effect of organic acids on renal clearance of methotrexate in man, Clin. Pharmacol. Ther. **10:**849, 1969.
45. Mandel, M. A.: The synergistic effect of salicylates on methotrexate toxicity, Plast. Reconstr. Surg. **57:**733, 1976.
46. Allison, J.: Methotrexate and smallpox vaccination (letter), Lancet **2:**1250.
47. Rosenbaum, E. H., et al.: Vaccination of a patient receiving immunosuppressive therapy for lymphosarcoma, J.A.M.A. **198:**737, 1966.
48. Kaplan, S. R., and Calabresi, P.: Immunosuppressive agents (first of two parts), N. Engl. J. Med. **289:**952-955, 1973.
49. DeVita, V. T., et al.: Monoamine oxidase inhibition by a new carcinostatic agent, N-isopropyl-a-(2-methylhydrazine)-p-toluamide (MIH), Proc. Soc. Exp. Biol. Med. **120:**561, 1975.
50. Matulane product information, Roche Laboratories, Nutley, N.J., 1979.
51. The Medical Letter: Cancer Chemother. **20:**81-88, 1978.

52. Mann, A. M., and Hutchison, J. L.: Manic reaction associated with procarbazine hydrochloride therapy of Hodgkin's disease, Can. Med. Assoc. J. **97**:1350, 1967.
53. Siber, G. R., et al.: Impaired antibody response to pneumococcal vaccine after treatment for Hodgkin's disease, **299**:442-448, 1978.
54. Capizzi, R. L., et al.: Improvement in the therapeutic index of methotrexate by L-asparaginase, Cancer Chemother. Rep., part 3, **6**:37-41, 1975.

Appendix

TABLES AND NOMOGRAMS

Body surface area (m^2)* as a function of height (inches) and weight (pounds)

Height (in)	Weight (lb)										
	10	**15**	**20**	**25**	**30**	**35**	**40**	**45**	**50**	**55**	**60**
20	0.27	0.33	0.38	0.43	0.47	0.51	0.55	0.58	0.62	0.65	0.68
22	0.28	0.34	0.40	0.45	0.49	0.53	0.57	0.61	0.64	0.67	0.70
24	0.29	0.30	0.41	0.47	0.51	0.55	0.59	0.63	0.66	0.70	0.73
26	0.30	0.37	0.43	0.48	0.53	0.57	0.61	0.65	0.69	0.72	0.76
28	0.31	0.38	0.44	0.50	0.55	0.59	0.63	0.67	0.71	0.75	0.78
30	0.32	0.39	0.46	0.51	0.56	0.61	0.65	0.69	0.73	0.77	0.80
32	0.33	0.40	0.47	0.53	0.58	0.62	0.67	0.71	0.75	0.79	0.82
34	0.34	0.41	0.48	0.54	0.59	0.64	0.69	0.73	0.77	0.81	0.85
36	0.34	0.42	0.49	0.55	0.61	0.66	0.70	0.75	0.79	0.83	0.87
38	0.35	0.43	0.50	0.57	0.62	0.67	0.72	0.76	0.81	0.85	0.89
	30	**35**	**40**	**45**	**50**	**55**	**60**	**65**	**70**	**75**	**80**
40	0.63	0.69	0.74	0.78	0.82	0.87	0.91	0.94	0.98	1.02	1.05
42	0.65	0.70	0.75	0.80	0.84	0.88	0.92	0.96	1.00	1.04	1.07
44	0.66	0.71	0.77	0.81	0.86	0.90	0.94	0.98	1.02	1.06	1.09
46	0.67	0.73	0.78	0.83	0.88	0.92	0.96	1.00	1.04	1.08	1.11
48	0.69	0.74	0.79	0.84	0.89	0.94	0.98	1.02	1.06	1.10	1.13
50	0.70	0.75	0.81	0.86	0.91	0.95	1.00	1.04	1.08	1.12	1.15
52	0.71	0.77	0.82	0.87	0.92	0.97	1.01	1.05	1.10	1.14	1.17
54	0.72	0.78	0.83	0.89	0.94	0.98	1.03	1.07	1.11	1.15	1.19
56	0.73	0.79	0.85	0.90	0.95	1.00	1.04	1.09	1.13	1.17	1.21
58	0.74	0.80	0.86	0.91	0.97	1.01	1.06	1.10	1.15	1.19	1.23
	50	**60**	**70**	**80**	**90**	**100**	**110**	**120**	**130**	**140**	**150**
60	0.98	1.08	1.16	1.25	1.32	1.40	1.47	1.54	1.60	1.66	1.72
62	0.99	1.09	1.18	1.26	1.34	1.42	1.49	1.56	1.62	1.69	1.75
64	1.01	1.11	1.20	1.28	1.36	1.44	1.51	1.58	1.65	1.71	1.77
66	1.02	1.12	1.21	1.30	1.38	1.46	1.53	1.60	1.67	1.73	1.79
68	1.03	1.13	1.23	1.31	1.40	1.47	1.55	1.62	1.69	1.75	1.82
70	1.04	1.15	1.24	1.33	1.41	1.49	1.57	1.64	1.71	1.78	1.84
72	1.06	1.16	1.26	1.35	1.43	1.51	1.59	1.66	1.73	1.80	1.86
	90	**100**	**110**	**120**	**130**	**140**	**150**	**160**	**170**	**180**	**190**
74	1.45	1.53	1.61	1.68	1.75	1.82	1.88	1.96	2.01	2.07	2.13
76	1.46	1.55	1.62	1.70	1.77	1.84	1.90	1.97	2.03	2.09	2.15
78	1.48	1.56	1.64	1.72	1.79	1.86	1.93	1.99	2.05	2.11	2.17
80	1.50	1.58	1.66	1.73	1.81	1.88	1.95	2.01	2.08	2.14	2.20
82	1.51	1.60	1.68	1.75	1.83	1.90	1.97	2.03	2.10	2.16	2.22
84	1.53	1.61	1.69	1.77	1.85	1.92	1.99	2.05	2.12	2.18	2.24
86	1.54	1.63	1.71	1.79	1.86	1.94	2.01	2.07	2.14	2.20	2.27

*From Gehan, E. A., and George, S. L.: Cancer Chemother. Rep. **54**:225-35, 1970.

Weight (lb)												
65	**70**	**75**	**80**	**85**	**90**	**95**	**100**	**105**	**110**	**115**	**120**	**125**
0.70	0.73	0.76	0.78	0.81	0.83	0.86	0.88	0.90	0.92	0.94	0.97	0.99
0.73	0.76	0.79	0.82	0.84	0.87	0.89	0.92	0.94	0.96	0.98	1.01	1.03
0.76	0.79	0.82	0.85	0.87	0.90	0.93	0.95	0.97	1.00	1.02	1.04	1.07
0.79	0.82	0.85	0.88	0.90	0.93	0.96	0.98	1.01	1.03	1.06	1.08	1.10
0.81	0.84	0.87	0.90	0.93	0.96	0.99	1.01	1.04	1.06	1.09	1.11	1.14
0.84	0.87	0.90	0.93	0.96	0.99	1.02	1.04	1.07	1.10	1.12	1.15	1.17
0.86	0.89	0.92	0.96	0.99	1.02	1.04	1.07	1.10	1.13	1.15	1.18	1.20
0.88	0.92	0.95	0.98	1.01	1.04	1.07	1.10	1.13	1.16	1.18	1.21	1.23
0.90	0.94	0.97	1.00	1.04	1.07	1.10	1.13	1.16	1.18	1.21	1.24	1.26
0.92	0.96	0.99	1.03	1.06	1.09	1.12	1.15	1.18	1.21	1.24	1.27	1.29
85	**90**	**95**	**100**	**105**	**110**	**115**	**120**	**125**	**130**	**135**	**140**	**145**
1.08	1.12	1.15	1.18	1.21	1.24	1.27	1.29	1.32	1.35	1.38	1.40	1.43
1.11	1.14	1.17	1.20	1.23	1.26	1.29	1.32	1.35	1.38	1.40	1.43	1.46
1.13	1.16	1.19	1.23	1.26	1.29	1.32	1.35	1.38	1.40	1.43	1.46	1.49
1.15	1.18	1.22	1.25	1.28	1.31	1.34	1.37	1.40	1.43	1.46	1.49	1.51
1.17	1.21	1.24	1.27	1.31	1.34	1.37	1.40	1.43	1.46	1.49	1.51	1.54
1.19	1.23	1.26	1.30	1.33	1.36	1.39	1.42	1.45	1.48	1.51	1.54	1.57
1.21	1.25	1.28	1.32	1.35	1.38	1.41	1.45	1.48	1.51	1.54	1.57	1.59
1.23	1.27	1.30	1.34	1.37	1.41	1.44	1.47	1.50	1.53	1.56	1.59	1.62
1.25	1.29	1.32	1.36	1.39	1.43	1.46	1.49	1.52	1.55	1.59	1.62	1.64
1.27	1.31	1.34	1.38	1.41	1.45	1.48	1.51	1.55	1.58	1.61	1.64	1.67
160	**170**	**180**	**190**	**200**	**210**	**220**	**230**	**240**	**250**	**260**	**270**	**280**
1.78	1.84	1.89	1.95	2.00	2.05	2.10	2.15	2.19	2.24	2.29	2.33	2.38
1.81	1.86	1.92	1.97	2.03	2.08	2.13	2.18	2.23	2.27	2.32	2.36	2.41
1.83	1.89	1.94	2.00	2.05	2.11	2.16	2.21	2.26	2.30	2.35	2.40	2.44
1.85	1.91	1.97	2.03	2.08	2.13	2.18	2.24	2.28	2.33	2.38	2.43	2.47
1.88	1.94	2.00	2.05	2.11	2.16	2.21	2.26	2.31	2.36	2.41	2.46	2.50
1.90	1.96	2.02	2.08	2.13	2.19	2.24	2.29	2.34	2.39	2.44	2.49	2.54
1.92	1.98	2.04	2.10	2.16	2.21	2.27	2.32	2.37	2.42	2.47	2.52	2.57
200	**210**	**220**	**230**	**240**	**250**	**260**	**270**	**280**	**290**	**300**	**310**	**320**
2.18	2.24	2.29	2.35	2.40	2.45	2.50	2.55	2.60	2.64	2.69	2.74	2.78
2.21	2.26	2.32	2.37	2.43	2.48	2.53	2.58	2.63	2.67	2.72	2.77	2.81
2.23	2.29	2.34	2.40	2.45	2.50	2.55	2.61	2.65	2.70	2.75	2.80	2.84
2.26	2.31	2.37	2.42	2.48	2.53	2.58	2.63	2.68	2.73	2.78	2.83	2.87
2.28	2.34	2.39	2.45	2.50	2.56	2.61	2.66	2.71	2.76	2.81	2.86	2.90
2.30	2.36	2.42	2.48	2.53	2.58	2.64	2.69	2.74	2.79	2.84	2.89	29.3
2.33	2.39	2.44	2.50	2.56	2.61	2.66	2.71	2.77	2.82	2.87	2.91	2.96

Body surface area (m^2)* as a function of height (cm) and weight (kg)

Height (cm)	Weight (kg)										
	4	**6**	**8**	**10**	**12**	**14**	**16**	**18**	**20**	**22**	**24**
50	0.25	0.31	0.36	0.40	0.44	0.48	0.51	0.54	0.57	0.60	0.63
55	0.26	0.32	0.37	0.42	0.46	0.50	0.53	0.57	0.60	0.63	0.66
60	0.27	0.33	0.39	0.43	0.48	0.52	0.55	0.59	0.62	0.65	0.68
65	0.28	0.34	0.40	0.45	0.49	0.53	0.57	0.61	0.64	0.67	0.70
70	0.29	0.36	0.41	0.46	0.51	0.55	0.59	0.63	0.66	0.69	0.73
75	0.30	0.37	0.42	0.48	0.52	0.57	0.61	0.64	0.68	0.71	0.75
80	0.31	0.38	0.44	0.49	0.54	0.58	0.62	0.66	0.70	0.73	0.77
85	0.31	0.39	0.45	0.50	0.55	0.60	0.64	0.68	0.72	0.75	0.79
90	0.32	0.40	0.46	0.51	0.56	0.61	0.65	0.70	0.73	0.77	0.81
95	0.33	0.40	0.47	0.53	0.58	0.63	0.67	0.71	0.75	0.79	0.83
	12	**14**	**16**	**18**	**20**	**22**	**24**	**26**	**28**	**30**	**32**
100	0.59	0.64	0.68	0.73	0.77	0.81	0.84	0.88	0.91	0.95	0.98
105	0.60	0.65	0.70	0.74	0.78	0.82	0.86	0.90	0.93	0.97	1.00
110	0.61	0.67	0.71	0.76	0.80	0.84	0.88	0.92	0.95	0.99	1.02
115	0.63	0.68	0.73	0.77	0.81	0.86	0.89	0.93	0.97	1.00	1.04
120	0.64	0.69	0.74	0.79	0.83	0.87	0.91	0.95	0.99	1.02	1.06
125	0.65	0.70	0.75	0.80	0.84	0.89	0.93	0.97	1.00	1.04	1.07
130	0.66	0.71	0.77	0.81	0.86	0.90	0.94	0.98	1.02	1.06	1.09
135	0.67	0.73	0.78	0.83	0.87	0.92	0.96	1.00	1.04	1.07	1.11
140	0.68	0.74	0.79	0.84	0.89	0.93	0.97	1.01	1.05	1.09	1.13
145	0.69	0.75	0.80	0.85	0.90	0.94	0.99	1.03	1.07	1.11	1.14
	30	**34**	**38**	**42**	**46**	**50**	**54**	**58**	**62**	**66**	**70**
150	1.12	1.20	1.27	1.34	1.40	1.46	1.52	1.58	1.63	1.69	1.74
155	1.14	1.21	1.29	1.35	1.42	1.48	1.54	1.60	1.65	1.71	1.76
160	1.15	1.23	1.30	1.37	1.44	1.50	1.56	1.62	1.68	1.73	1.78
165	1.17	1.25	1.32	1.39	1.46	1.52	1.58	1.64	1.70	1.75	1.81
170	1.18	1.26	1.34	1.41	1.48	1.54	1.60	1.66	1.72	1.78	1.83
175	1.20	1.28	1.35	1.43	1.49	1.56	1.62	1.68	1.74	1.80	1.85
180	1.21	1.29	1.37	1.44	1.51	1.58	1.64	1.70	1.76	1.82	1.88
	40	**44**	**48**	**52**	**56**	**60**	**64**	**68**	**72**	**76**	**80**
185	1.42	1.49	1.56	1.63	1.69	1.75	1.81	1.87	1.93	1.98	2.03
190	1.44	1.51	1.58	1.65	1.71	1.77	1.83	1.89	1.95	2.00	2.06
195	1.45	1.53	1.60	1.67	1.73	1.79	1.85	1.91	1.97	2.02	2.08
200	1.47	1.54	1.62	1.68	1.75	1.81	1.87	1.93	1.99	2.05	2.10
205	1.49	1.56	1.63	1.70	1.77	1.83	1.89	1.95	2.01	2.07	2.12
210	1.50	1.58	1.65	1.72	1.79	1.85	1.91	1.97	2.03	2.09	2.14
215	1.52	1.59	1.67	1.74	1.80	1.87	1.93	1.99	2.05	2.11	2.17
220	1.53	1.61	1.68	1.75	1.82	1.89	1.95	2.01	2.07	2.13	21.9

*From Gehan, E. A., and George, S. L.: Cancer Chemother. Rep. **54:**225-35, 1970.

Weight (kg)												
26	**28**	**30**	**32**	**34**	**36**	**38**	**40**	**44**	**48**	**52**	**56**	**60**
0.66	0.68	0.71	0.73	0.75	0.78	0.80	0.82	0.86	0.90	0.94	0.97	1.01
0.68	0.71	0.74	0.76	0.78	0.81	0.83	0.85	0.90	0.94	0.98	1.01	1.05
0.71	0.74	0.76	0.79	0.81	0.84	0.86	0.88	0.93	0.97	1.01	1.05	1.09
0.73	0.76	0.79	0.82	0.84	0.87	0.89	0.91	0.96	1.00	1.05	1.09	1.13
0.76	0.79	0.81	0.84	0.87	0.89	0.92	0.94	0.99	1.04	1.08	1.12	1.16
0.78	0.81	0.84	0.87	0.89	0.92	0.95	0.97	1.02	1.07	1.11	1.16	1.20
0.80	0.83	0.86	0.89	0.92	0.95	0.97	1.00	1.05	1.10	1.14	1.19	1.23
0.82	0.85	0.88	0.91	0.94	0.97	1.00	1.02	1.08	1.13	1.17	1.22	1.26
0.84	0.87	0.91	0.94	0.97	0.99	1.02	1.05	1.10	1.15	1.20	1.25	1.29
0.86	0.89	0.93	0.96	0.99	1.02	1.05	1.07	1.13	1.18	1.23	1.28	1.32
34	**36**	**38**	**40**	**42**	**44**	**48**	**52**	**56**	**60**	**64**	**68**	**72**
1.01	1.04	1.07	1.10	1.13	1.15	1.21	1.26	1.30	1.35	1.40	1.44	1.48
1.03	1.06	1.09	1.12	1.15	1.18	1.23	1.28	1.33	1.38	1.43	1.47	1.52
1.05	1.08	1.11	1.14	1.17	1.20	1.25	1.31	1.36	1.41	1.45	1.50	1.55
1.07	1.10	1.13	1.16	1.19	1.22	1.28	1.33	1.38	1.43	1.48	1.53	1.58
1.09	1.12	1.15	1.19	1.22	1.24	1.30	1.36	1.41	1.46	1.51	1.56	1.60
1.11	1.14	1.17	1.21	1.24	1.27	1.32	1.38	1.43	1.49	1.54	1.58	1.63
1.13	1.16	1.19	1.23	1.26	1.29	1.35	1.40	1.46	1.51	1.56	1.61	1.66
1.15	1.18	1.21	1.25	1.28	1.31	1.37	1.43	1.48	1.53	1.59	1.64	1.69
1.16	1.20	1.23	1.26	1.30	1.33	1.39	1.45	1.50	1.56	1.61	1.66	1.71
1.18	1.22	1.25	1.28	1.32	1.35	1.41	1.47	1.53	1.58	1.64	1.69	1.74
74	**78**	**82**	**86**	**90**	**94**	**98**	**102**	**106**	**110**	**114**	**118**	**122**
1.79	1.84	1.88	1.93	1.98	2.02	2.07	2.11	2.15	2.19	2.23	2.27	2.31
1.81	1.86	1.91	1.96	2.00	2.05	2.09	2.14	2.18	2.22	2.26	2.30	2.34
1.84	1.89	1.94	1.98	2.03	2.08	2.12	2.17	2.21	2.25	2.29	2.34	2.38
1.86	1.91	1.96	2.01	2.06	2.10	2.15	2.19	2.24	2.28	2.32	2.37	2.41
1.88	1.94	1.99	2.04	2.08	2.13	2.18	2.22	2.27	2.31	2.35	2.40	2.44
1.91	1.96	2.01	2.06	2.11	2.16	2.20	2.25	2.30	2.34	2.38	2.43	2.47
1.93	1.98	2.04	2.09	2.13	2.18	2.23	2.28	2.32	2.37	2.41	2.45	2.50
84	**88**	**92**	**96**	**100**	**104**	**108**	**112**	**116**	**120**	**124**	**128**	**132**
2.08	2.13	2.18	2.23	2.28	2.33	2.37	2.42	2.46	2.50	2.55	2.59	2.63
2.11	2.16	2.21	2.26	2.31	2.35	2.40	2.44	2.49	2.53	2.58	2.62	2.66
2.13	2.18	2.23	2.28	2.33	2.38	2.43	2.47	2.52	2.56	2.60	2.65	2.69
2.15	2.21	2.26	2.31	2.36	2.40	2.45	2.50	2.54	2.59	2.63	2.68	2.72
2.18	2.23	2.28	2.33	2.38	2.43	2.48	2.52	2.57	2.62	2.66	2.70	2.75
2.20	2.25	2.30	2.36	2.41	2.45	2.50	2.55	2.60	2.64	2.69	2.73	2.77
2.22	2.27	2.33	2.38	2.43	2.48	2.53	2.58	2.62	2.67	2.71	2.76	2.80
2.24	2.30	2.35	2.40	2.45	2.50	2.55	2.60	2.65	2.69	2.74	2.79	2.83

BODY SURFACE AREA OF ADULTS*

Nomogram for determination of body surface area from height and weight:

A straightedge placed from the patient's height (left column) to his weight (right column) will give his body surface area (middle column).†

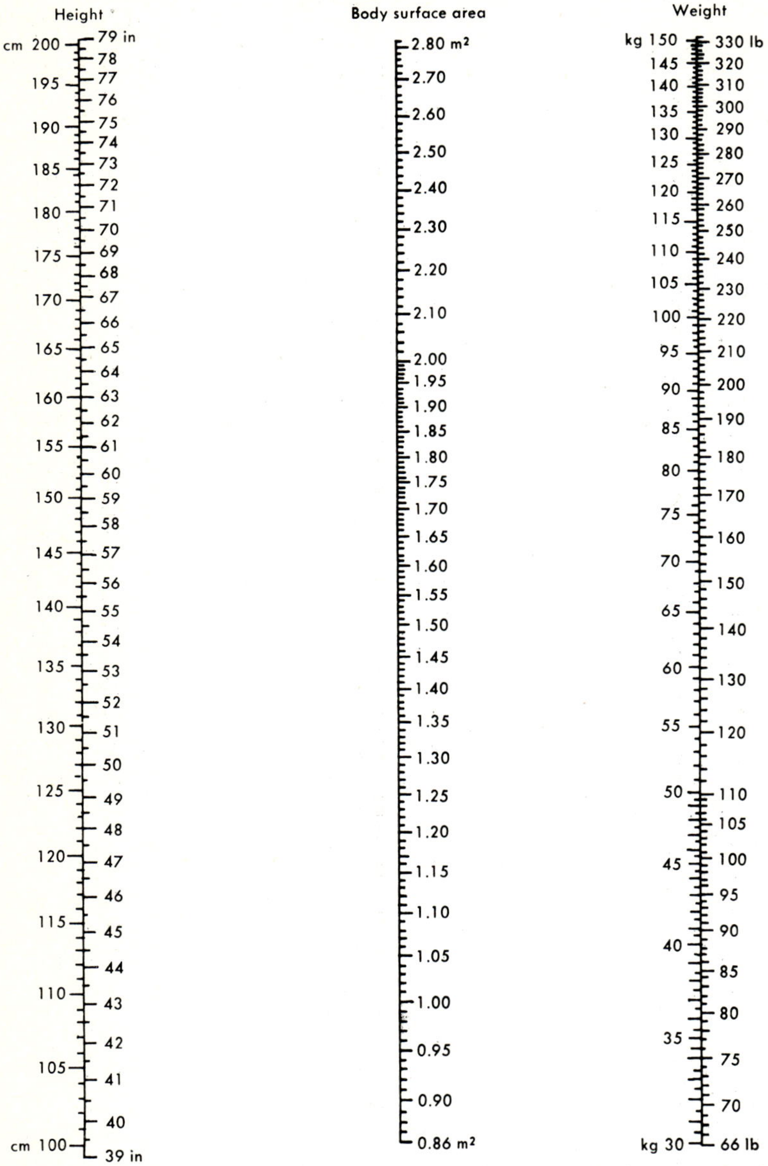

*From Documenta Geigy scientific tables, ed. 7, courtesy CIBA-Geigy Limited, Basle, Switzerland.
†From the formula of Du Bois and Du Bois, Arch. Intern. Med. **17**:863, 1916. $S = W^{0.425} \times H^{0.725} \times 71.84$, or $\log S = \log W \times 0.425 + \log H \times 0.725 + 1.8564$ (S = body surface in cm^2, W = weight in kg, H = height in cm)

BODY SURFACE AREA OF CHILDREN*

Nomogram for determination of body surface area from height and weight:

A straightedge placed from the patient's height (left column) to his weight (right column) will give his body surface area (middle column).†

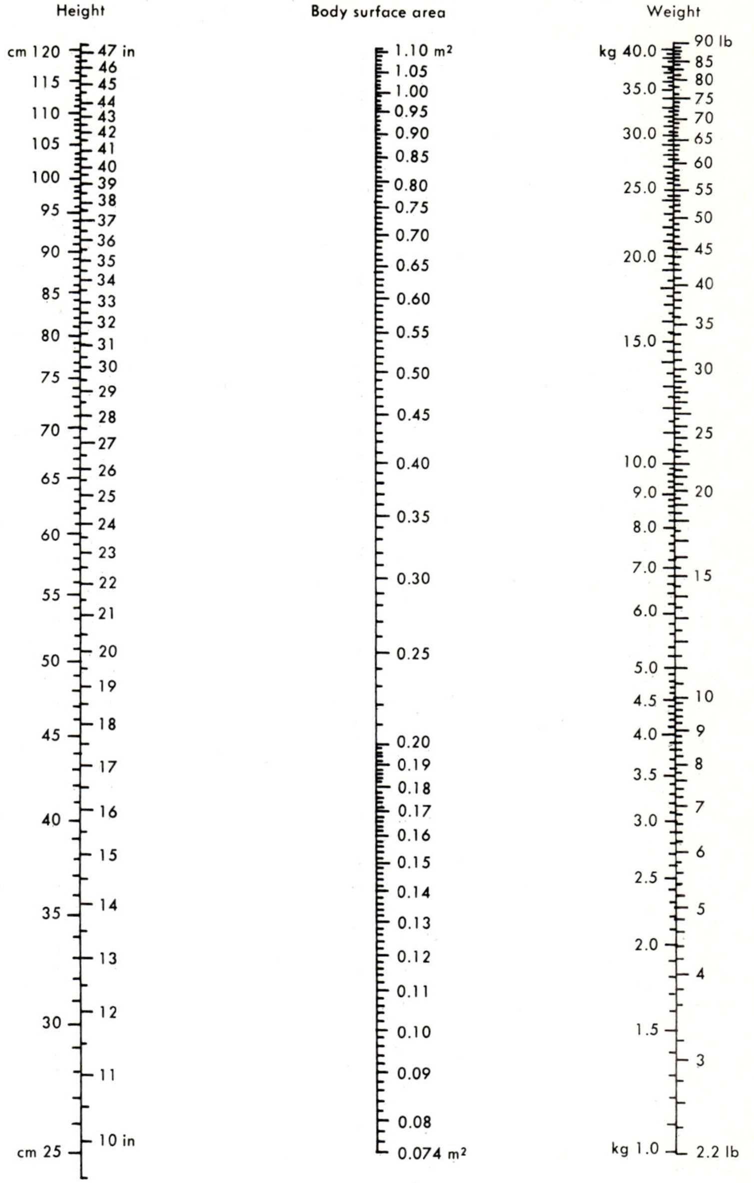

*From Documenta Geigy scientific tables, ed. 7, courtesy CIBA-Geigy Limited, Basle, Switzerland.

†From the formula of Du Bois and Du Bois, Arch. Intern. Med. **17**:863, 1916. $S = W^{0.425} \times H^{0.725} \times 71.84$, or $\log S = \log W \times 0.425 + \log H \times 0.725 + 1.8564$ (S = body surface in cm^2, W = weight in kg, H = height in cm)

Average weights of adults*

Height (in shoes)		Average weights in pounds and kilograms (in indoor clothing)															
		15-16 years		17-19 years		20-24 years		25-29 years		30-39 years		40-49 years		50-59 years		60-69 years	
ft in	cm	lb	kg	lb	kg	lb	kg	lb	kg	lb	kg	lb	kg	lb	kg	lb	kg
Men																	
5 0	152.4	98	44.5	113	51.3	122	55.3	128	58.1	131	59.4	134	60.8	136	61.7	133	60.3
5 0½	153.7	100	45.4	114.5	51.9	123.5	56	129.5	58.7	132.5	60.1	135.5	61.5	137.5	62.4	134.5	61
5 1	154.9	102	46.3	116	52.6	125	56.7	131	59.4	134	60.8	137	62.1	139	63	136	61.7
5 1½	156.2	104.5	47.4	117.5	53.3	126.5	57.4	132.5	60.1	135.5	61.5	138.5	62.8	140.5	63.7	137.5	62.4
5 2	157.5	107	48.5	119	54	128	58.1	134	60.8	137	62.1	140	63.5	142	64.4	139	63
5 2½	158.8	109.5	49.7	121	54.9	130	59	136	61.7	139	63	142	64.4	143.5	65.1	140.5	63.7
5 3	160	112	50.8	123	55.8	132	59.9	138	62.6	141	64	144	65.3	145	65.8	142	64.4
5 3½	161.3	114.5	51.9	125	56.7	134	60.8	139.5	63.3	143	64.9	146	66.2	147	66.7	144	65.3
5 4	162.6	117	53.1	127	57.6	136	61.7	141	64	145	65.8	148	67.1	149	67.6	146	66.2
5 4½	163.8	119.5	54.2	129	58.5	137.5	62.4	142.5	64.6	147	66.7	150	68	151	68.5	148	67.1
5 5	165.1	122	55.3	131	59.4	139	63	144	65.3	149	67.6	152	68.9	153	69.4	150	68
5 5½	166.4	124.5	56.5	133	60.3	140.5	63.7	146	66.2	151	68.5	154	69.9	155	70.3	152	68.9
5 6	167.6	127	57.6	135	61.2	142	64.4	148	67.1	153	69.4	156	70.8	157	71.2	154	69.9
5 6½	168.9	129.5	58.7	137	62.1	143.5	65.1	149.5	67.8	155	70.3	158.5	71.9	159.5	72.3	156.5	71
5 7	170.2	132	59.9	139	63	145	65.8	151	68.5	157	71.2	161	73	162	73.5	159	72.1
5 7½	171.5	134.5	61	141	64	147	66.7	153	69.4	159	72.1	163	73.9	164	74.4	161	73
5 8	172.7	137	62.1	143	64.9	149	67.6	155	70.3	161	73	165	74.8	166	75.3	163	73.9
5 8½	174	139.5	63.3	145	65.8	151	68.5	157	71.2	163	73.9	167	75.8	168	76.2	165.5	75.1
5 9	175.3	142	64.4	147	66.7	153	69.4	159	72.1	165	74.8	169	76.7	170	77.1	168	76.2
5 9½	176.5	144	65.3	149	67.6	155	70.3	161	73	167.5	76	171.5	77.8	172.5	78.2	170.5	77.3
5 10	177.8	146	66.2	151	68.5	157	71.2	163	73.9	170	77.1	174	78.9	175	79.4	173	78.5
5 10½	179.1	148	67.1	153	69.4	159	72.1	165	74.8	172	78	176	79.8	177.5	80.5	175.5	79.6
5 11	180.3	150	68	155	70.3	161	73	167	75.8	174	78.9	178	80.8	180	81.6	178	80.8
5 11½	181.6	152	68.9	157.5	71.4	163.5	74.2	169.5	76.9	176.5	80.1	180.5	81.9	182.5	82.8	180.5	81.9
6 0	182.9	154	69.9	160	72.6	166	75.3	172	78	179	81.2	183	83	185	83.9	183	83
6 0½	184.2	156.5	71	162	73.5	168	76.2	174.5	79.2	181	82.1	185	83.9	187	84.8	185.5	84.1
6 1	185.4	159	72.1	164	74.4	170	77.1	177	80.3	183	83	187	84.8	189	85.7	188	85.3
6 1½	186.7	161.5	73.3	166	75.3	172	78	179.5	81.4	185.5	84.1	189.5	86	191.5	86.9	190.5	86.4
6 2	188	164	74.4	168	76.2	174	78.9	182	82.6	188	85.3	192	87.1	194	88	193	87.5
6 2½	189.2	166.5	75.5	170	77.1	176	79.8	184	83.5	190.5	86.4	194.5	88.2	196.5	89.1	195.5	88.7
6 3	190.5	169	76.7	172	78	178	80.8	186	84.4	193	87.5	197	89.4	199	90.3	198	89.8
6 3½	191.8	—	—	174	78.9	179.5	81.4	188	85.3	196	88.9	200	90.7	202	91.6	201	91.2
6 4	193	—	—	176	79.8	181	82.1	190	86.2	199	90.3	203	92.1	205	93	204	92.5

Women

4 10	147.3	97	44	99	44.9	102	46.3	107	48.5	115	52.2	122	55.3	125	56.7	127	57.6
4 10½	148.6	98.5	44.7	100.5	45.6	103.5	46.9	108.5	49.2	116	52.6	123	55.8	126	57.2	128	58.1
4 11	149.9	100	45.4	102	46.3	105	47.6	110	49.9	117	53.1	124	56.2	127	57.6	129	58.5
4 11½	151.1	101.5	46	103.5	46.9	106.5	48.3	111.5	50.6	118.5	53.8	125.5	56.9	128.5	58.3	130	59
5 0	152.4	103	46.7	105	47.6	108	49	113	51.3	120	54.4	127	57.6	130	59	131	59.4
5 0½	153.7	105	47.6	107	48.5	110	49.9	114.5	51.9	121.5	55.1	128.5	58.3	131.5	59.6	132.5	60.1
5 1	154.9	107	48.5	109	49.4	112	50.8	116	52.6	123	55.8	130	59	133	60.3	134	60.8
5 1½	156.2	109	49.4	111	50.3	113.5	51.5	117.5	53.3	124.5	56.5	131.5	59.6	134.5	61	135.5	61.5
5 2	157.5	111	50.3	113	51.3	115	52.2	119	54	126	57.2	133	60.3	136	61.7	137	62.1
5 2½	158.8	112.5	51	114.5	51.9	116.5	52.8	120.5	54.7	127.5	57.8	134.5	61	138	62.6	139	63
5 3	160	114	51.7	116	52.6	118	53.5	122	55.3	129	58.5	136	61.7	140	63.5	141	64
5 3½	161.3	115.5	52.4	118	53.5	119.5	54.2	123.5	56	130.5	59.2	138	62.6	142	64.4	143	64.9
5 4	162.6	117	53.1	120	54.4	121	54.9	125	56.7	132	59.9	140	63.5	144	65.3	145	65.8
5 4½	163.8	119	54	122	55.3	123	55.8	127	57.6	133.5	60.6	141.5	64.2	146	66.2	147	66.7
5 5	165.1	121	54.9	124	56.2	125	56.7	129	58.5	135	61.2	143	64.9	148	67.1	149	67.6
5 5½	166.4	123	55.8	125.5	56.9	127	57.6	131	59.4	137	62.1	145	65.8	150	68	151	68.5
5 6	167.6	125	56.7	127	57.6	129	58.5	133	60.3	139	63	147	66.7	152	68.9	153	69.4
5 6½	168.9	126.5	57.4	128.5	58.3	130.5	59.2	134.5	61	140.5	63.7	149	67.6	154	69.9	155	70.3
5 7	170.2	128	58.1	130	59	132	59.9	136	61.7	142	64.4	151	68.5	156	70.8	157	71.2
5 7½	171.5	130	59	132	59.9	134	60.8	138	62.6	144	65.3	153	69.4	158	71.7	159	72.1
5 8	172.7	132	59.9	134	60.8	136	61.7	140	63.5	146	66.2	155	70.3	160	72.6	161	73
5 8½	174	134	60.8	136	61.7	138	62.6	142	64.4	148	67.1	157	71.2	162	73.5	163	73.9
5 9	175.3	136	61.7	138	62.6	140	63.5	144	65.3	150	68	159	72.1	164	74.4	165	74.8
5 9½	176.5	—	—	140	63.5	142	64.4	146	66.2	152	68.9	161.5	73.3	166.5	75.5	—	—
5 10	177.8	—	—	142	64.4	144	65.3	148	67.1	154	69.9	164	74.4	169	76.7	—	—
5 10½	179.1	—	—	144.5	65.5	146.5	66.5	150.5	68.3	156.5	71	166.5	75.5	171.5	77.8	—	—
5 11	180.3	—	—	147	66.7	149	67.6	153	69.4	159	72.1	169	76.7	174	78.9	—	—
5 11½	181.6	—	—	149.5	67.8	151.5	68.7	155.5	70.5	161.5	73.3	171.5	77.8	177	80.3	—	—
6 0	182.9	—	—	152	68.9	154	69.9	158	71.7	164	74.4	174	78.9	180	81.6	—	—

*Insured persons in the United States (Society of Actuaries, Build and Blood Pressure Study, vol. 1, Chicago, 1959, page 16, with interpolations by the editors of these scientific tables). Reproduced from Documental Geigy scientific tables, ed. 7, courtesy Ciba-Geigy Limited, Basle, Switzerland.

Average weights of children*

Age	Male		Female	
	Height (cm)	Weight (kg)	Height (cm)	Weight (kg)
Birth	50.8	3.4	50.8	3.2
1/12	53.6	4.3	54.6	4.1
2/12	56.4	5.1	57.2	5.0
3/12	59.2	6.0	59.7	5.9
4/12	61.7	6.8	62.0	6.6
5/12	64.5	7.6	64.0	7.3
6/12	67.3	8.5	65.5	7.7
7/12	68.8	8.9	67.1	8.2
8/12	70.4	9.3	68.6	8.6
9/12	71.9	9.6	70.1	9.0
10/12	73.2	10.0	71.4	9.3
11/12	74.7	10.4	72.9	9.6
12/12	76.2	10.8	74.2	10.0
1 & 1/12	77.2	11.0	75.2	10.2
2/12	78.0	11.3	76.2	10.5
3/12	79.0	11.5	77.2	10.7
4/12	79.8	11.8	78.2	10.9
5/12	80.8	12.0	79.2	11.1
6/12	81.8	12.2	80.0	11.4
7/12	82.8	12.4	81.0	11.6
8/12	83.8	12.6	82.0	11.8
9/12	84.6	12.8	83.1	12.0
10/12	85.6	12.9	84.1	12.2
11/12	86.6	13.1	85.1	12.4
12/12	87.4	13.3	86.1	12.5
2 & 6/12	92.2	14.3	91.2	13.7
3	96.5	15.2	95.5	14.8
3 & 6/12	100.8	16.3	99.6	15.9
4	103.9	17.3	103.4	16.9
4 & 6/12	107.2	18.2	107.2	18.2
5	110.7	19.5	110.5	19.2
5 & 6/12	114.3	20.7	114.0	20.6
6	117.6	21.9	117.6	22.0
6 & 6/12	120.7	23.2	120.7	23.4
7	123.7	24.6	123.7	24.8
7 & 6/12	126.7	26.2	126.7	26.5
8	129.8	27.7	129.8	28.1
8 & 6/12	132.6	29.4	132.6	29.9
9	135.4	31.1	135.4	31.6
9 & 6/12	138.2	33.0	138.2	33.5
10	141.0	34.9	141.0	35.5
10 & 6/12	143.3	36.9	144.3	37.8

*Reproduced with permission from Johns Hopkins Hospital: The Harriet Lane Handbook, ed. 7, edited by Dennis L. Headings. Copyright © 1975 by Year Book Medical Publishers, Chicago.

Average weights of children—cont'd

Age	Male		Female	
	Height (cm)	Weight (kg)	Height (cm)	Weight (kg)
11	145.8	38.9	147.6	40.2
11 & 6/12	148.6	41.1	150.9	42.9
12	151.4	43.3	154.2	45.6
12 & 6/12	154.4	45.7	157.0	47.9
13	157.5	48.0	159.5	50.2
13 & 6/12	161.3	51.1	161.0	52.4
14	164.8	54.1	162.8	54.6
14 & 6/12	167.9	57.1	163.8	56.3
15	171.2	60.1	164.8	57.5
15 & 6/12	173.2	62.3	165.1	58.4
16	175.3	64.5	165.6	59.3
16 & 6/12	176.0	65.8	165.6	60.0
17	176.5	67.1	165.6	60.7

ADULT LABORATORY VALUES

Common serum chemistries*

Test	Units	S.I. units
Albumin	3.5-4.8 gm/dl	0.54-0.74 mmol/l
Ammonia (plasma)	0-60 μg/dl	0-35.2 μmol/l
Bilirubin		
Total	.3-1.5 mg/dl	5.1-25.6 μmol/l
Direct	0-.2 mg/dl	0-3.4 μmol/l
Blood gases (arterial, whole blood)		
pH	7.35-7.45	7.35-745.
Po_2	80-105 mm Hg	10.6-14.0 kPa
Pco_2	35-45 mm Hg	4.7-6.0 kPa
Calcium		
Total	9.0-10.3 mg/dl	2.25-2.57 mmol/l
Free	4.5-5.0 mg/dl	1.12-1.25 mmol/l
Carbon dioxide content	24-32 mEq/l	24-32 mmol/l
β-Carotene	.70-2.50 μg/ml	1.3-4.6 μmol/l
Ceruloplasmin	23-50 mg/dl	1.5-3.3 μmol/l
Chloride	95-105 mEq/l	95-105 mmol/l
Copper	68-143 μg/dl	10.7-22.5 μmol/l
Complement (total)	150-250 CH50	150-250 arb. units
C_3	101-189 mg/dl	1.0-1.9 g/l
C_4	10-75 mg/dl	0.10-0.75 g/l
Creatinine		
Male	.8-1.3 mg/dl	70-110 μmol/l
Female	.6-1.1 mg/dl	50-100 μmol/l
Fibrinogen	150-360 mg/dl	1.5-3.6 g/l
Folate		
Serum	3-15 ng/ml	7-34 nmol/l
Red cell	117-541 ng/ml	265-1230 nmol/l
Glucose, fasting (plasma)	65-110 mg/dl	3.57-6.05 mmol/l
Haptoglobin	100-300 mg/dl	1.0-3.0 g/l
Immunoglobulin		
IgA	65-395 mg/dl	0.65-3.9 g/l
IgM	65-360 mg/dl	0.65-3.6 g/l
IgG	620-1540 mg/dl	6.2-15.4 g/l
Iron		
Male	80-160 μg/dl	14.3-28.6 μmol/l
Female	60-135 μg/dl	10.7-24.2 μmol/l
Binding cap.	250-350 μg/dl	44.7-62.6 μmol/l
Saturation	20-45%	0.20-0.45 arb. units
Lactate (plasma)	.3-1.3 mmol/l	0.3-1.3 mmol/l
Lipids		
Total	450-1000 mg/dl	4.5-10.0 g/l
Cholesterol	165-310 mg/dl	4.27-8.0 mmol/l
Triglyceride	65-200 mg/dl	0.65-2.0 g/l
Magnesium	1.5-2.4 mEq/l	0.75-1.20 mmol/l

*From Manual of medical therapeutics, ed. 22, Boston, 1977, Little, Brown and Co.

Common serum chemistries—cont'd

Test	Units	S.I. units
Osmolality	270-290 mOsm/kg	270-290 mOsm/kg
Phosphorus, inorganic	2.5-5.5 mg/dl	0.81-1.78 mmol/l
Potassium (plasma)	3.5-4.5 mEq/l	3.5-4.5 mmol/l
Protein, electrophoresis		
Albumin	3.5-4.8 gm/dl	35-48 g/l
Alpha-1-globulin	0.1-0.5 gm/dl	1-5 g/l
Alpha-2-globulin	0.3-1.2 gm/dl	3-12 g/l
Beta globulin	0.7-1.7 gm/dl	7-17 g/l
Gamma globulin	0.7-2.7 gm/dl	7-27 g/l
Protein, total	6.5-8.5 gm/dl	65-85 g/l
Pyruvate (whole blood)	30-70 μmol/l	30-70 μmol/l
Sodium	135-145 mEq/l	135-145 mmol/l
Urea nitrogen	12-25 mg/dl	4.3-8.9 mmol/l
Uric acid	4.0-8.0 mg/dl	0.24-0.47 mmol/l
Vitamin A	30-65 μg/dl	1.04-2.26 μmol/l
Vitamin B_{12}	250-1200 pg/ml	185-885 pmol/l

Common serum enzymatic activities*

Test	Units	S.I. units
Aldolase	1.5-8.1 mU/ml	25.0-135.0 nmol/l · s
Amylase	15-90 U/l	15-90 U/l
Creatinine phosphokinase	25-145 mU/ml	.42-2.42 μmol/l · s
Hydroxybutyric dehydrogenase	95-245 mU/ml	1.58-4.09 μmol/l · s
Lactic dehydrogenase	110-250 mU/ml	1.83-4.17 μmol/l · s
Lipase	Up to 1.0 STU/ml	Up to 1000 arb. units
Phosphatase, acid	Up to .7 U/l	Up to .7 U/l
Phosphatase, alkaline	30-95 mU/ml	0.50-1.58 μmol/l · s
Transaminase		
Alanine amino (SGPT)	5-35 mU/ml	0.083-0.751 μmol/l · s
Aspartate amino (SGOT)	10-40 mU/ml	0.167-0.67 μmol/l · s

*From Manual of medical therapeutics, ed. 22, Boston, 1977, Little, Brown and Co.

Common serum hormone values*

Test	Units	S.I. units
ACTH	20-100 pg/ml	20-100 ng/l
Aldosterone	3-10 ng/dl	83.1-277 nmol/l
Cortisol (plasma)	8-24 μg/dl	0.22-0.67 μmol/l
FSH, male	Up to 20 mU/ml	Up to 20 U/l
Gastrin, fasting	25-250 pg/ml	25-250 ng/l
Growth hormone, fasting	<5 pg/ml	<5 ng/l
Insulin, fasting	7-34 μU/ml	7-34 mU/l
LH, male	Up to 20 mU/ml	Up to 20 U/l
Parathyroid hormone	0-10 U/ml	0-10 arb. units
Prolactin	<30 ng/ml	<30 μg/l
Renin activity (plasma)	1.0-4.8 ng/ml/hr	0.3-1.3 ng/l · s
Testosterone		
Male	380-980 ng/dl	13-34 nmol/l
Female	20-80 ng/dl	1-3 nmol/l
Thyroxine, total (T_4)	5.0-11.0 μg/dl	64-142 nmol/l
T_3 Resin uptake	35-45%	0.35-0.45 arb. units
Triiodothyronine (T_3)	60-190 ng/dl	0.92-2.93 nmol/l
TSH	Up to 8 μU/ml	Up to 8 mU/l

*From Manual of medical therapeutics, ed. 22, Boston, 1977, Little, Brown and Co.

Common urinary chemistries*

Test	Units	S.I. units
Calcium	100-250 mg/day	2.5-6.25 mmol/d
Catecholamines	Up to 100 μg/day	Up to 100 μg/d
Epinephrine	Up to 20 μg/day	Up to 110 nmol/d
Norepinephrine	10-80 μg/day	59-472 nmol/d
Copper	0-30 μg/day	0.0.472 μmol/d
Cortisol	16-80 μg/day	4-221 nmol/d
Creatinine	15-25 mg/kg/day	0.13-0.22 mmol/kg/d
17-Hydroxycorticosteroids, male	3-15 mg/day	8.3-41.4 μmol/d
5-Hydroxyindoleacetic acid	1-7 mg/day	5.3-37.1 μmol/d
17-Ketosteroids, male	6-18 mg/day	20.7-62.3 μmol/d
Protein	Up to 150 mg/day	Up to 150 mg/d
Vanillylmandelic acid (VMA)	5-7 mg/day	2.5-35.3 μmol/d

*From Manual of medical therapeutics, ed. 22, Boston, 1977, Little, Brown and Co.

Common hematologic studies*

Test		Units	S.I. units
Coagulation studies			
Bleeding time		<8 min	<.481 ks
Partial thromboplastin time		24-36 sec	24-36s
Prothrombin time		70-100%	.7-1.0 arb. units
Thrombin time		11.9-18.5 sec	11.9-18.5s
Complete blood count			
Hematocrit			
Male		42-52%	0.42-0.52
Female		37-47%	0.37-0.47
Hemoglobin			
Male		14.0-18.0 gm/dl	8.68-11.16 mmol/l
Female		12.0-16.0 gm/dl	7.44-9.92 mmol/l
Erythrocyte count			
Male		4.6-6.2 $\times$ 10^6/cu mm	4.6-6.2 $\times$ 10^{12}/l
Female		4.2-5.4 $\times$ 10^6/cu mm	4.2-5.4 $\times$ 10^{12}/l
Leukocyte count	100%	4.8-10.8 $\times$ 10^3/cu mm	4.8-10.8 $\times$ 10^9/l
Segmented neutrophils	40-60%	2500-6000/cu mm	
Lymphocytes	20-40%	1000-4000/cu mm	
Eosinophils	1-3%	50-300/cu mm	
Basophils	0-1%	0-100/cu mm	
Monocytes	4-8%	200-800/cu mm	
Myelocytes	0%	0/cu mm	
Juvenile neutrophils	0-1%	0-100/cu mm	
Band neutrophils	0-5%	0-500/cu mm	
Platelet count		150-400 $\times$ 10^3/cu mm	150-400 $\times$ 10^9/l
Erythrocyte indices			
Mean corpuscular hemoglobin		27-31 pg	1.7-2.0 fmol
Mean corpuscular hemoglobin conc.		32-36	20.0-22.3 mmol/l
Mean corpuscular volume		81-99 cu microns	81-99 fl
Erythrocyte			
Sedimentation rate			
Male		Up to 9 mm/hr	Up to 9 arb. units
Female		Up to 20 mm/hr	Up to 20 arb. units

*From Manual of medical therapeutics, ed. 22, Boston, 1977, Little, Brown and Co.

Bone marrow cells*

Normal myelogram	Percent
Hemocytoblasts	0-0.5
Early normoblasts	1-5
Intermediate normoblasts	12-20
Late normoblasts	6-10
Myeloblasts	0.3-2
Promyelocytes	1-8
Neutrophil myelocytes	5-20
Neutrophil metamyelocytes	13-32
Neutrophil polymorphonuclears	7-30
Eosinophils (total)	0.5-4
Basophils (total)	0-1
Lymphocytes	3-20
Monocytes	0.5-5
Plasma cells	0-2
Megakaryocytes	Occasional
Pro-erythroblasts	0.5-4

*Israels, M. C. G.: An atlas of bone-marrow pathology, ed. 3, London, 1966, William Heinemann Medical Books Ltd., p. 25.

Cerebral spinal fluid and tumor specific antigens (TSA)

Cerebral spinal fluid		Tumor specific antigens (TSA)	
Cells	Fewer than 5 per cu mm, all mononuclear	*Serum carcinoembryonic antigen (CEA)**	
		0-2.5 ng/ml	Normal value
Chloride	120-130 mEq/L (20 mEq/L higher than in serum)	5-10 ng/ml	Moderately suspicious of an active tumor
Colloidal gold test	Not more than 1 in any tube	≥-10 ng/ml	Strongly suggestive of tumor present
Gamma globulin	1.3-4.7 mg/100 ml 4.3-12.3% of total protein		
Glucose	50-75 mg/100 ml (20 mg/100 ml less than in blood)	*Alpha fetoprotein (AFP)*†	
		<40 ng/ml	Normal value
Pressure	70-180 mm water		
Protein	15-45 mg/100 ml		

*Data from page 405 of Clinical laboratory medicine, ed. 3, by Richard Ravel. Copyright © 1978 by Year Book Medical Publishers, Chicago.

†From Interpretation of diagnostic tests, ed. 3, Boston, 1978, Little, Brown and Company, p. 83.

PEDIATRIC LABORATORY VALUES

Common serum chemistries*

Alkaline phosphatase	
(1 King-Armstrong unit = 7.08 milli-International Unit [mIU])	
Birth	35-105 mIU/ml
1 month-1 year	70-250 mIU/ml
1-3 years	70-210 mIU/ml
3-10 years	70-180 mIU/ml
10-16 years	100-275 mIU/ml
Acid phosphatase (total)	
(1 King-Armstrong unit = 1.77 milli-International Unit [mIU])	
Birth	3-6 mIU/ml
1 month-1 year	6.5-11 mIU/ml
1-3 years	6.5-11 mIU/ml
3-10 years	3.5-9 mIU/ml
10-16 years	3-10 mIU/ml
Aldolase	<11 mU/ml
Ammonia	<150 μg% (Seligson blood ammonia)
Amylase, serum	<160 caraway units/100 ml
Ascorbic acid	Over 0.3 mg%
Bicarbonate (CO_2 capacity or combining power	22-30 mEq/l
Bilirubin	
Cord	Up to 1.8 mg%
2-4 days	Mean peak 7 mg%, Range 2-12 mg%
After newborn period	Less than 0.8 mg% total
Bromsulphalein retention (at 45 minutes)	
Newborn	Up to 20%
Thereafter	Less than 5%
Calcium	9.0-11.5 mg%
Carotene	
Newborn	25 μg%
Thereafter	60-180 μg%
Chloride	94-106 mEq/l
Cholesterol	150-275 mg%, 65-76% esterified
Copper	
1 month	50-100 μg%
1 year	110-175 μg%
5-17 years	80-280 μg%
Adult	80-180 μg%
Creatinine phosphokinase	<50 mU/ml
Creatinine	0.7-1.5 mg%
Fibrinogen, plasma	200-400 mg/ml
Glucose (fasting)	55-100 mg%
Haptoglobin	1:32-1:256

*Reproduced with permission from Johns Hopkins Hospital: The Harriet Lane handbook, ed. 7, edited by Dennis L. Headings. Copyright © 1975 by Year Book Medical Publishers, Chicago.

Common serum chemistries—cont'd

Iodine, protein bound			
Newborn	6-10.7 μg%		
1 week	9-14 μg%		
1-12 weeks	5.6-9.2 μg%		
3-12 months	5.3-7.3 μg%		
Thereafter	3.5-8.0 μg%		

Butanol extractable iodine averages 0.5 μg lower.

Iron

	Mean serum Fe	Total Fe binding capacity	Percent saturation
1 week	148 μg%	262 μg%	65
3 months	50	350	15
6-12 months	106	429	25
1-2 years	95	414	22
2-6 years	116	395	28
6-12 years	127	340	38

Ketones	Up to 3 mg%
Lactic acid (fasting)	Up to 10 mg% if precipitated STAT, otherwise, up to 20 mg%
Lactic dehydrogenase	0-300 mU/ml
Lead	Under 0.04 mg%
Lipids	
Total	450-1000 mg%
Phospholipids	Mean 225 mg% (usually slightly higher than cholesterol)
Magnesium	1.5-2.5 mEq/l
Mucoproteins (as tyrosine)	1.9-4.5 mg%
pH (arterial whole blood	7.35-7.45 (0.03 lower in venous blood)
Pco_2 (arterial)	35-45 mm Hg
Po_2 (arterial)	75-100 mm Hg
Phenylalanine	<3 mg%
Phosphorus, inorganic	
1st year	4-7 mg%
1-12 years	5-6 mg%
Adult	3-4.5 mg%
Porcelain	8-20 mEq/l
Potassium	
0-10 days	Up to 7 mEq/l
Thereafter	3.5-5.0 mEq/l
Proteins	
Total	6-8 g%
Albumin	4.7-5.7 g%
Globulin	1.3-2.5 g%

Proteins — Average (range) in grams

Age	Total	Albumin	Globulin	Gamma globulin
Premature	5.5 (4.6)	3.7 (2.5-4.5)	1.8 (1.2-2)	0.7 (0.5-0.9)
FT Newborn	6.4 (5-7.1)	3.4 (2.5-5)	3.1 (1.2-4)	0.8 (0.7-0.9)
1-3 months	6.6 (4.7-7.4)	3.8 (3-4.2)	2.5 (1-3.3)	0.3 (0.1-0.5)
3-12 months	6.8 (5-7.5)	3.9 (2.7-5)	2.6 (2-3.8)	0.6 (0.4-1.2)
1-15 years	7.4 (6.5-8.6)	4.0 (3.2-5)	3.1 (2-4.4)	0.9 (0.6-1.2)

Common serum chemistries—cont'd

Sodium	136-145 mEq/l
Tocopherol (vitamin E)	
Premature	0.05-0.35 mg%
FT newborn	0.1-0.35 mg%
2-5 months	0.2-0.6 mg%
6-24 months	0.35-0.8 mg%
2-12 years	0.55-0.9 mg%
Adult and breast-fed babies	0.6-1.1 mg%
Transaminases	
SGOT	<19 mU/ml
SGPT	<17 mU/ml
Urea nitrogen	
Non-protein nitrogen	6-23 μg%
Uric acid	2.9-8.0 mg%
Vitamin A	>40 μg%
Zinc turbidity	
Newborn	Less than 10
1-8 months	Less than 3
9-12 months	Less than 5
Thereafter	Less than 8

Bone marrow cells*

	Normal % and range
WBC	
"Blasts"	2.0 (0.3-5.8)
Undiff. myelocytes (A & B)	5.0 (1.0-8.0)
Diff. myelocytes (0)-neutrophils	12.0 (5.0-19.0)
Diff. myelocytes (0)-eosinophils	1.5 (0.5-3.0)
Diff. myelocytes (0)-basophils	0.3 (0-0.5)
Metamyelocytes-neutrophils	22.0 (13.0-32.0)
Metamyelocytes-eosinophils	
P.M.N. neutrophils	20.0 (7.0-30.0)
P.M.N. eosinophils	2.0 (0.5-4.0)
P.M.N. basophils	0.2 (0-0.7)
Monocytes	2.0 (0.5-5.0)
Lymphocytes	10.0 (3.0-17.0)
Plasma cells	0.4 (0-2.0)
Reticulum cells & macrophages	0.2 (0.2-2.0)
Mitotic figures	
Unclassified cells	
RBC	
Megaloblasts	0
Pronormoblasts	4.0 (1.0-8.0)
Basophilic normoblasts	
Polychromatophilic norm.	18.0 (7.0-32.0)
Orthochromatic norm.	

*Reproduced with permission from Johns Hopkins Hospital: The Harriet Lane handbook, ed. 7, edited by Dennis L. Headings. Copyright © 1975 by Year Book Medical Publishers, Chicago.

Common hematologic studies*†

	Gm Hgb	% Hct	WBC/mm³	% Polys	% Retics
1 day	16-22‡	53-73‡	18,000 (7-35,000)	45-85	2.5-6.5
1 week	13-20‡	43-66‡	10,000 (4-20,000)	30-50	0.1-4.5
1 month	16	53	10,000 (6-18,000)	30-50	0.1-1.0
3 months	11.5	38	10,000 (6-17,000)	30-50	0.7-3.0
6 months	12	40	10,000 (6-16,000)	30-50	0.7-2.3
1 year	12	40	10,000 (6-15,000)	30-50	0.6-1.7
2-6 years	13	43	9,000 (7-13,000)	35-55	0.5-1.0
7-12 years	14	46	8,500 (5-12,000)	40-60	0.5-1.0

*Reproduced with permission from Johns Hopkins Hospital: The Harriet Lane handbook, ed. 7, edited by Dennis L. Headings. Copyright © 1975 by Year Book Medical Publishers, Chicago.
†Absolute eosinophil count: 100-600/mm³, average 250
‡Under the age of 1 month capillary Hgb and Hct exceed venous:
1 hour: 3.6 g average difference
5 days: 2.2 g average difference
3 weeks: 1.1 g average difference

Normal blood pressure values at various ages*

Age in years†	Mean systolic	Range in 95% of normal children	Age in years†	Mean diastolic	Range in 95% of normal children
½-1 year	90	±25	½-1 year	61	±19
1-2 years	96	±27	1-2 years	65	±27
2-3 years	95	±24	2-3 years	61	±24
3-4 years	99	±23	3-4 years	65	±19
4-5 years	99	±21	4-5 years	65	±15
5 years	94	±14	5 years	55	±9
6 years	100	±15	6 years	56	±8
7 years	102	±15	7 years	56	±8
8 years	105	±16	8 years	57	±9
9 years	107	±16	9 years	57	±9
10 years	109	±16	10 years	58	±10
11 years	111	±17	11 years	59	±10
12 years	113	±18	12 years	59	±10
13 years	115	±19	13 years	60	±10
14 years	118	±19	14 years	61	±10
15 years	121	±19	15 years	61	±10

*Reproduced with permission from Johns Hopkins Hospital: The Harriet Lane handbook, ed. 7, edited by Dennis L. Headings. Copyright © 1975 by Year Book Medical Publishers, Chicago.
†Data for ½-5 years from Allen-Williams, G. M.: Arch. Dis. Child **20**:125, 1945. Data for 5-15 years from Graham, A. W.; Hines, E. A., Jr; and Gage, R. P.: Am. J. Dis. Child **69**:203, 1945.

Cerebral spinal fluid*

Amount (obtainable by LP)	
Newborn	Up to 5 ml
Adult	10-150 ml
Initial pressure	
Newborn	50-90 mm CSF
Infant	40-150 mm
Child	70-200 mm
Specific gravity	1.005-1.009
pH at 38° C	7.33-7.42
Calcium	4.5-5.5 mg% (approximates ionized serum Ca)
Cell count	
Newborn	Up to 25 WBC (average 8) and up to 650 RBC/mm^3
After 1st month	Up to 7 lymphocytes
Glucose	40-80 mg% (at least ½ of blood sugar)
Pandy (mainly globulin)	0 (may be positive in newborn)
Protein (80% albumin)	
Ventricular	5-15 mg%
Cisternal	5-25 mg%
Lumbar	5-40 mg% Up to 150 mg% in newborn†
G-O transaminase	4-14 units, often about ½ of SGOT

*Reproduced with permission from John Hopkins Hospital: The Harriet Lane handbook, ed. 7, edited by Dennis L. Headings. Copyright © 1975 by Year Book Medical Publishers, Chicago. Ref: Wyers, H. J. G., and Bakker, J. C. W.: Neederland Tijdschrift voor Kindergeneeskunde, **22:**253, 1954.

†There is too little data available on newborn CSF to define normal limits or to allow fine diagnostic distinctions.

Temperature equivalents*

Centigrade	Fahrenheit	Centigrade	Fahrenheit
34.0	93.2	38.6	101.4
34.2	93.6	38.8	101.8
34.4	93.9	39.0	102.2
34.6	94.3	39.2	102.5
34.8	94.6	39.4	102.9
35.0	95.0	39.6	103.2
35.2	95.4	39.8	103.6
35.4	95.7	40.0	104.0
35.6	96.1	40.2	104.3
35.8	96.4	40.4	104.7
36.0	96.8	40.6	105.1
36.2	97.1	40.8	105.4
36.4	97.5	41.0	105.8
36.6	97.8	41.2	106.1
36.8	98.2	41.4	106.5
37.0	98.6	41.6	106.8
37.2	98.9	41.8	107.2
37.4	99.3	42.0	107.6
37.6	99.6	42.2	108.0
37.8	100.0	42.4	108.3
38.0	100.4	42.6	108.7
38.2	100.7	42.8	109.0
38.4	101.1	43.0	109.4
$F = 32 + (9/5 \times \text{temp.})$		$C = (\text{temp.} - 32) \times 5/9$	

*Reproduced with permission from Johns Hopkins Hospital: The Harriet Lane handbook, ed. 7, edited by Dennis L. Headings. Copyright © 1975 by Year Book Medical Publishers, Chicago.

Converting mg/kg → mg/M²*

Adult	mg/kg × 37 = mg/M^2	Monkey	mg/kg × 12 = mg/M^2
Child	mg/kg × 25 = mg/M^2	Rat	mg/kg × 5.9 = mg/M^2
Dog	mg/kg × 20 = mg/M^2	Mouse	mg/kg × 3.0 = mg/M^2

*From Freireich, E. J., Gehan, E. A., Rall, D. P., et al.: Cancer Chemother. Rep. **50**(4):219-244, 1966.

Factor table for converting dose equivalents from one species to another, mg/kg units*

FORMULA: Species dose (mg/kg) × factor = equivalent dose (mg/kg) in other species

Species	Factor	Other species	Species	Factor	Other Species
Mouse	1/2	Rat	Dog	6	Mouse
	1/4	Monkey		4	Rat
	1/5	Dog		5/3	Monkey
	1/12	Man		1/2	Man
Rat	2	Mouse	Man	12	Mouse
	1/2	Monkey		7	Rat
	1/4	Dog		3	Monkey
	1/7	Man		2	Dog
Monkey	4	Mouse			
	2	Rat			
	3/5	Dog			
	1/3	Man			

*From Freireich, E. J., Gehan, E. A., Rall, D. P., et al.: Cancer Chemother. Rep. **50**(4):219-244, 1966.

INDEX

C

D

N

R

S

T

U

V